COMPUTATIONAL APPROACHES IN DRUG DISCOVERY, DEVELOPMENT AND SYSTEMS PHARMACOLOGY

COMPUTATIONAL APPROACHES IN DRUG DISCOVERY, DEVELOPMENT AND SYSTEMS PHARMACOLOGY

Edited by

RUPESH KUMAR GAUTAM
Department of Pharmacology, Indore Institute of Pharmacy, IIST Campus, Indore, Madhya Pradesh, India

MOHAMMAD AMJAD KAMAL
King Fahd Medical Research Center (KFMRC), King Abdulaziz University, Jeddah, Saudi Arabia

POOJA MITTAL
Chitkara College of Pharmacy, Chitkara University, Rajpura, Punjab, India

ELSEVIER

ACADEMIC PRESS
An imprint of Elsevier

Academic Press is an imprint of Elsevier
125 London Wall, London EC2Y 5AS, United Kingdom
525 B Street, Suite 1650, San Diego, CA 92101, United States
50 Hampshire Street, 5th Floor, Cambridge, MA 02139, United States
The Boulevard, Langford Lane, Kidlington, Oxford OX5 1GB, United Kingdom

ISBN 978-0-323-99137-7

For information on all Academic Press publications
visit our website at https://www.elsevier.com/books-and-journals

Publisher: Stacy Masucci
Acquisitions Editor: Andre G. Wolff
Editorial Project Manager: Samantha Allard
Production Project Manager: Sajana Devasi P K
Cover Designer: Miles Hitchen

Typeset by STRAIVE, India

Contents

Contributors

Athanasios Alexiou
Novel Global Community Educational Foundation, Hebersham, NSW, Australia; AFNP Med, Wien, Austria

Sakshi Bhardwaj
Krupanidhi College of Pharmacy, Bangalore, Karnataka, India

Shabana Bibi
Department of Biosciences, Shifa Tameer-e-Millat University, Islamabad, Pakistan; Yunnan Herbal Laboratory, College of Ecology and Environmental Sciences, Yunnan University, Kunming, China

Maheshkumar Borkar
SVKM's Dr. Bhanuben Nanavati College of Pharmacy, Mumbai, Maharashtra, India

Bhawna Chopra
Guru Gobind Singh College of Pharmacy, Yamuna Nagar, Haryana, India

Hitesh Chopra
Chitkara College of Pharmacy, Chitkara University, Rajpura, Punjab, India

Anna Chiara Corriero
Anglia Ruskin University—Rivermead Campus, Chelmsford, United Kingdom

Ashwani K. Dhingra
Guru Gobind Singh College of Pharmacy, Yamuna Nagar, Haryana, India

Rupesh Kumar Gautam
Department of Pharmacology, Indore Institute of Pharmacy, IIST Campus, Indore, Madhya Pradesh, India

Rajat Goyal
MM College of Pharmacy, Maharishi Markandeshwar (Deemed to be University), Mullana, Ambala, Haryana, India

Ajmer Singh Grewal
Guru Gobind Singh College of Pharmacy, Yamuna Nagar, Haryana, India

Kumar Guarve
Guru Gobind Singh College of Pharmacy, Yamuna Nagar, Haryana, India

Gaurav Gupta
School of Pharmacy, Suresh Gyan Vihar University, Jaipur, Rajasthan, India

Mohammad Mehedi Hasan
Department of Biochemistry and Molecular Biology, Faculty of Life Science, Mawlana Bhashani Science and Technology University, Tangail; Division of Computer-Aided Drug Design, The Red-Green Research Centre, BICCB, Dhaka, Bangladesh

Md. Shahadat Hossain
Department of Biochemistry and Molecular Biology; Department of Pharmacy, Faculty of Life Science, Mawlana Bhashani Science and Technology University, Tangail, Bangladesh

Thet Thet Htar
School of Pharmacy, Monash University Malaysia, Bandar Sunway, Selangor, Malaysia

Fahadul Islam
Department of Pharmacy, Faculty of Allied Health Sciences, Daffodil International University, Dhaka, Bangladesh

Shikha Joon
Institutes for Systems Genetics, Frontiers Science Center for Disease-Related Molecular Network, West China Hospital, Sichuan University, Chengdu, China; iGlobal Research and Publishing Foundation, New Delhi, India

Mohammad Amjad Kamal
Department of Pharmacy, Faculty of Allied Health Sciences, Daffodil International University, Dhaka, Bangladesh; Institutes for Systems Genetics, Frontiers Science Center for Disease-related Molecular Network, West China Hospital, Sichuan University, China; King Fahd Medical Research Center, King Abdulaziz University, Jeddah, Saudi Arabia; Enzymoics; Novel Global Community Educational Foundation, Hebersham, NSW, Australia

Abhishek Kanugo
SVKM's NMIMS School of Pharmacy and Technology Management, Shirpur, Dhule, Maharashtra, India

Ramit Kapoor
Clarivate India Pvt. Ltd, Noida, Uttar Pradesh, India

Gurjeet Kaur
Department of Pharmacology, Postgraduate Institute of Medical Education and Research, Chandigarh, India

Komal Preet Kaur
Northeastern University Toronto, Toronto, ON, Canada

Ashraf Ullah Khan
Faculty of Pharmaceutical Sciences, Abasyn University Peshawar, Peshawar; Pharmacological Sciences Research Lab, Department of Pharmacy, Faculty of Biological Sciences, Quaid-I-Azam University, Islamabad, Pakistan

Muhammad Saad Khan
Department of Biosciences, Faculty of Sciences, COMSATS University Islamabad, Sahiwal, Pakistan

Shafi Ullah Khan
Product & Process Innovation Department, Qarshi Brands (Pvt) Ltd, Hattar Industrial Estate, Haripur; Faculty of Pharmaceutical Sciences, Abasyn University Peshawar, Peshawar, Pakistan

J. Kumaravel
Department of Pharmacology, Postgraduate Institute of Medical Education and Research, Chandigarh, India

Bikash Medhi
Department of Pharmacology, Postgraduate Institute of Medical Education and Research, Chandigarh, India

Anurag Mishra
NIMS Institute of Pharmacy, NIMS University, Jaipur, Rajasthan, India

Pooja Mittal
Chitkara College of Pharmacy, Chitkara University, Rajpura, Punjab, India

Dimitrios V. Moysidis
Faculty of Medicine, Aristotle University of Thessaloniki, Thessaloniki, Greece

Mukesh Nandave
Department of Pharmacology, Delhi Pharmaceutical Sciences and Research University, New Delhi, India

Andreas S. Papazoglou
Faculty of Medicine, Aristotle University of Thessaloniki, Thessaloniki, Greece

Ketan C. Parmar
Department of Chemistry, Sir P.T. Sarvajanik College of Science, Veer Narmad South Gujarat University, Surat, India

Sachchidanand Pathak
Kashi Institute of Pharmacy, Varanasi, Uttar Pradesh; School of Pharmacy, Suresh Gyan Vihar University, Jaipur, Rajasthan, India

Arati Prabhu
SVKM's Dr. Bhanuben Nanavati College of Pharmacy, Mumbai, Maharashtra, India

Ajay Prakash
Department of Pharmacology, Postgraduate Institute of Medical Education and Research, Chandigarh, India

Abhay Raizaday
Department of Pharmceutics, College of Pharmacy, JSS Academy of Technical Education, Noida, Uttar Pradesh, India

Sarita Rawat
Faculty of Pharmacy and Sciences, Amrapali Group of Institutes, Nainital, Uttarakhand; School of Pharmacy, Suresh Gyan Vihar University, Jaipur, Rajasthan, India

Rehab A. Rayan
Department of Epidemiology, High Institute of Public Health, Alexandria University, Alexandria, Egypt

Kalicharan Sharma
Department of Pharmaceutical Chemistry, Delhi Pharmaceutical Sciences and Research University, New Delhi, India

Priyanka Sharma
Department of Pharmacology, Delhi Pharmaceutical Sciences and Research University, New Delhi, India

Saurabh Sharma
Department of Pharmacology, Postgraduate Institute of Medical Education and Research, Chandigarh, India

Bairong Shen
Institutes for Systems Genetics, Frontiers Science Center for Disease-Related Molecular Network, West China Hospital, Sichuan University, Chengdu, China

Santosh Kumar Singh
School of Pharmacy, Suresh Gyan Vihar University, Jaipur, Rajasthan, India

Rajeev K. Singla
Institutes for Systems Genetics, Frontiers Science Center for Disease-Related Molecular Network, West China Hospital, Sichuan University, Chengdu, China; iGlobal Research and Publishing Foundation, New Delhi, India

Ganesh Sonawane
SND College of Pharmacy, Yeola, Maharashtra, India

Kajal Sonawane
SND College of Pharmacy, Yeola, Maharashtra, India

Enty Tjoa
Department of Microbiology, School of Medicine and Health Sciences, Atma Jaya Catholic, University of Indonesia, Jakarta, Indonesia

Christos Tsagkaris
Novel Global Community Educational Foundation, Hebersham, NSW, Australia

Qudsia Yousafi
Department of Biosciences, Faculty of Sciences, COMSATS University Islamabad, Sahiwal, Pakistan

Editors biography

Dr. Rupesh Kumar Gautam is currently working as Professor and Head, Department of Pharmacology, Indore Institute of Pharmacy, Rau, Indore, India. He has more than 14 years of teaching and research experience. He has more than 65 research and review articles to his credit in various journals of repute. He has also published 10 books and 18 book chapters with Elsevier, Springer, Wiley, Scrivener, Bentham, NOVA, etc. He has filed 2 patents and registered 42 copyrights. He has supervised 21 M. Pharm scholars. Dr. Gautam has also received grants from various government agencies/associations for conducting FDP/seminars/conferences/workshops. He has attended and organized several International and National seminar, conferences, and workshops as a team member and organizing secretary/coordinator. He has been Guest Editor of Phytomedicine, Current Pharmaceutical Design, Neuroscience and Biobehavioral Reviews, Evidence-Based Complementary and Alternative Medicine, and Biomed Research International.

Mohammad Amjad Kamal is Distinguished Adjunct Professor at King Fahd Medical Research Center, King Abdulaziz University, Saudi Arabia. Professor Kamal's overall biochemical research output has culminated in more than 600 publications in journals of international repute and 61 abstracts in international conferences. His research was pivotal in supporting the development of the novel anti-Alzheimer agents from the laboratory to the clinic via collaboration with Dr. Nigel H. Greig (United States). He migrated to Australia in 1998 and was awarded a prestigious U2000 Postdoctoral Fellowship in 2000 by the University of Sydney, School of Molecular and Microbial Biosciences.

Pooja Mittal is currently working as an Associate Professor at Chitkara College of Pharmacy, Chitkara University, Rajpura, Punjab, India. She has 9+ years of experience in teaching and research. Prior to this, she worked at RIMT University, Mandi Gobindgarh (Punjab), Maharishi Markandeshwar University (Sadopur), Ambala (Haryana), and at Baddi University of Emerging Sciences and Technology, Baddi (Solan). She received the travel grant from DST-SERB in 2016 to attend the International Convention of

Controlled Release Society, held at Seattle, USA. She received her Ph.D. degree from Department of Pharmaceutical Engineering and Technology, IIT (BHU) Varanasi in 2018. She also received the Young Scientist Award-WF from SPER in 2017.

CHAPTER 1

In silico pharmacology

Sachchidanand Pathak[a,f], Anurag Mishra[b], Ganesh Sonawane[c], Kajal Sonawane[c], Sarita Rawat[d,f], Abhay Raizaday[g], Santosh Kumar Singh[e], and Gaurav Gupta[e]
[a]Kashi Institute of Pharmacy, Varanasi, Uttar Pradesh, India
[b]NIMS Institute of Pharmacy, NIMS University, Jaipur, Rajasthan, India
[c]SND College of Pharmacy, Yeola, Maharashtra, India
[d]Faculty of Pharmacy and Sciences, Amrapali Group of Institutes, Nainital, Uttarakhand, India
[e]School of Pharmacy, Suresh Gyan Vihar University, Jaipur, Rajasthan, India
[f]School of Pharmacy, Suresh Gyan Vihar University, Jaipur, Rajasthan, India
[g]Department of Pharmceutics, College of Pharmacy, JSS Academy of Technical Education, Noida, Uttar Pradesh, India

1. Introduction to in silico studies

In the drug development process, it is crucial to assess the medication's potential toxicological risk as quickly as feasible to save time and money. A wide range of in vivo and in vitro methods are used to evaluate a drug candidate's toxicological risk. Many alternatives in silico techniques for toxicity estimation have been developed since the 1970s. In silico approaches have been established and are extensively employed to develop and evaluate pharmacological hypotheses. Databases, quantitative structure-activity relationships (QSARs), molecular search engines, homology models, machine learning, and many more software programs are all used in digital simulation, also known as computer-based modeling. Computational pharmacology (also called computational therapeutics or in silico) refers to an extremely expansive discipline that focuses on developing new software tools to extract, analyze, and integrate the data produced by biological and medical experiments [1,2].

In silico techniques relate to methods or predictions that use computational methodologies. It is a computer component known as silicium that is referred to by the phrase in silico. The speed and high throughput of in silico methods allow for the rapid prediction of a huge number of molecules. An in silico experiment is carried out on a computer or through computer simulation in bioscience and another experimental discipline. In silico medical research can accelerate the speed of findings while eliminating the necessity for costly lab, labor, and clinical trials. One approach to accomplish this is to

Computational Approaches in Drug Discovery, Development and Systems Pharmacology
https://doi.org/10.1016/B978-0-323-99137-7.00006-X

increase the efficiency with which drug candidates are produced and screened [3–5].

The phrase "in silico," which is connected to the more generally used biological words "in vivo" and "in vitro," refers to computer-assisted experiments. The origins of the phrase "in silico" are unknown, with several researchers claiming to have had a hand in its development. However, Sieburg and Danchin et al. are among the first authors to use the term in print. Computer-aided drug design, also known as in silico pharmacology, computational pharmacology, or computational therapeutics encompasses a wide range of tools for capturing, analyzing, and integrating biological and medical data from a wide range of sources. Further, it describes the building of computer models or simulations using this data to generate predictions, offer hypotheses, and eventually lead to medical discoveries or treatment advancements [6–9]. Managing information as a valuable resource has been cited as a key to industrial success time and time again. It is possible to apply this to drug discovery, which is a very sophisticated information handling and interpretation process There is a lot of data to go through, and we need to find the shortcuts or criteria that will help us swiftly identify the targets and compounds that are most likely to progress through clinical trials and eventually to the marketplace. The pharmaceutical sector is becoming more closely aligned with engineering-based disciplines as a result of advances in computational or in silico approaches [10–12].

If we want to build on the achievements of the human genome, we must also combine computational and experimental data. All data types must be connected before in silico drug development can commence. Beyond genes and proteins, we may still be missing a lot of information that might have a significant influence on the pharmaceutical industry's capacity to discover novel medicines. Molecular models of ligand-receptor interactions in neuropharmacology, for example, need to be connected to network techniques if they are going to be used to explain neurological illnesses adequately. The effect of the compound on the biosystem and the effect of the biosystem on the compound may be summarized as "what the compound and the biosystem do to each other." A pharmacodynamic PD event occurs when a medication affects a biological system and causes a pharmacological and toxic reaction. The xenobiotic is absorbed, distributed, metabolized, and excreted by the biological system in a symbiotic way [13,14]. Pharmacokinetic (PK) events are what we are referring to here. However, it is important to understand that these two characteristics of the behavior of xenobiotics are intertwined. The metabolites produced during biotransformation may have their unique PD effects and hence influence the potency and frequency of PD effects. For example, hemodynamic changes and changes in enzyme activity are PD impacts that may have an impact on the organism's condition and its ability to cope with outside substances. The worldwide scope of this connection can only be grasped via a systemic approach, such as in PK/PD modeling and clinical pharmacology. Many biological components that generate PD events when they come into contact with a drug or another xenobiotic should be named targets for the sake of thoroughness [15,16]. In addition to anabolic and catabolic enzymes, nucleic acids, and ion channels, these are examples of targets. Drug-metabolizing enzymes, transporters, and circulating proteins are examples of agents in the body that metabolize or transport, distribute, or excrete drugs. Didier Rognan's evaluation of chemogenomics, in which a lead therapy against one gene family member is used for another analogous target, will be thoroughly examined in this publication (personal communication). Despite this, there have been a lot of efforts to establish links between molecular structure and extensive biological activity and repercussions that should be explored. Proteome cross-sectional biological spectra, for example, have been documented. Hierarchical clustering of spectra similarity enabled the connection between structure and bioactivity to be established. Despite the dearth of pharmacological target data, much research on agonist and antagonist profiles at multiple receptors have shown equal functional activity. When using IC50 data as affinity fingerprints to identify functional activity similarities among drugs, a pharmacophoric bias was expected to be introduced. Similar probabilistic methods have also been used by the same authors to connect medicine labeling information with biological spectra, employing a similar probabilistic approach. It was discovered that related drugs showed comparable biological spectra when side-effect profiles were grouped, for example [17,18]. In this work, it is possible to predict the biospectra of a new molecule by comparing it to a known one. With further testing on a huge number of drug-like chemicals that were not included in the original signature database, this method can be much more certain [19,20].

This polypharmacology network of drugs with varied protein-targeting abilities was also published by another Pfizer team as part of the global pharmacological space mapping. More than 200,000 molecules with biological data (from their collection and the literature) were used to develop Bayesian binary models (for molecules active at or inactive at 10 M or less) for 698 different targets, suggesting that these models could be useful for predicting primary pharmacology. Several oral medications with molecular weights above 500 and cLog*P* values over 5 were found in a 2D molecular property space examination of 617 authorized drugs. As of this writing, they have yet to realize their full potential as pharmacological targets. It is possible that this research has to be combined with others like Fliri to achieve its full potential, which would then allow for the simultaneous understanding and prediction of the target, proteome, functional activity, and side effects. Analysis of more than 12,000 anticancer compounds utilizing 48 chemical 2D descriptors and principal component analysis (PCA) found that they occupied an entirely separate space from the "hit-like" and "oral drug-like" spaces [21–24]. This suggests that new methods than those commonly employed for drug likeness are needed to locate compounds for anticancer targets in commercial databases, since they may, unfortunately, exclude out potential clinical prospects.

Based on their chemical structure, many methods have been devised to predict the likely biological targets of chemicals. One study used probabilistic neural networks with 24 atom-type descriptors to categorize compounds that operate against one of seven targets to classify 799 substances from the MDDR database (G-protein-coupled receptors, kinases, enzymes, nucleic hormone receptor, and zinc peptidases). Classification models for 21 depression-related targets based on atom-type descriptors were generated using MDDR database molecules. Between 45% and 90% of the time, these models were accurate in predicting and recalling a molecule's molecular weight, with the compounds retrieved on average having a molecular weight of less than 300 (and some being active against several models). Because of their speed, general-purpose SVM filters were recommended for use in virtual screening. It has been shown that modest numbers of reference inhibitors for a variety of targets in the MDDR database can provide varied enrichment factors larger than random. Small molecule-protein interactions can be studied by flexibly docking molecules into a variety of proteins. Researchers have utilized the inverse docking technique INVDOCK on a database of 147 proteins known to be hazardous (DART). DNA polymerase beta and DNA topoisomerase I, two of the most regularly used anti-HIV drugs, were shown to be relatively accurate targets for this method in recent investigations [25–27].

2. History and evolution of in silico approaches

For drug design and allied disciplines in the field of drug discovery, informatics was not a prerequisite for their existence or growth as scientific fields. A lot of the first ideas on structure-activity relationships may be found in the

19th century, as Albert (1971, 1985) summarizes so well. For example, Corwin Hansch's pioneering work in drug design opened the path for the acknowledgement of lipophilicity and electronic characteristics as key factors in therapeutic efficacy and PKs (PD and PK) [28,29].

When it came to medicinal effectiveness, Crum brown and Fraser found that the chemical structure (the kind and connection of atoms inside molecules; the 2D structure (2D) of substances was also a key determinant. The discovery of conformational effects on bioactivity in the middle of the 20th century broadened this approach.

As early as the 19th century, visionary scientists like John Langley, Paul Ehrlich, and Alfred Clark presented the concept of receptors as a way to pinpoint the precise locations where a medicinal agent may work. The similarities and differences between receptors and enzymes were discussed by Alberto in detail [30–32].

Biological and chemical advances intertwined, creating a deluge of data and knowledge that could not be handled by the brain alone, spurring the birth and growth of computer science. With his pioneering work in the 1950s, Hansch was a pioneer in the use of calculators and statistics to arrive at quantitative links between structure (in fact, parameters, descriptors, and metrics) and activity. Following this development, computer graphics and molecular modeling were introduced in the 1980s and 1990s, paving the way for QSAR. In the field of drug development and pharmacology, computer science has transformed from a basic instrument to a major force. Pharmacology is being elevated to new levels thanks to the chemistry-biology-informatics trinity, as this brief overview will demonstrate [33,34].

3. In silico local QSAR modeling

The first computers were employed to analyze connections between chemical properties and biological activity in the early 1960s, and in silico pharmacology was born. The field progressed into what is now known as QSAR, which became an important part of medicinal chemistry and pharmacology rapidly. Computational chemistry-based drug development was revolutionized by the introduction of QSAR modeling. Similar molecules with little structural differences can have radically diverse biological activities. QSAR modeling focuses on this type of connection between molecular structure and changes in biological activity. The chemical structure or physicochemical characteristics of a sequence of chemicals are compared in QSARs. QSAR is a way of mapping the way a molecule is linked with a process, such as biological activity or chemical reactivity. In QSAR investigations, a wide range of descriptors can be used. Descriptors are mathematical representations of biological properties. These descriptors are a group or subset of descriptors that may be used to predict ADME/Tox characteristics and characterize the structure of a pharmaceutical molecule without organisms. ADME stands for absorption, distribution, metabolism, and excretion in PKs and pharmacology. Predicting the ADME property of any compound is a key element in the design of the drug. It is useful for predicting the toxicity of certain chemicals [35,36]. To decrease the number of descriptors in each molecule, a process called feature selection is employed in silico QSAR modeling. Good descriptor selection is essential for successful data mining. If incorrect descriptors are used to represent molecules, no reasonable predictions can be made. Selecting the right descriptor will depend on understanding the computational issue you are trying to solve. Understanding this connection may need relevant analysis and correlation analysis methods. When picking descriptors, look for these things: bioactivity-relevant descriptors, descriptors that have highly varied and/or ambiguous value distributions, descriptors that are independent of one another, unambiguous descriptors, and descriptors that are easy to convey to scientists and make distinctions between relevant patterns (specificity). Researchers that are employed by a variety of firms have examined data mining capabilities as they relate to speed and reliability [37,38].

4. Quantitative structure-activity relationships

Computational methods began to reveal quantifiable correlations between chemical structure and PK and PD properties in biological systems as early as the 1960s. Since then, current medicinal chemistry and pharmacology rely heavily on QSAR analysis and identification. It was first aimed at giving computer estimations for the bioactivity of compounds. As a result, the term "QSAR" would be used to describe any endeavor to create a link between chemical composition and a biological repercussion (i.e., toxicity (ADME/Tox) or physicochemical properties). The largest definition of QSARs is the creation of a mathematical model that links the microstructure to a chemical characteristic or biological impact using a statistical method. A QSAR model cannot account for outliers caused by different molecules acting in different ways or binding to receptors in different ways, and this is a difficult task due to the inherent noise in the original data and the particular methodological aspects involved in building a QSAR model. It is ultimately possible to predict biological effects for additional molecules by using a model that has been trained on an appropriate collection of training molecules, but there are several restrictions to model applicability that need to be taken into account. As a result of these efforts, hundreds of QSAR models have been developed and kept in the C-QSAR database for over 40 years [39–41].

5. Descriptor-based methods

Chemical structures are quantitatively expressed using molecular descriptors in quantitative structure-activity relationships. It is crucial to identify the most relevant molecular descriptors for modeling the biological effect of interest since the number and variation are so vast. Classifying molecular descriptors according to the chemical representation from which they are formed is a typical practice. One-dimensional descriptors store numerically generic properties such the molecular weight, molar refractive index, and the octanol/water partition coefficient. Some of these descriptors are often employed as physiologically relevant descriptors in the QSAR equations, despite their low dimensionality. The molecules' topological representations are used to generate 2D descriptions. 2D-QSAR descriptors are routinely employed to generate these models and are a widely utilized technique for both predicting physical and chemical properties and giving quantitative estimates of various biological consequences [42,43].

However, 3D descriptors are directly obtained from molecules' 3D structures, resulting in so-called three-dimensional quantitative structural analysis techniques (QSAR). Since they are dependent on the conformation of the molecule, 3D descriptors are one of a kind. Therefore, when experimentally validated structural information about the target protein is available, molecule alignment is a precondition for many 3D-QSAR techniques. Different methods and tactics have been devised for arranging molecules, either directly via the superposition of molecules or through docking chemicals into protein active sites as the situation may need. When using 3D QSAR, the most widely used comparative molecular field and similarity index analysis should be taken into consideration. New 3D-QSAR techniques based on surface-based feature distributions were developed to solve this limitation. When it comes to 3D-QSAR techniques, the descriptors used are theoretically more representative of the molecular features that are disclosed when interacting with proteins, compared to 2D-QSAR methods. Unfortunately, based on decades of experience in a broad range of applications, this is not always the case [44,45].

6. Rule-based methods

To create statistically significant QSAR models, a few dozen molecules to be evaluated are utilized as training sets, and the second set of molecules is employed as a second set. Several novel techniques have been developed because of the increasing availability of biological data on ligands and protein-ligand complexes. Maximizing this information to extract knowledge and build guidelines that may later be used to quantitatively analyze the putative biological effects of substances from a structure is the focus of these studies Excellent examples of rule-based techniques in drug metabolism prediction are derived from human knowledge of ligand biotransformation. Rule-based algorithms search for targeted cells (functional groups) in the request molecule first, then list all conceivable metabolic transformations these target sites may undergo, and lastly prioritize the resultant metabolites according to criteria that have been utilized in previous studies. MetabolExpert and METEOR are examples of existing systems of this sort [46,47]. There are about 300 response rules and over 800 reasoning rules in the METEOR system's biotransformation lexicon. Instead of being basic entries in a reaction database, metabolic reactions describe general reactions. Absolute and relative rules may be found in the reasoning engine. Relative and absolute reasoning are two different approaches to evaluating the likelihood of biotransformations taking place. Rules of absolute reasoning prioritize the oxidation of primary alcohols above the oxidation of secondary alcohols, for example. The laws of relative reasoning assign equal precedence when a preference is unknown. Using the nonnumerical Logic of Argumentation, the reasoning engine may then evaluate the likelihood of a certain answer occurring in the query substrate using reasons for and against the hypothesis. An external log P predictor may affect the likelihood of biotransformation depending on the global association between drug metabolism and lipophilicity, which the reasoning engine is linked to. To avoid a combinatorial explosion of results from unconstrained searches, the reasoning engine adds additional limits. A variety of search levels are possible, and only responses that are more likely than the set threshold will be presented. Galantamine's biotransformations predicted in silico matched those seen in vivo in rats, dogs, and humans in recent use of this method [48,49].

7. In silico pharmacology in target identification

One of the most time-consuming parts of drug development is the identification of drug targets, which is a very lengthy process. Large-scale data analyses are not as common since traditional approaches, such as in vivo and in vitro, might be unreliable at times. Pharmaceutical companies have a huge advantage in identifying new possible drug targets due to sophisticated in silico methods, which impacts the effectiveness and timeliness of clinical work for ascertaining novel drug targets. For the discovery of targeted medicines, the building of drug-target interface networks, and the study of small-molecule regulatory networks, it is critical to creating quick and precise target identification and prediction methods. The discovery of a possible therapeutic medication target's function and knowledge of its involvement in the illness process is the first stage in target-based drug development. A single molecule, such as a gene or protein, that plays a function in a certain ailment is referred to as a target. A therapeutic target is a specific molecule within a metabolic or signaling pathway that is essential to the survival or virulence of a disease or a microbe. To combat the symptoms of illness, several approaches target the pathway's operation by cutting off a critical molecule's operation. This essential molecule's activity can be inhibited by binding drugs to its active site. A potential solution is to repair the existing route by boosting certain molecules which were maybe damaged by the disease [50,51] (Fig. 1).

To find the right target and the demographic most likely to benefit from the drug, several scientific techniques (including techniques for big data analysis) are utilized. Table 1 gives an explanation of in silico pharmacology simulations for several proteins.

8. In silico identification of drug-target interactions

Discovering novel drug targets, one of the most essential phases in new drug development, is crucial for identifying existing protein targets and their interactions (or potential interactions) in the field. Identifying DTIs will help to uncover their role in many biological mechanisms, including several functions critical to several biological systems. It is possible to improve how medicines interact with different parts of the body when scientists map the human genome and molecular medicine progress. Despite considerable effort in recent years, the FDA has only approved a small number of drug candidates. The major reason is that such medication candidates have unacceptable toxicity and severe side effects. Recent research shows that pharmacological interactions with specific protein targets have a significant impact on the toxicity and side effects of therapeutic candidates. Several public databases were established in response to the huge quantity of information about interactions between drugs and targets, such as the

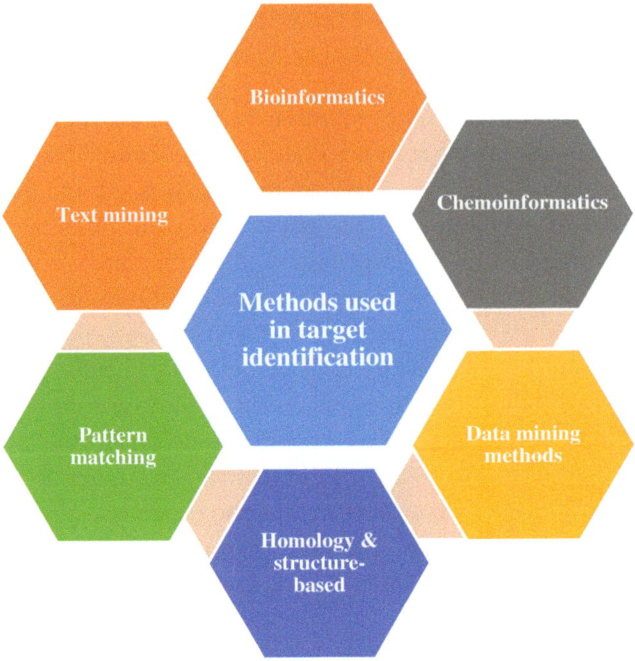

Fig. 1 Methods used in target identification.

Table 1 New high-affinity molecules discovered via a combination of computational methods and in silico pharmacology methods.

Targeted class	Targeted name
Enzyme	Renin, COX-1, COX-2, Farnesyl transferase, a serine protease, AChE, Tyrosine-protein phosphatase nonreceptor type 1, Factor-Xa, Deubiquitinating enzyme, Aromatase (CYP19), Cathepsin D, Sirtuin type 2, Glycogen phosphorylase
Transporter	ADME-related (e.g., P-gp), Na^+/D-glucose co-transporter
Receptor	Dopamine, CCR5 antagonist, Estrogen receptor, 5-HT_{1A}, Endothelial differentiation gene receptor antagonists, AMPA receptor, Urotensin antagonists, 5-HT_{2B}
Drug metabolizing enzymes	UDP-glucuronosyltransferases, Catechol *O*-methyltransferase, Cytochrome P450s, Sulfotransferases
Kinases	BCR-ABL tyrosine kinase CK2 and PKD, Syk C-terminal, Protein kinase C CDK1, ERK2, EFGR tyrosine kinase, SH2 domain, Lck SH2 domain
Channels	Potassium, sodium, and calcium
Transcription factors	AP-1 transcription factor
Other therapeutic targets	Prion diseases, Mesangial cell proliferation inhibitor

DrugsBank, SuperTarget, and Matador, as well as the Kyoto Encyclopedia of Genes and Genomes and the Therapeutic Target Database (TTD), have been created. A few empirically confirmed interactions that are important for DTI prediction are held in the databases, and they are seen as gold standards. Due to the high costs, extended time requirements, and ineffectiveness of experimental approaches to detect DTIs, drug firms will likely find it very difficult to do all needed trials to ensure that the toxicity and side-effects of a pharmacological molecule are uncovered. To streamline the process of detecting DTIs, new computational methods must be designed to verify them, giving experimental investigations more meaningful information, thereby increasing the chances of discovering novel drug candidates and targets. Many different in silico techniques have been explored to deal with the difficulties of DTI prediction. The ligand-based and receptor-based techniques, often known as conventional computational methodologies, govern a lot of computational drug discovery work [52,53]. Chemical structural similarity is used in the ligand-based virtual screening approach to predict DTIs. Another side, the ligand-based method might not be successful for target proteins with few identified ligands. In DTI prediction, a receptor-based method termed reverse docking has been utilized to link a pharmaceutical chemical with a target protein. On the other side, this approach could not be utilized on targets with unknown 3D features. As a consequence, it appears that efficient computational approaches based on protein sequence rather than protein 3D structure are successful in predicting DTIs. Several machine learning-based computational methods for predicting DTIs have recently been developed, with each drug-target combination being treated as a separate sample in the classification model. The work is predicated on the idea that drugs would bind to identical target proteins in the same way. Negative samples are randomly connected pairings of a drug-target bind with recognized contacts, whereas positive samples are drug-target pairs with known interactions (noninteracting). A mixture of drug and protein feature vectors make up each sample. Francisco et al. proposed a 2D molecular descriptor for pharmacological feature extraction. This was used to construct a multi-target QSAR model to predict DTIs. The BLM-NII method was introduced by Mei et al. to forecast the fresh target probability of a certain medication, and it has shown to be quite precise in predicting DTIs. Chen et al. utilized a machine learning technique to locate chemical-chemical similarities and chemical-protein connections that serve as possible drug targets [54–56].

9. Software-based calculations of molecular descriptors

Because molecular descriptors are becoming increasingly relevant in a variety of scientific disciplines, DRAGON software for calculating molecular descriptors has become a valuable tool for scientists. Molecular descriptors are utilized to analyze the physical and chemical characteristics of substances (in addition to being used in QSAR/QSPR predictions), including how molecules operate in pharmaceuticals and environmental conservation. These descriptors are additionally utilized to examine the compound libraries, which is important for improving quality control, in chemistry, pharmaceutical sciences, and health research. They are created when molecules, which are conceived of as actual objects, are converted into a molecular representation that allows for mathematical manipulation. Several molecular descriptors showed in recent years, based on various theories and techniques. "The molecular descriptor is the final result of a logic and mathematical procedure which transforms chemical information encoded within a symbolic representation of a molecule into a useful number or the result of some standardized experiment" [57,58]. Depending on the molecular depiction, the informative density of a molecular descriptor is evident and the method employed to calculate it. All molecular descriptors should have details on the chemical, meet some fundamental invariance features and general criteria, and be generated using well-established techniques that allow molecular descriptors to be computed for any collection of molecules. In addition to a particular understanding of the topic, knowledge of statistics, chemometrics, and the concepts of the QSAR/QSPR methods are required for the application of molecular descriptors. The goal of the DRAGON program is to offer the user a choice of molecular descriptors generated from various molecular representations, allowing the user to select the molecular descriptors that are most appropriate for his or her study. The initial version of DRAGON, dubbed "WHIM/3D QSAR" by Milano Chemometrics and QSAR Research Group, was released in 1994 and was designed specifically for the computation of WHIM descriptors. Following that, many more descriptors were added, resulting in new software called DRAGON, which supplied around 600 descriptors and was published in 1997. Since 1997, DRAGON has been continuously updated to include novel molecular descriptors and new algorithms for improving precision and time efficiency, as well as its capacity to read various molecular file formats, to promote research in QSAR. DRAGON can calculate 1664 chemical descriptors and is intended to run on both Windows and Linux computers [59,60]. For Windows, there are two versions: DRAGON professional, which can only be used in stand-alone mode, and DRAGON plus, which can be used in both stand-alone and background mode. There is just one version for Linux, named dragon, and it only runs in background mode using a command line. DRAGON is not intended to be used as a QSAR program; it simply gives molecular descriptors and does not conduct QSAR analysis or geometry optimization. DRAGON, on the other hand, allows you to combine computed molecular descriptors and user-defined characteristics for a collection of molecules, resulting in a full output file that can be loaded by any correlation analysis tool. In addition, DRAGON now includes a menu that allows for the calculation of pair correlations between chemical descriptors and experimental characteristics, as well as a graphical study of the distribution of molecules in the descriptor and response space [61,62].

10. Knowledge-based approaches

It is possible to estimate the molecular-free energy of interactions between molecules using databases of ligand-protein complexes when ligands dock into protein cavities. Interatomic distance contributions discovered in complexes are converted into pair-potential functions for each pair of ligand/protein atom types in this knowledge-based technique. To derive an estimate of the ligand-protein interaction's free energy, ligand/protein atom pairs that are close to one another are added together. One of the advantages of this method is that it implicitly takes into account contributions to ligand-protein interaction that are not well known. Different potentials were used for different complexes, depending on their ligand and protein atom types, the range of interatomic distances they scanned, and the width of distance bins they used. BLEEP, PMF, and SMoG2001, three knowledge-based potentials, were recently tested to see if they could predict protein ligand-binding affinities in a set of 77 complexes. Knowledge-based possibilities fail to surpass the others constantly. A lot depends on the type of ligand-protein complexes being researched even if previous knowledge prospects are far from universally relevant. Efforts to improve protein-ligand potentials have been considered as a method of harmonizing time and efficiency while getting the most of data and optimizing transferability [63,64].

11. Testing of virtual ligands

Molecules in large biochemical libraries are scored and ranked according to their likelihood of having affinities for a specific target, a technique known as "virtual screening." QSAR's original focus on tiny sets of congeneric compounds might be seen as an attempt to expand this notion to the chemical dimension characterized by synthesized molecules as well as those that could be synthesized. Late in the 1990s, computer-based approaches had matured enough to provide an alternative to high-throughput screening experiments, which surprisingly low performance and greater costs than initially anticipated. The word itself was established at this time. Virtual screening technologies have been accepted by the pharmaceutical industry throughout the years as an effective supplement to HTS to the point that they have unquestionably become a vital element of today's lead generating process.

Instead of relying on technology for HTS, virtual screening relies on knowledge about the target of interest and its bioactive ligands and its structure. When it comes to discovering new bioactive scaffolds using virtual screening, information about the target derived from existing bioactive ligands is as useful as information about the target structures. A decision on which strategy is best will be based on the available information rather than a priori on how well it performs [65,66].

12. Methods based on ligands

Virtual screening approaches based on ligands are many. It all depends on the type of structural information that is being employed, and hence the complexity of the algorithm and the computing cost. Chemical similarity calculations are at the heart of ligand-based virtual screening since they are based on the primary similarity-property idea. Thus, a database may be used to rank all compounds in the database based on how similar they are to one or several bioactive ligands. It is common for these strategies to outperform the random selection of molecules in databases in terms of enrichment. Drug development programs can prioritize experimental testing of high-scoring compounds after this approach, which is a cost-effective technique.

When it comes to virtual screening, topological fingerprints that encode the existence of substructure pieces in molecules have been the most often utilized representation of the structure. The usage of distributions of atom-centered feature pairs in virtual screening applications has also been demonstrated to be extremely successful at the topological level. These methods can be used instead of topological approaches to study molecular structures. In virtual screening, one of the most often used techniques is the superposition of molecules onto one or more conformations of a reference bioactive ligand [67,68].

Using 3D structural representations of chemicals based on pharmacophore similarity is arguably the most used strategy. The pharmacophore has been defined as the three-dimensional arrangement of molecular properties necessary for bioactivity since its beginnings. Although the industry had a slow start, pharmacophore approaches are currently employed to evaluate a broad variety of therapeutic targets for the virtual screening of chemical databases. Many targets have been found using pharmacophores as part of virtual screening methods, such as the protein kinase C and farnesyltransferase, as well as the HIV integrase and antagonists of the endothelium differentiation gene receptor as well as the CCR5 antagonist. Pharmacophores have been produced by several ADME/Tox-related proteins. We can see the vast spectrum of applications of pharmacophore-based approaches in these projects, which include a wide range of biological challenges. Newer methods for extracting ligand pharmacophores from protein cavities have been developed recently for the production of pharmacophores for diverse targets and simultaneous pharmacophore selectivity screening [69,70].

13. Target-based methods

Target-based virtual screening approaches need to have structural knowledge about the target, either through experiments or by homology modeling. While these approaches are aimed at providing an accurate representation of what's likely to happen in terms of docking, they also attempt to provide an accurate estimate of how much binding affinity the ligand will have with the protein (scoring after more than two decades of study, docking and scoring ligands in target sites remains a difficult task. Cummings et al. To remove ligand-dependent biases in scoring functions, many active site adjustments and multiple scoring functions (consensus scoring) have been recommended by Charifson et al. Many docking approach now utilizes all of the information generated from ligand conformation to rectify some of the limitations of current scoring systems and actively direct ligand orientations into the protein cavity. A virtual screening method known for its ability to find and generate new bioactive chemicals has overcome several of these constraints. An example of this is the discovery of novel picomolar ligands for the human carbonic anhydrase II by using a knowledge-based potential (SMoG) in protein-ligand docking. Many kinase targets have also been discovered by docking approaches, including those of the cyclin-dependent kinases, the epidermal growth factor receptor kinase and the vascular endothelial growth factor receptor 2 kinases. Finally, docking approaches have attracted a lot of interest in recent years, notably for the many GPCR targets of therapeutic importance. This is due to the lack of empirically determined structures for these GPCRs. Modeling the target of interest's structure using a template of another target, typically containing knowledge about ligand constraints, is used in these circumstances to produce structural information computationally. Successfully identifying new antagonists for neurokinin-1 and 1A-adrenergic receptors have been a result of these tactics [71–73].

14. Affinity profiling

Aside from the chemical dimension, current advancements in virtual affinity profiling have added a biological component to the QSAR model. Recently, a flurry of novel approaches for evaluating the pharmacological profile of compounds across a variety of targets has been published. In drug discovery, these might have a significant impact by allowing researchers to identify possible side effects of compounds during the optimization process due to off-target affinities. Our ability to extract pharmacological data from molecules and proteins, as well as to acquire structural information about proteins, has made significant contributions to the present growth of these technologies [74,75].

15. Ligand-based methods

For oligonucleotide affinity profiling, annotated chemical libraries, which include pharmacological data in conventional chemical archives, have proved beneficial. Chemicals that have been published in medical chemistry journals during the last 30 years may be found inside the database of WOMBAT. Information on more than 132,000 compounds may be found in the MDL Drug Data Report, which was compiled from patent literature, industry publications, and conferences. The AurSCOPE databases include annotations on more than 38,500 chemicals with over 1,300,000 biological activities linked to members of therapeutically relevant protein families. GVK Biosciences' MedChem and Target Inhibitor databases include more than 2,000,000 compounds culled from more than 20,00,000 academic papers. The end-user can link small compounds to particular proteins as a consequence of all of these huge annotation activities. Consequently, virtual affinity profiling may be performed using protein models based on ligands, which can subsequently be utilized to construct protein models [76,77].

The PASS computer system analyses structure-activity relationships for the training set using 35,000 physiologically active compounds from the literature. More than 500 distinct biological processes can have their chemical activity spectra predicted by the system. Other groundbreaking research examined the molecular structures of 48 compounds in connection to their pharmacological profile about a collection of more than 70 receptors, transporters, and channels in the central nervous system. This was done by grouping 1567 drugs based on the % inhibition values that were obtained for an assay set of 92 based on the single high-ligand concentration. Previously, MDDR was shown to be a valuable tool for the study of four distinct target types: enzymes, GPCRs, nuclear receptors, and channels that are activated by ligands. Then, using dopamine D2-binding molecules as a reference set, we searched for structures that bind to dopamine D2, as well as all other dopamine receptors and class A GPCRs. The naive Bayesian multiple-category Laplacian model was trained on 964 target classes using WOMBAT's extensive connection-fingerprint database. According to the MDDR database, the algorithm correctly identified the top three most likely targets for chemicals with an average accuracy rate of 77%. There are more than 500 biological endpoints annotated to hundreds of structures in a database that include pharmacological end points (cell-based, animal model-based, ADME, and therapeutic outcomes). Substructures found in molecules that are connected to a certain end point in the database are then marked for future examination. To better understand the affinities of the molecules that incorporate each topological scaffold, new datasets have just been created. This approach may be used to find scaffolds that show statistical enrichment in specific biological activity. A literature-based chemical library has 1426 molecules connected with 27 members of the nuclear receptor family, and this information was used to extract the library's most promiscuous scaffolds. Ontology-based pattern identification discovered nearly 1500 scaffold families with statistically significant structure-activity characteristics. The pharmacological profile of 100 antiviral medicines was also assessed using a ligand-based affinity profiling approach employing different structure-based pharmacophore models developed for diverse viral targets. Ninety per cent of the substances tested in the trial were successfully profiled using virtual activity. An accurate descriptor model for the nuclear receptor family profiling was created by employing a novel set of topological atom center distributions and a library of 2033 compounds annotated to 25 nuclear receptors. Using ligand-based nuclear receptor profiling, researchers used this strategy to the second database of 2944 medications and revealed off-target affinity [78,79].

16. Methods based on the goal

There has been a growth in the number of experimentally characterized protein structures, which has led to the development of affinity profiling methods based on target-based coverage of protein families. Due to technical restrictions, several therapeutically important protein families are presently underrepresented in 3D structures (e.g., membrane-bound proteins). More than 20,000 structural members make up the enzyme family, which is the largest. GPCRs have just a few structures, while nuclear receptors and ligand-gated ion channels have over 200. In the latter case, computationally generated structural models are needed to augment the current low levels of coverage of empirically obtained structures [80,81].

Despite its computationally high cost, target-based virtual profiling (also known as inverse docking) has seen some recent applications in the industry. As a result of sequence docking against trypsin, chymotrypsin, and the S1-specificity preferences of serine proteases, different combinatorial libraries were able to predict the preferences of serine proteases. Finding micromolar inhibitors for the human-specific GPRT from *Giardia lamblia* was made possible by screening three libraries against a panel of six PRTs from different species. Virtual screening of a library of 5000 random compounds and 78 known active ligands was also performed against 19 distinct protein structures representing 10 nuclear receptors. Only one of the receptors showed enrichments of 33 to 100 times, showing that a particular ligand may be utilized to locate the exact receptor in a family of receptors. Despite this, the capacity to discriminate between closely related receptor isoforms remained a significant challenge. Half of the computer-identified potential protein targets were confirmed by inverse docking experiments, which entails aligning a molecule to the protein cavity utilizing multiple conformer shape-matching conformers on two pharmaceutical compounds. Additionally, it was used to forecast prospective toxicity concerns and to discover protein targets connected to small-molecule side effects, with an estimated prediction success rate of 83% The sc-PDB contains all 6415 3D structures from the Protein Data Bank. Using this database of binding sites, four unrelated ligands might be found in the top 1% of scored binding sites, with an enrichment of 70 to 100 times greater than random screening. In addition, it has been shown that the relative affinities of inhibitors for different kinase members may be readily calculated. Inhibitor kinase targets and experimental patterns in binding affinities were both found using this way of examining kinase inhibitors. Small compounds may now be tested against 698 protein structures, covering 15 therapeutic areas, using an internet service that was only made public last month [82,83].

17. Data visualization

Many various qualities can be predicted using computational techniques, which necessitates the use of multidimensional approaches and potentially advanced visualization tools for data mining in the examination of such data. There are widely viable tools such as Diva and Spotfire that can be incorporated into internally developed decision support systems, while modern techniques are also obtainable with comparable 3D graphing and filtering possibilities for ADME and physicochemical property data clustering algorithms based on 2D structural similarity, recursive partitioning, Sammon maps, and self-organizing maps, such as agglomerative hierarchical clustering, can also be integrated with computational predictions.

A thorough understanding of medication interactions with the proteome is essential since they might have several off-target effects at the same time. Proteins and small molecules may be connected by connections in networks when information is transferred at a specific affinity threshold, or proteins can be highlighted in networks that are based on targets when they interact with small molecules. To better understand transcriptional factor pathways, network analysis has long been the traditional approach for doing so. To study the connections between endogenous molecules, commercially available technologies may be used to establish a channel of just molecules. These techniques can also be used to visualize gene expression data for nuclear receptors that regulate drug metabolism and toxicity [84–86].

A network method may also be used to create medications that have a high affinity for numerous targets or to prevent anti-targets. In one recent example, an annotated chemical library encompassing 2033 compounds and representing the interactions of 25 nuclear receptors was developed. Small molecule side-effect prediction might be improved by identifying possible cross-pharmacology between members of this class. There are many hurdles ahead for network techniques, such as comparing several networks. We've already covered some of these issues. When using this sort of technique to visualize the influence of a compound on the linked proteome and compare the effects of related compounds or various dosages, this might be essential. The use of more complicated network biology models may also be necessary to better target, dose, and frequency. An in silico modeling of inhibitor effects on the NF-B pathway (incorporating PK data) has demonstrated that inhibition upstream of this protein has a larger potential for protein oscillatory behavior than for direct inhibition. This type of behavior is prevalent in networks that get negative feedback, and it should be taken into consideration and understood to maximize the therapeutic effect [87,88].

18. Examples of in silico pharmacology

All the proteins that have been modeled in silico under the umbrella of in vitro pharmacology would be impossible to cover in this overview. Here is a summary of the protein types and modeling techniques used. New ligands have been found as a result of virtual screening, and we will go through them as well. Highly recommended reading for anybody interested in learning more about the successes of various computer-aided design processes is a comprehensive assessment of the many proteins that have been successfully targeted by various in silico approaches. As a means of enhancing the efficiency of drug discovery and development, computational techniques have been used to practically all major proteins involved in absorption, distribution, metabolism, and toxicity (ADME/Tox). All proteins and protein families that have been researched utilizing current state-of-the-art in silico drug development tools will be examined in this study [89,90].

The following is a list of drug targets.

18.1 Enzymes

The ubiquitin regulatory system, which controls how ubiquitin is attached to and deconjugated from substrate proteins, may hold therapeutic possibilities for cancer and other diseases. Even though its substrate is made up of amino acids rather than polypeptides, the enzyme HAUSP that de-ubiquitinates the p53 protein may help in the identification of new medications. P53 and other ubiquitinated proteins may be de-ubiquitinated by a nonpeptidic inhibitor of the protein-degrading enzyme that has been demonstrated to be effective. IC50 values are in the micromolar range and trigger cell death in the absence of the tumor suppressor p53, which is mutated in half of all cancer cases (hence, p53 inhibition per se may not represent an optimal target for modulation). These compounds highlight the importance of the sterically accessible ketones for bioactivity: Dibenzylidenacetone (SUB), curcumin, the punaglandin compounds from coral, and the inhibitory effects of shikonin. For additional chemical optimization, these compounds may be utilized.

The cytochrome P450 (CYP)19 enzyme aromatase has been demonstrated to be a valuable target in the battle against breast cancer. Nonsteroidal anti-inflammatory medications were used to create a ligand-based pharmacophore. This model's detection of known inhibitors from an in-house library was further improved by including molecular structure. Searching the NCI database for chemicals was done using a 16-compound model created by Accelrys Inc. (San Diego, CA, USA). Toxicology-related proteins were also tested for in the hits utilizing various pharmacophores before testing. Two of the three compounds had their micromolar inhibitors found [91,92].

Structure-based pharmacophores for acetylcholine esterase were developed and then used in a search for natural compounds in a database. The approach identified scopoletin and scopolin as potential hits, and both showed some in vivo activity. Searches for known COX-1 and COX-2 pharmacophore inhibitors were conducted using similar databases. Examples of ethnopharmacological and computational strategies working together to discover novel medications are shown below.

To study 5-LOX in humans, a combination of ligand-based and structure-based approaches were used. A five-feature pharmacophore was developed using a Catalyst qualitative HipHop model and 16 different compounds. An enzyme homology model was constructed using two LOX enzymes from soybean and one from the rabbit. The four-feature pharmacophore of the 5-LOX homology model was updated and improved using molecular docking once all of the data had been obtained. Virtual screening was recommended for compounds having phenylthiourea or 5-pyrimidine groups as candidates for aminoacid residues at the binding site. More than 50,000 compounds were virtual screened using human 12- and 15-LOX homology models using Schrödinger Inc.'s Glide docking software. There was an inhibitory effect on eight of the 20 medicines examined [93,94].

It's been more than 30 years since any renin inhibitor has been developed for the market. Despite this, hypertension researchers continue to be intrigued by renin as a potential target. Nonpeptidic inhibitors of human renin have been found using a structure-based design. Piperidines, such as Ro-0661168 and related 3,4-substituted piperidines, are among these chemicals. Unlike aliskiren, which only attaches to the protein in its "closed renin" form, these piperidines bind to and stabilize a different form of the protein known as "openrenin.". These early efforts to build novel renin inhibitors using computer-aided design have been surprisingly sparse in number. Angiotensinogen peptide analogs with chain modifications might be identified using a single QSAR. Although Kier's first-order molecular connection index descriptor and molecular weight were shown to correlate, log *P* did not show a correlation. A whole new approach to design shows that GrowMol can regenerate 3,4-disubstituted piperidines in 1% of the produced structures, a computational technique for the synthesis of renin inhibitors. Novel renin inhibitors were discovered in the early 1990s using a Catalyst pharmacophore. Many novel substances that mapped to renin pharmacophores were found in Pomona (an early 3D database of compounds) but had not been tested in vitro. Using a consensus scoring system, LigandFit docking experiments discovered 10 known inhibitors in the top 8.4% of a library of 1000 compounds having an open renin crystal structure. Four high-scoring compounds that were not considered as inhibitors had excluded volumes and four hydrophobes, a hydrogen bond donor or a positive ionizable feature. Another study found enrichment factors that were 17 times greater than chance while scanning the MDDR database for more than 100,000 drugs containing 10 renin inhibitors. Genetic algorithms have been used to discriminate between renin inhibitors and noninhibitors in a small area of the MDDR using just a few interpretable characteristics. Renin inhibitors were shown to have much more amide bonds, molecular weights, and hydrogen bond donors than their nonrenin inhibitor equivalents. Novel renin inhibitors, for example, have lately been the subject of an extensive study that gives a wealth of new data that may be used to improve QSAR models and search databases in search of new starting scaffolds for optimization [95,96].

Cathepsin D may be an Alzheimer's disease target if it is found in lysosomes, where it might be implicated in the release of -amyloid precursor protein. Cancers such as breast and ovarian may benefit from Cathepsin D if it is shown to be hyperactive. Protease inhibitors were thoroughly reviewed, and Cathepsin D was discussed just briefly in the discussion. Structure-based design and combinatorial chemistry were used to find cathepsin D nanomolar replacement compounds. For a little more than a seventh of the structures, researchers turned to Pepstatin, a 3.8-pM inhibitor. These chemicals suppressed the formation of hyperphosphorylated Tau fragments in human hippocampus slices. Few computational studies have been done on cathepsin D and other aspartic proteases like renin and -secretase. To find new Cathepsin D inhibitors, several researchers have used molecular dynamics and free energy analysis (MM-PBSA). Additionally, Cathepsin D molecules have been rediscovered using ADAPT, which places necessary components in the right places. An algorithmic design program is used here. Computational models may be used to identify nonpeptidic and selective compounds for protease inhibition. Based on eight Cathepsin D inhibitors ($r=0.98$), a pharmacophore for Cathepsin D inhibitors has been created. The 11,441 substances in the database could only be narrowed down to 10 using pharmacophore. As a result of a 95% similarity search conducted by ChemFinder (CambridgeSoft, Cambridge, MA, USA), 16 unique compounds were identified. All of them were subjected to in vitro testing. More than 40% inhibition of the target was suggested by at least one match in both pharmacophore and similarity searches. ADME properties of active medicines were expected to be well absorbed, while solubility and CYP2D6 inhibition concerns were predicted for some [97,98].

Pharmacophore and structure-based approaches have been used to optimize the acyl urea hit for human glycogen phosphorylase. It was possible to construct additional analogs using the Catalyst HypoGen pharmacophore. There was a high ($r=0.71$) correlation between the use of these substances and the capacity to predict future events. An X-ray structure of a single molecule was used to confirm the predicted binding arrangement. Final results were obtained utilizing all the molecules synthesized and verified to be following the X-ray structure using a CoMFA model. In rats, this chemical was shown to reduce blood glucose levels in vivo and to have a strong cellular effect.

High-resolution crystals of the human sirtuin type 2 deacetylation of -tubulin have been found; this enzyme may be used to regulate aging and certain cancers. The Maybridge docking database provided a small hit list from which 15 compounds were examined, five of which displayed micromolar pharmacological activity.

Since its crystal structure can be used to create a homology model of the human enzyme, catechol *O*-methyltransferase has emerged as a possible drug target for Parkinson's disease. To further understand the structure-activity connection of these catechins and their metabolites, FlexX software was used to dock them (SAR). Lys 144 distance from responsive catechol hydroxy group, as well as enzyme catalytic tail length, were all shown to block catechins [99,100].

18.2 Kinases

In the pharmaceutical sector, the more than 500 kinases provide an appealing family of targets. To build chemogenomic dendrograms, small-molecule selectivity data were used to map the kinase space, and the highly homologous kinases were shown to be inhibited by small molecules in the same way. For kinases, virtual screening approaches have been used extensively. Using the apo CDK2 and olomoucine as starting points, the structure-based design strategy was able to create novel and powerful CDK1 inhibitors. For the CDK1 sequence, just a few amino acid substitutions were made. A visual study of the ligand's molecular structure led to the discovery of potential molecular modification locations. Design work prompted ligand optimization to enhance activity from 4.5 M to 25 nM very fast. Alsterpaullone has an IC50 of 35 nM, however, this could be reduced to 0.23 nM by using a CDK1/cyclin B homology model that was manually docked.

For the Syk C-terminal SH2 domain, a structure based in silico screening technique was used to locate low molecular weight fragments with millimolar binding affinity for each binding site. A starting point for further lead optimization was reached by linking the fragments, resulting in molecules with a molecular weight in the 38–350 M range.

Pseudoreceptors were constructed using the flexible atom receptor model approach with 27 EGFR tyrosine kinase inhibitors. High r2 and q2 values were found in the top 15 models, which were also tested using a six-molecule test set. Also, a crystal structure of CDK2 was found in agreement with the pseudoreceptor's structure [101,102].

For this study, DOCK was used in conjunction with the crystal structure of the Lck SH2 domain to screen 2 million commercially available chemicals. Extensive filtering was required to come up with a list of viable targets. In vitro, two compounds were inhibitory at 10 and 40 M and 34 substances inhibited at 100 M. KD values were found to be in the micromolar range in some instances using fluorescence titration. The same team found ERK2 inhibitors by screening 800,000 compounds computationally and assessing 80 of them in vitro. When fluorescence was titrated against ERK2, cell proliferation was reduced in five of these compounds, and two of them had KD values in the low micromolar range. Docking of the active molecules predicted both molecular orientations, and X-ray crystallography confirmed those predictions.

STI-571 (imatinib, Gleevec) was discovered in a single and multiple conformation database utilizing the Ligand Scout method. A hydrophobic pocket in the binding site of STI-571 may be favorable to the 3-substituted benzamidine derivative when docked into the binding site and the energy lowered. These two proteins are members of the COP9 signalosome, which regulates the stability of p53 (a tumor suppressor gene) and c-Jun (a cancer-promoting gene). Other than ubiquitin isopeptidase inhibitor and activator protein-1 activator protein-1 inhibitor, curcumin has also been shown to have anti-CK2, anti-PKD, and anti-PKD properties. In a library of over a million compounds, 2D and 3D similarity searches found 35 molecules using curcumin and emodin as reference structures. Seven of them were inhibitory in action. Piceatannol, for example, had IC50 values of 2.5 and 0.5 M against CK2 and PKD that were higher than those of curcumin. However, it is noteworthy to note that few of these studies account for selectivity for other kinases, which suggests that kinase activation molecules have been found. Ultimately, for therapeutic effectiveness, some kinases may have to be activated (while others are selectively inhibited) [103,104].

It was pioneering work by Hansch et al. that used a few chemical descriptors and small groups of similar compounds to correlate quantitative structure-metabolism correlations. For human CYPs, Lewis and colleagues have developed multiple QSAR and homology models and have seen an increase in the number of models and the number of data sets due to the advent of more complex computational modeling techniques. Lewis and colleagues: When docking molecules into these enzymes, water molecules may also be key hydrogen bond mediators, since some recent techniques incorporate water molecules in the binding sites. Drugs may be discovered by the use of docking approaches, for example. Metoclopramide was docked with a CYP2D6 homology model, along with 19 other drugs, and an $r^2=0.61$ association between IC50 and docking score was discovered. The major metabolite was discovered and confirmed in vitro to be a novel aromatic N-hydroxy metabolite. In comparison to previous computer models of mammalian CYPs that have been made available, they are very accurate. For enzymes like CYP3A4, certain computational approaches, such as docking utilizing known crystal structures, may have difficulty producing meaningful predictions. As others have argued in recent years, there may be more than one way to look at this enzyme and others [105,106].

Phase II enzymes, such as UDP-glucuronosyltransferases, catalyze the conjugation of glucuronic acid to substrates containing an appropriate functional group, therefore aiding in the removal of medicines. Several QSAR and pharmacophore models for rat and human enzymes have been built using relatively modest data sets. Hydrophobes and the glucuronidation feature are shared by the human UGT1A1, UGT1A4, and UGT1A9, but UGT1A9 has an extra hydrogen bond accepting characteristic. First, sulfotransferases, another family of conjugating enzymes, have been crystallized and a QSAR technique has been utilized to predict substrate affinity to SULT1A3. Other isozymes have not yet had computer models constructed, as far as we know. For in silico models, conjugating enzymes have been less common than other enzymes. They have not been used as much in the industry because there are not as many in vitro studies and compounds examined.

Several organizations have already studied the computational modeling of drug transporters in great detail. In vitro screening and enrichment may be improved by using several models of the transporter system to explore databases for novel targets and inhibitors. Co-transporters of Na + and D-glucose in the renal proximal tubules were modeled using phlorizin analogs and the DISCO program. In this way, it was possible to make an educated guess of the binding site's size. In contrast to current research on transporter pharmacophores, this model was neither tested nor used in database searches [107,108].

18.3 Receptors

On the cellular membranes, there are many more than 20 families of receptors that constitute over 1000 proteins of the receptorome. As a therapeutic target, receptors have a vast range of ligands to choose from. Aside from this limited fraction of the receptorome, we have only identified or defined a small number of the receptors. Anticonvulsant and neuroprotectant ligands have been developed for the -amino-3-hydroxy-5-methyl-4-isoxazole propionate receptor, which is implicated in a wide range of CNS disorders. A four-point catalyst HIP-HOP pharmacophore with 14 antagonists was constructed because there is presently no 3D structural information. Using this, eight compounds were selected for testing from the May bridge database and six were proven to be active in vivo as anticonvulsants.

From the central nervous system to the gut wall, serotonin plays an important function in many physiological processes. To regulate cardiovascular development, it has a large number of receptors along with its diverse functions. It's thought that the 5-HT2 receptors are G protein-coupled 7-transmembrane-spanning receptors that are found in the heart, intestine, and brain, as well as in human carcinoid tumors. Individuals with valvular heart disease defects were treated with the now-banned "fen-phen" medication that was connected to this receptor in recent years. The major metabolite, norfenfluramine, has a strong impact on 5-HT2B. The computer modeling of this receptor has been constrained up to this point in its development. The 5-HT2B contractile receptor antagonists tetrahydro-ß carboline compounds were employed in an old-fashioned QSAR investigation in the rat stomach fundus. The poor model statistics were likely caused by the model's inability to handle the complex functional response and the limited range of activity that was examined in QSAR GRID-GOLPE using 38 (aminoalkyl) benzo and heterocycloalkanone antagonists of the human receptor. There was no way to evaluate any of these theories since there were no outside predictions. Bacteriorhodopsin and rhodopsin have been used to build homology models for the 5-HT2B receptors in mice and humans. The bacteriorhodopsin structure confirmed an aromatic box theory for the ligand interaction between transmembrane domains 3, 6, and 7 with serotonin. An updated 5-HT2B homology model, based on the rat 5-HT2A rhodopsin model, was used to determine the interaction sites for norfenfluramine after molecular dynamics simulations Using van der Waals contacts and methyl groups, Val 2.53 was discovered to have a function in high-affinity ligation. QSAR models for this receptor might be created to speed up the screening process for excessively strong inhibitors [109–111].

Extensive modeling of the 5-HT1A serotonin receptor has occurred. SYBYL was used as an example for defining antagonist site pharmacophores. Active analog modeling was used to predict stereospecificity in molecules. This iteration used FlexX docking to fine-tune 700 homology models based on the crystal structure of bovine rhodopsin to better reflect the actual binding properties of ligands. The completed model was used to execute a virtual screening simulation, and the authors concluded that it might be used for a real virtual screening. A library of 10,000 molecules, seeded with 34 5-HT1A ligands, was also screened by DOCK. Ninety per cent of these active chemicals made it into the top 1000 compounds, indicating a substantial enrichment. Only one of the 78 tested compounds had an affinity of less than 1 nM, according to the same model. A structure based in silico optimization was performed to boost selectivity with additional GPCRs and optimize the PK profile. Because these compounds were discovered to have an affinity for hERG, they were then computationally analyzed using the homology model, which indicated that hydrophobicity may be altered. It was determined that the clinical candidate had excellent selectivity for both targets and antitargets and that the backup compounds were selected in the same manner.

SYBYL was used to construct a pharmacophore for 5-HT1D agonists with selectivity against 5-HT2A, a 5-HT2A antagonist connected to undesired changes in blood pressure, as an early computer-aided pharmacophore [112,113].

Antipsychotic drugs that target 5-HT6 receptors include a broad range of medications. The bovine rhodopsin structure was used to generate human and rat 5-HT6 receptor homology models, which were used to dock ligands that differed across species. Analysis of ligand binding was carried out using docking techniques to identify amino acid residues that should be modified. Using the in vitro data, new compounds may be developed using the models established. This research used computational, molecular biology, and traditional pharmacology approaches.

The Na^+, K^+-ATPase receptor mediates the inhibition of the Na+, K+-ATPase and cation transport and ionotropic effects of cardiotonic steroids. A molecular understanding of Digitalis' actions has only recently been developed. A homology model based on the SERCA1a crystal structure was put to the test using nine cardiac glycosides. The model's capacity to reproduce the receptors of rats and mice may have explained Obain's attraction for multiple species. To test the idea of identifying a binding site, models suggested changing amino acids, although this has not yet been tested.

Parkinson's disease and schizophrenia have been linked to the dopamine receptors in the brain. To find novel antagonists, researchers have relied on QSAR models because there is yet no crystal structure. For each of the 48 chemicals studied, four distinct QSAR approaches (CoMFA, PLS, kNN, and SVM) were utilized, and training and testing statistics were obtained for each method. More than 750,000 molecules had been mined using SVM and kNN models, resulting in 54 consensus hits. In the training set, five of these hits were known to bind the receptor, whereas other proposed hits did not include the catechol group often seen in most dopamine inhibitors [114,115].

Antihypertensive medicines can benefit from targeting the 1A receptor, which regulates vascular tone. Multi-feature tree (MTree) defines the training set molecules as feature tree descriptors that are produced from a topological molecular network and are then aligned pairwise for the ligand-based screen. With the help of a collection of six antagonists, a pharmacophore model for Catalyst was created and tested. An ionizable feature at the center of both methods was found to be bordered by hydrophobic areas. A database of more than 47,500 molecules was ranked using these two approaches. MTree's enrichment factor was more than twice as high as Catalyst's in the top 1% of the database.

For the pharmaceutical business, nuclear receptors are a critical class of ligand-activated transcription factors that are sometimes referred to as "double-edged swords." On the other hand, mutations in nuclear receptors have been linked to a wide range of common human disorders, including cancer, diabetes, and osteoporosis, and hence they are regarded as extremely relevant therapeutic targets for the treatment of these diseases. When it comes to CYP enzymes and drug transporters that might assist medication efficacy, nuclear receptors are also regarded as possible therapeutic antitargets because of their role in regulating the metabolism of pharmaceutically important substances.

Virtual screening has recently discovered novel small-molecule modulators of nuclear receptors. Homology models of the retinoic acid receptor were constructed utilizing the known structure of the estrogen receptor subtype in the antagonist configuration. New RAR antagonists in the micromolar range were uncovered through virtual screening of a chemical library. A similar approach resulted in the discovery of 14 novel antagonists of the micromolar thyroid hormone receptors. To find novel ER antagonists, researchers focused on the estrogen receptor's peptide-binding surface LxxLL. Some of these medications may represent new ER antagonists that can be used as an alternative to current anti-estrogen treatment. Three low micromolar hits with >100 times the binding selectivity for ER were also recently discovered by screening databases. Researchers developed a new family of partial agonists for the peroxisome proliferator-activated-receptor-a that showed a remarkable selectivity profile against other subtypes of the same nuclear receptor group [116,117].

18.4 Ion channels

Among the most important therapeutic channels are the voltage-gated ion channels for potassium, sodium, and calcium that are located in the outer membranes of several cell types. Effectiveness has been shown in the treatment of anesthesia, cardiovascular illness, and the central nervous system CoMFAs and SVMs, 2D-QSARs, Genetic Programming and Self-Organization Maps have been applied to most ion channels. Recursive partitioning has also been used. These two channels appear to have been most intensively researched in this area thus far. The sodium channel, on the other hand, has significantly fewer instances of computational models. As either therapeutic targets or ant targets to avoid, these three types of ion channels have been extensively researched.

For example, a model for the hERG potassium channel has contrasted three distinct approaches for training and testing with the same collection of molecules. Atom path lengths were partitioned using recursive partitioning, Sammon maps, and Kohonen maps. For both training and testing, the classification quality was excellent. External test chemicals were better classified by Sammon mapping than by Kohonen mapping. To exclude molecules that differed significantly from the training set from the quantitative predictions for recursive partitioning, one may apply a Tanimoto similarity filter. The path length descriptors may also be used to show how similar the molecules in the training set are to each other. An additional subset of molecules, marked in blue for close neighbors and red for distant ones, can also be compared [118–120].

18.5 Involved in the transcription process

Nonpeptidic compounds with low-energy conformations were compared to a 3D pharmacophore drawn from the activity of a cyclic decapeptide against the AP-1 transcription factor. In a lead hopping strategy, new 1-thia-4-azaspiro[4,5]decane and benzophenone compounds with binding and cell-based action were found as AP-1 inhibitors.

18.6 Antibacterials

The catalyst program was used to build a pharmacophore for Mycobacterium TB thymidine monophosphosphate kinase inhibitors using 20 deoxythymidine monophosphate analogs and docking. Finally, the completed model was utilized to filter a vast database including known inhibitors. High significance has been assigned to the model's enrichment factor of 17. It was also used to quickly screen half a million chemicals to uncover novel inhibitors [121,122].

18.7 Antivirals

Influenza virus has a large amount of neuraminidase on its surface. Catalyst pharmacophores were generated using a structure-based technique, and these pharmacophores were then employed in a database search to find known inhibitors. Selective hit lists were also a feature of the game.

Protease from the human rhinovirus 3C is a target for antirhinitis therapy. Initially, a pharmacophore based on the structure of AG 7088 was designed; however, this proved to be too limiting. To create a second pharmacophore, we utilized the catalyst HIP-HOP method. It was beneficial to search the World Drug Index database for known and tested antiviral compounds, as well as other databases for new compounds that meet the pharmacophore, indicating that they should be tested, despite the lack of final testing validation data. Another antirhinitis target is the coat protein of the human rhinovirus. PCA-based clustering was employed in conjunction with a pharmacophore and docking technique. The structure and form of a known inhibitor were used to construct a pharmacophore, which was evaluated for its capacity to locate known inhibitors in a database. In the end, 10 substances were identified after analyzing the Maybridge database. Viral growth was inhibited by six different substances that were investigated. Most of them were found to be poisonous or insoluble, though. To locate known inhibitors for the rhinovirus serotype 16, the Ligand Scout technique was tested and found in the PDB.

Efforts have been made to identify and target the SARS coronavirus 3C-like proteinase as an attractive drug design target. Docking chemical databases into a homology model was accomplished. Drug-like criteria and a pharmacophore model were employed to narrow down the list of suspects. In a study including a total of 40 compounds, three were found to have micromolar activity, with the best-being calmidazolium at a concentration of 61 M [123,124].

Pharmacophores have predicted the suppression of hepatitis C RNA-dependent RNA polymerase by diketo acid derivatives. A five-feature pharmacophore model was developed using 40 chemicals with activity levels spanning three logarithmic orders. According to the study, the predicted and experimental results for nine diketo acid derivatives and 19 additional compounds were in good agreement.

Asthma and rheumatoid arthritis are connected to the integrin VLA-4, as are other inflammatory and autoimmune diseases. Catalyst pharmacophores have been employed in the search for antagonists based on the crystal structure of a peptidic inhibitor. The available chemicals directory's reagents were used to search a library of possible compounds. They then produced 12 compounds, with activity levels ranging from 0.13 to 20 micrograms per milliliter. It was, therefore, possible to produce inhibitors that were active in the Vivo using nonpeptides. One group employed CoMFA with a collection of 29 antagonists with an activity range of 1 to 662 nM to develop an internal model with strong validation statistics, which was then used to identify favorable locations for molecular substitution modifications. It is not apparent if the CoMFA model worked for designing additional compounds [125,126].

It is feasible to begin the process of developing new pharmaceuticals for a variety of illnesses by using existing medications. As an example, researchers have used Tanimoto similarity of 3D searching using known inhibitors to look for prion disease leads in the WHO essential medication list. Several compounds have been suggested in this study, but they have not been tested, therefore the technique has not been thoroughly tested yet. The selective disruption of protein-protein interactions is a sought after therapeutic approach to control many illnesses, as they are essential components of cellular signaling cascades. It has proven challenging to find small-molecule inhibitors for pharmacological targets because of their shallow binding sites. Several signaling proteins can be influenced by the G-protein G complex through protein-protein interactions. G-protein-protein interactions have been studied using FlexX docking and consensus scoring of 1990 molecules from the NCI diversity set database. It was observed that only nine of the 85 substances that had been tested as inhibitors of the G12-SIRK peptide had IC50 values of 100 nM or less. Substructure searching was used to find similar compounds to one of the most potent inhibitors to construct a SAR. We may see more potent lead compounds in the future because of these efforts.

19. Complex property modeling

Although in vitro testing and database searches have typically been used to find biologically active compounds for target proteins, we are now looking at in silico models which contain molecules that have previously been recognized as having biological activity for the target protein. In this part, we will look at some of the more complex properties that have been simulated in silico. It is important to remember that although many physicochemical features like clog*P* and water solubility have been extensively studied, the training sets for these models contain thousands or tens of thousands of molecules.

A molecule's half-life may be calculated, for example, by measuring its clearance rate. The intrinsic clearance, which may comprise many enzymes, has therefore been used to quantify the activity of enzymes toward a drug. One of the earliest models for this trait was the CYP-mediated metabolism of chlorinated volatile organic compounds, which is likely suggestive of CYP2E1. Analysis of hepatocyte-derived compounds has yielded multiple linear regression, PCA, PLS, and Neural Networks with leave-one-out cross-validation to predict human clearance in vivo. A catalyst pharmacophore has also been constructed by separating the clearance data from microsomes and hepatocytes before predicting the other data set. Intrinsic pharmacophore characteristics are thought to impact intrinsic clearance in this method [127,128].

Numerous attempts have been made to anticipate the quantity of medication that is partitioned into tissue vs plasma. Combined with the drug's half-life in the circulation, this characteristic helps determine the ideal dose. Sammon and Kohonen mapping techniques, for example, used eight chemical descriptors to map 253 distinct drugs from the literature. These algorithms were able to correctly classify around 80% of the compounds. Recently, a random forest approach and 31 molecular descriptors were utilized to develop a prediction model using a sample of 384 medicines and steady-state literature volume data. This model's geometric mean fold error with 23 molecules was expected to be 1.78 by comparison with earlier models that employed animal or in vitro techniques.

To predict the plasma half-life of various ADME features, data from 458 medications in the literature and four chemical descriptors were used to build Sammon and Kohonen maps. Similar to volume distribution models, these models accurately classified around 80% of the chemicals they investigated. It is possible to assess the metabolization of medicine using renal clearance, which assumes that all of a medication's excretion is unchanged. The last and most difficult feature to grasp is this one. In a published QSAR model, more than 130 molecules and 62 Volsurf or 37 Molconn-Z descriptors were used. To successfully identify between the two classes of drugs tested (0%–20% and 20%–100%), only one model employed soft independent modeling of the analogies and Molconn-Z descriptors.

Computational structure-based design techniques employ them to choose the most probable virtual molecules to bind the protein with the greatest affinity as a fifth example of a complex property that has been developed utilizing many ways such as force fields, empirical and knowledge-based approaches. A genetic algorithm feature selection approach and the Kernel partial least squares (K-PLCs) QSAR methodology were used to describe the binding affinity data for the small molecule training sets that include binding affinity data and the proteins they bind to. Combining bootstrapping, scrambling the data, and external test sets, the models were tested. The essential chemical descriptors associated with the most powerful interactions may be discovered using K-PLS QSAR models covering a large number of proteins. It will be interesting to see whether these models can be developed using the much larger binding affinity data sets that are now available [129,130].

As with the enzyme's highest catalytic activity (V_{max}), this is also an example of a complex property. This value is influenced by the steric properties of the active site and the ease with which the leaving group may be evicted from the active site. A neural network technique was used to predict the V_{max} data for N-dealkylation mediated by CYP2D6 and CYP3A4 and included whole molecules, the reaction centroid, and group-related characteristics. These models may also be used to predict molecules that were not included in the training. To finish the investigation, other reactions and enzymes must be investigated. To obtain greater confidence in the models' usefulness and applicability, larger test sets are needed.

20. Establishing the boundaries of a computer model's usefulness

Comparable to models used in other fields, certain in silico pharmacology approaches have similar limitations, such as those used to predict physicochemically or ADME/Tox features. Examples of models include those created using a small homologous sequence of pharmacologically relevant compounds (local model) or a wide variety of molecules with various structural variations (global model). Their advantages and disadvantages may be seen in each of these methods. The application domain of the local model may be substantially smaller than for the global model, such that moving to a different chemical series might result in prediction failure. As an example, a global model may fail to predict a molecule if it is too far away from the training set's representative molecules. QSAR models have special restrictions in this area. Although global models may be more effective for this characteristic, many of the previously discussed in silico examples show how QSAR models tend to be local, making it more difficult for them to jump to new structural series. The application scope of models and techniques to compute this attribute has been detailed extensively in several works. Similarity to training set chemicals may be an accurate indicator of prediction quality for a hERG model. According to our knowledge, no explicit investigation of the application domain for in silico pharmacology models has been done to the same extent as has been done for physicochemical parameters such as solubility and log P. Although statistical QSAR approaches have been the primary emphasis, the application area of pharmacophore models is not being addressed [131,132].

It is feasible to offer prediction confidence by consensus using hybrid or meta-computational methods (that include many modeling methodologies and algorithms) for forecasting the likely physicochemical and pharmacological characteristics of molecules. If QSAR or pharmacophore models are also available, the docking approaches using homology models for particular proteins of pharmacological relevance might be applied. Homology models and QSARs have been employed together and to validate each other on several occasions in the research of drug-metabolizing enzymes.

In drug metabolism, several outputs (metabolites, for example) are common, a scenario not generally observed in other pharmacological experiments in which a single set of conditions generates a single consequence. Fig. 2 shows how local and comprehensive approaches may be categorized, with local methods being relevant to small biological systems such as a single enzyme or a single enzymatic activity, while comprehensive methods can be used to more complex biological systems. For example, regioselective metabolites are normally foreseeable from such approaches, but the synthesis of alternative pathways (e.g., oxidation vs glucuronidation) isn't. Because they can account for the vast majority of metabolic processes and provide predictions that are considerably closer to what happens in the body, global algorithms (i.e., algorithms that can be applied to a wide variety of biological systems) can be very helpful here [133].

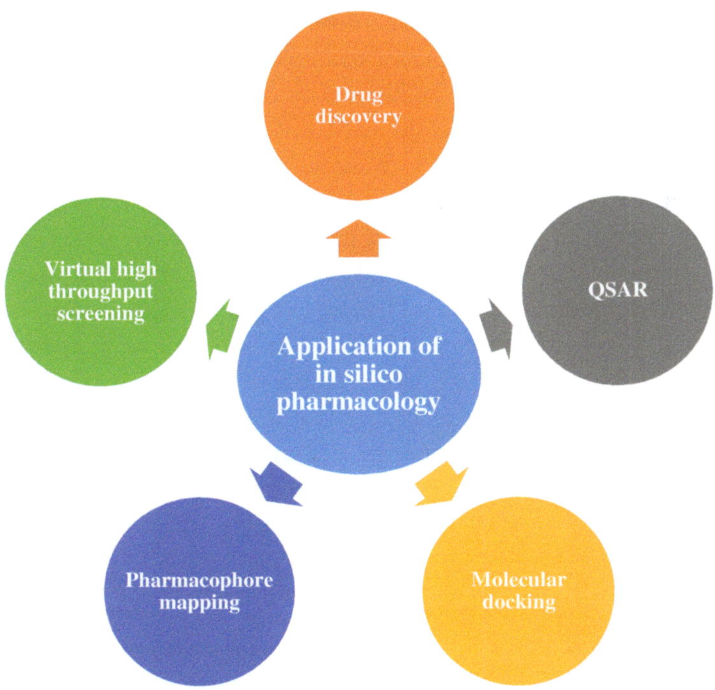

Fig. 2 Application of in silico pharmacology.

21. Anecdotes and cautionary tales

No more proof of biological activity was provided by the authors of a few studies in which computational approaches were employed to forecast the lead compounds for testing. Computational studies have traditionally been undertaken after the molecules have been synthesized, and they have typically offered images and explanations of the findings. Pharmacological activity predictions seem to be going the other way, since they are being published without evident experimental proof, as long as the models are validated in some manner. To determine how far predictions can be extended, future conversations may include a discussion of predicted molecules and their distance from the training set, or some other way.

Because many of the molecules detected by virtual screening procedures have not been investigated in vitro, it is impossible to know for sure whether they are false positives or are part of molecular aggregation. Many proteins' small molecular weights have led to the designation of these molecules as "promiscuous inhibitors." To locate these potentially promiscuous inhibitors, a preliminary computational model was built. Our examination of the scientific literature suggests that it would be worthwhile to conduct extensive experimental testing of their projected bioactive chemicals to rule out this possibility. The number of examples of computational technique failures that are reported may be limited by publication bias. The presence of tough objectives for modeling with diverse methodologies would be really helpful since this appears to be a try and error process for each researcher today.

As described in an earlier study, we believe that the current state of in silico pharmacology, as well as how the field has progressed up to this point, can be used to discover new molecules with bioactive properties and diverse binding sites, as well as to better understand metabolic interactions and pathways. In this study, we have not directly explored PK/PD or full organ/cell/disease simulations; nonetheless, we recognize that they are an essential part of the computer-aided drug design strategy and maybe more broadly integrated with other in silico pharmacology methodologies [134,135].

22. Scope, limitations, and current trends

An in silico pharmacology framework has been proposed that illustrates some of the major functions played by computational technologies in pharmacology. Finding novel antagonists or agonists for a target utilizing a variety of approaches, whether or not there is a structure for the target, is one of these responsibilities. Signaling cascades based on annotated data can also aid in the understanding of biology by using networks and pathways, determining the connectivity of a drug in the form of a network with targets for selectivity, integrating with other models for PD, and eventually emerge of systems in silico pharmacy. This technique may be utilized to find novel chemical probes for academic pharmacologists, rather than lead compounds for optimization to become pharmaceutical products, notwithstanding our pharmaceutical bias. Many advantages of using in silico pharmacology include a reduction in the number of molecules created and evaluated, a rise in the pace of tests, and a reduction in animal and reagent usage as a result of a good prediction of most pharmacological qualities. Take into account the many anticipated qualities, such as assessing in-silico models (or data) on their relevance to pharmacology (or confidence in the model or data). Also, we must address the shortcomings of in silico pharmacology techniques, such as the elasticity and promiscuity of proteins and their molecular structure. Although crystal structures for various mammalian drug-metabolizing enzymes have recently been available, it remains difficult to predict drug metabolism. Animal testing and in vitro experiments with subcellular preparations generated from many species are common in pharmaceutical research, thus we need models from other species to help us better understand and scale-up variations across species. We will talk more about in silico approaches' applicability now, which has been a common criticism leveled at them [136,137].

23. Applications of in silico pharmacology

23.1 Drug discovery

Developing drugs is a complicated, lengthy process that takes many skills and many types of effort. Usually shown as a linear, sequential method that begins with target and prime identification, then progresses through lead optimization and preclinical in vitro and in vivo investigations to see if drugs meet a set of pre-determined criteria before moving forward with clinical development. For quick and precise target identification and prediction in drug discovery, the in silico methodology is preferred.

23.2 QSAR

QSAR is a statistical method for attempting to link a molecule's physical and chemical characteristics to its biological activity. The goal of QSAR is to predict molecule characteristics from their structure without the necessity for an in vitro or in vivo investigation. The QSAR method is focused on the idea that a chemical molecule's activity is connected to its structure. QSAR models are frequently presented as a means for the industry to save money on toxicological research or to avoid using animals in testing.

23.3 Molecular docking

It is one of the most important tools in structural molecular biology, which helps in the determination of binding affinity between molecules. To investigate the binding energy of the protein/ligand combination, the two are joined and then disengaged. Docking or computer-assisted drug design is divided into two categories: "Receptor-based techniques," which utilize the target protein's structure, and "Ligand-based methods," which use existing inhibitors [73,138].

23.4 Pharmacophore mapping

The process of making a three-dimensional pharmacophore is known as pharmacophore design. The characteristics found in a pharmacophore include hydrogen bond donors and acceptors, positively and negatively charged groups, hydrophobic areas, and aromatic rings. These are said to be the basis of a pharmacophore's ability to be a successful link between the biological target and a drug. A pharmacophore map may be made by superimposing active chemicals to find out what they have in common. De novo design or 3D database searching both are done using the pharmacophore map. Micromolecules with very different 2D configurations commonly displace one another from the binding domain of macromolecules. Pharmacophore mapping is a technique for converting 2D structure-activity data into 3D-binding supplies for a target biomolecule.

23.5 Virtual high-throughput screening

This approach assesses huge chemical pools for the possibility of binding to proteins and utilizing a computer to identify well-matched molecules. The technology of virtual screening is a computerized approach to help and explore new drugs. Fast, massive database searches are performed to look for binding targets such as proteins and enzymes, where different chemical structures are given as input (Table 2) [116,125].

Table 2 Sources for commercial ADMET software.

Software	Distributor	Uses
QikProp	Schrodinger	Predicts ADME for medication candidates in a short time
q-TOX	Accelrys(Pharmacopeia)	Calculates the toxicity of substances purely based on their molecular composition
VolSurf	Tripos	Quantify ADME Characteristics and build ADME Models for ADME Properties
Metabolizer Preview	ChemAxon	Anticipates key metabolites and assesses metabolic stability by the consideration of all potential metabolites and their resultant metabolites. It can be used for the discovery of metabolically sensitive functionalities and toxicity prediction
ACD/PhysChem Suite	ACD/Labs	I can instantly identify simple characteristics like pK_a, log P, log D, and aqueous solubility in a fragment-based method
ACD/ADME Suite	ACD/Labs	It can perform things like inferring information like whether or not a drug is specific to P-gp, or if a medication will cross

Continued

Table 2 Sources for commercial ADMET software—cont'd

Software	Distributor	Uses
		the blood-brain barrier and how much, and it also makes Conclusions on how a drug will interact with the P450 system
ACD/DMSO Solubility	ACD/Labs	Predicts solubility in DMSO solution
Sieve	Silicos	Molecular filter application
ADMET Predictor	Simulationsplus, Inc.	Sophisticated ADMET characteristics prediction modeling software
ClassPharmer	plu Simulation Plus, Inc.	ClassPharmer is a tool for the prioritizing, de novo design, scaffold hopping, and lead optimization of molecules with a focus on identifying leads
Discovery StudioTOPKAT Software	Accelrys	Models for assessing chemical toxicity using chemical molecular structure, verified by cross-validation
Discovery Studio ADMET Software	Accelrys	The ADMET Collection contains elements that may be used to determine ADMET characteristics of molecules
Adriana.code	Molecular Networks	Program to compute small molecule physicochemical characteristics (e.g., H-bonds, dipole moment, and polarizability)

Table 2 Sources for commercial ADMET software—cont'd

Software	Distributor	Uses
OncoLogic	USEnvironmentalProtection Agency (EPA)	To understand how chemicals might cause cancer, it examines whether or not a certain chemical has the potential to cause cancer, relying on data modeling, making expert decisions in a mimicked manner, and information on how substances produce cancer in both animals and people
HazardExpert Pro	CompuDrug	Uses hazardous fragments to anticipate the toxicity of organic compounds
Leadscope	Leadscope	Estimates toxicity using QSAR
META	MultiCASE	Analyzes how compounds will metabolize
PK-Sim	Bayer TechnologyServices	Predicts ADMET properties
SimCYP	SimCYP	A way to anticipate drug-drug interactions and clinical consequences
Cloe Predict	Cyprotex Discovery	The accuracy of pharmacokinetic predictions has significantly improved with the use of physiologically based pharmacokinetic

Continued

Table 2 Sources for commercial ADMET software—cont'd

Software	Distributor	Uses
		modeling (PBPK), in addition to intestinal absorption predictions based on solubility, pK_a, and Caco-2 permeability data
KnowItAll-ADME | ToxEdition.	Bio-Rad Laboratories	Use of consensus modeling to predict ADMET characteristics
MetaDrug	GeneGo	Makes predictions about a compound's toxicity and metabolism

24. Conclusion and future perspective

The recent applications of in silico pharmacology with extremely efficient and computational methods play a key role in chemical, biology, and drug development. With further advancements and wider validation criteria, a maturity stage is expected in the upcoming few years as well as computational drug research will progressively grow toward completeness.

In silico methods play an essential role in target and lead discovery and contribute considerably too early drug discovery. It is expected that the role of in silico methods in drug development will grow significantly in the future. To have a much larger impact, in silico approaches will need to become a part of every drug development researcher's toolkit.

In silico pharmacology's future is unclear at this time. Currently, computational and in vitro techniques are more closely linked than in vivo investigations, but will this trend continue in the future? Furthermore, would in silico methods ever eliminate the need for animal testing, as some animal rights advocates would want us to believe? For two indisputable reasons, the answer here must be a resounding "no" in the foreseeable future. Biological systems are chaotic because they are nonlinear. Consequently, there is no correlation between input and output, with even the tiniest variations between beginning circumstances translating into huge output differences. The intricacy of biological systems cannot be accurately modeled by any computer software, no matter how "complex and systems-like" it may be. Gregory Chaitin, the mathematician who coined the term "algorithmically incompressible" in the context of biological systems, is correct in his assertion.

It is conceivable that the integration of models will get more complicated, as we have seen with the coupled metabolic modeling techniques in silico pharmacology. A wide-ranging influence will only be achieved when in silico tools become an integral part of every pharmacologist's toolbox, and this will involve training in modeling and informatics, as well as training in vivo, vitro, and molecular. This should provide pharmacologists with a realistic sense of what in silico approaches can and cannot do when it comes to their goal of developing novel medicines The importance of rapid adaption and implementation of in silico techniques in pharmaceutical research has been recognized, and it is predicted to increase overall drug discovery efficiency even further. The complexity of the situation cannot be adequately modeled by a computer program at this time. However, once a medication has been fully identified using in silico approaches, it will be made available to patients for clinical usage with little or no confirming testing.

References

[1] J. Li, X. Zhang, C. Liu, The computational approaches of lncRNA identification based on coding potential: status quo and challenges, Comput. Struct. Biotechnol. J. 18 (2020) 3666–3677.
[2] B. Lim, M. Hwang, J.S. Song, A.J. Ryu, B. Joung, E.B. Shim, H. Ryu, H.N. Pak, Effectiveness of atrial fibrillation rotor ablation is dependent on conduction velocity: an in-silico 3-dimensional modeling study, PLoS One 12 (2017), e0190398.
[3] J.Y. Liu, K.F. Lee, C.W. Sze, Y. Tong, S.C. Tang, T.B. Ng, Y.B. Zhang, Intestinal absorption and bioavailability of traditional Chinese medicines: a review of recent experimental progress and implication for quality control, J. Pharm. Pharmacol. 65 (2013) 621–633.
[4] Q. Liu, H. Zhou, L. Liu, X. Chen, R. Zhu, Z. Cao, Multi-target QSAR modelling in the analysis and design of HIV-HCV co-inhibitors: an in-silico study, BMC Bioinform. 12 (2011) 294.
[5] A. Loewe, O. Dössel, Commentary: virtual in-silico modeling guided catheter ablation predicts effective linear ablation lesion set for longstanding persistent atrial fibrillation: multicenter prospective randomized study, Front. Physiol. 8 (2017) 1113.
[6] H. MacKay, A. Abizaid, A plurality of molecular targets: the receptor ecosystem for bisphenol-A (BPA), Horm. Behav. 101 (2018) 59–67.
[7] I.R. Mami, T.Z. Amina, J. Pérard, Z. Arrar, M.E.A. Dib, Hemisyntheses and in-silico study of new analogues of carlina oxide from Carthamus Caeruleus roots, Comb. Chem. High Throughput Screen. 24 (2021) 1503–1513.
[8] P. Mamoshina, K. Kochetov, F. Cortese, A. Kovalchuk, A. Aliper, E. Putin, M. Scheibye-Knudsen, C.R. Cantor, N.M. Skjodt, O. Kovalchuk, A. Zhavoronkov,

Blood biochemistry analysis to detect smoking status and quantify accelerated aging in smokers, Sci. Rep. 9 (2019) 142.
[9] S. Mani, S.N. Rao, M.V. Kranthi Kumar, Genetic heterogeneity of mitochondrial genome in thiamine deficient Leigh syndrome patients, J. Neurol. Sci. 404 (2019) 91–100.
[10] R. Mathiyalagan, S. Subramaniyam, S. Natarajan, Y.J. Kim, M.S. Sun, S.Y. Kim, Y.J. Kim, D.C. Yang, Insilico profiling of microRNAs in Korean ginseng (Panax ginseng Meyer), J. Ginseng Res. 37 (2013) 227–247.
[11] H.A. Mustafa, A.M.S. Albkrye, B.M. AbdAlla, M.A.M. Khair, N. Abdelwahid, H.A. Elnasri, Computational determination of human PPARG gene: SNPs and prediction of their effect on protein functions of diabetic patients, Clin. Transl. Med. 9 (2020) 7.
[12] B.J. Mylliemngap, A. Borthakur, D. Velmurugan, A. Bhattacharjee, Insilico analysis and molecular docking of resuscitation promoting factor B (RpfB) protein of Mycobacterium tuberculosis, Bioinformation 8 (2012) 646–651.
[13] P. Nauroy, S. Hughes, A. Naba, F. Ruggiero, The in-silico zebrafish matrisome: a new tool to study extracellular matrix gene and protein functions, Matrix Biol. 65 (2018) 5–13.
[14] S. Negi, H. Singh, A. Mukhopadhyay, Gut bacterial peptides with autoimmunity potential as environmental trigger for late onset complex diseases: in silico study, PLoS One 12 (2017), e0180518.
[15] A. Nikdel, H. Budman, Identification of active constraints in dynamic flux balance analysis, Biotechnol. Prog. 33 (2017) 26–36.
[16] H. Nikzad, M. Karimian, K. Sareban, M. Khoshsokhan, A.H. Colagar, MTHFR-Ala222Val and male infertility: a study in Iranian men, an updated meta-analysis and an in silico-analysis, Reprod. BioMed. Online 31 (2015) 668–680.
[17] R. Orecchia, P. Fossati, S. Zurrida, M. Krengli, New frontiers in proton therapy: applications in breast cancer, Curr. Opin. Oncol. 27 (2015) 427–432.
[18] G. Orlando, D. Raimondi, F. Tabaro, F. Codicè, Y. Moreau, W.F. Vranken, Computational identification of prion-like RNA-binding proteins that form liquid phase-separated condensates, Bioinformatics (Oxford, England) 35 (2019) 4617–4623.
[19] J. Ostmeyer, L. Cowell, B. Greenberg, S. Christley, Reconstituting T cell receptor selection in-silico, Genes Immun. 22 (2021) 187–193.
[20] L.C. Palacio, D.C. Pachajoa, G. Durango-Giraldo, C. Zapata-Hernandez, J.P. Ugarte, J. Saiz, R. Buitrago-Sierra, C. Tobón, Atrial proarrhythmic effect of lead as one of the PM10 metal components of air pollution. An in-silico study, PLoS One 16 (2021), e0258313.
[21] R.U. Palaniappan, S. Ramanujam, Y.F. Chang, Leptospirosis: pathogenesis, immunity, and diagnosis, Curr. Opin. Infect. Dis. 20 (2007) 284–292.
[22] A.K. Pandey, S. Verma, An in-silico evaluation of dietary components for structural inhibition of SARS-Cov-2 main protease, J. Biomol. Struct. Dyn. 40 (2022) 136–142.
[23] S. Pandey, B.K. Singh, De-novo drug design, molecular docking and in-silico molecular prediction of AChEI analogues through CADD approaches as anti-Alzheimer's agents, Curr. Comput. Aided Drug Des. 16 (2020) 54–72.
[24] V. Paramanik, H. Krishnan, M. Kumar Thakur, Estrogen receptor α- and β-interacting proteins contain consensus secondary structures: an in silico study, Ann. Neurosci. 25 (2018) 1–10.
[25] P.P. Parvatikar, S. Patil, J. Hoskeri, S. Swargam, R. Kulkarni, K.K. Das, Screening, development of transglutaminase-2 inhibitors and its derivative as anti-lung cancer agent by insilico and invitro approach, Curr. Comput. Aided Drug Des. (2021).
[26] A.D. Patel, R. Barot, I. Parmar, I. Panchal, U. Shah, M. Patel, B. Mishtry, Molecular docking, in-silico ADMET study and development of 1,6- dihydropyrimidine

derivative as protein tyrosine phosphatase inhibitor: an approach to design and develop antidiabetic agents, Curr. Comput. Aided Drug Des. 14 (2018) 349–362.
[27] V. Patel, J. Shah, A.K. Gupta, Design and in-silico study of bioimaging fluorescence Graphene quantum dot-Bovine serum albumin complex synthesized by diimide-activated amidation, Comput. Biol. Chem. 93 (2021), 107543.
[28] Y. Pathak, A. Mishra, G. Choudhir, A. Kumar, V. Tripathi, Rifampicin and Letermovir as potential repurposed drug candidate for COVID-19 treatment: insights from an in-silico study, Pharmacol. Rep. 73 (2021) 926–938.
[29] V.M. Pérez-García, L.E. Ayala-Hernández, J. Belmonte-Beitia, P. Schucht, M. Murek, A. Raabe, J. Sepúlveda, Computational design of improved standardized chemotherapy protocols for grade II oligodendrogliomas, PLoS Comput. Biol. 15 (2019), e1006778.
[30] V.C. Pezoulas, G.I. Grigoriadis, N.S. Tachos, F. Barlocco, I. Olivotto, D.I. Fotiadis, Generation of virtual patient data for in-silico cardiomyopathies drug development using tree ensembles: a comparative study, in: 2020 Annual International Conference of the IEEE Engineering in Medicine and Biology Society, 2020, pp. 5343–5346.
[31] S. Polak, B. Wisniowska, K. Fijorek, A. Glinka, M. Polak, A. Mendyk, The open-access dataset for insilico cardiotoxicity prediction system, Bioinformation 6 (2011) 244–245.
[32] P.K. Prasad, L.M. Goswami, V. Tandon, A. Chatterjee, PCR-based molecular characterization and insilico analysis of food-borne trematode parasites Paragonimus westermani, Fasciolopsis buski and Fasciola gigantica from Northeast India using ITS2 rDNA, Bioinformation 6 (2011) 64–68.
[33] S.F. Pravdin, T.I. Epanchintsev, A.V. Panfilov, Overdrive pacing of spiral waves in a model of human ventricular tissue, Sci. Rep. 10 (2020) 20632.
[34] P. Purohit, R.K. Mittal, K. Khatana, Quinoline-3-carboxylic acids "DNA minor groove-binding agent", Anti Cancer Agents Med. Chem. 22 (2021).
[35] J. Qiu, Y. Shang, Z. Ji, T. Qiu, In-silico antigenicity determination and clustering of dengue virus serotypes, Front. Genet. 9 (2018) 621.
[36] D. Rajesh, S. Muthukumar, G. Saibaba, D. Siva, M.A. Akbarsha, B. Gulyás, P. Padmanabhan, G. Archunan, Structural elucidation of estrus urinary lipocalin protein (EULP) and evaluating binding affinity with pheromones using molecular docking and fluorescence study, Sci. Rep. 6 (2016) 35900.
[37] S. Rajvanshi, K. Choudhary, N. Agrawal, Threading: a novel insilico indagation method for genetic characterization of some diplostomoid metacercariae (Digenea: Diplostomidae Poirier, 1886), Exp. Parasitol. 171 (2016) 71–76.
[38] S. Rajvanshi, J. Verma, A. Nirupama, Validation of Bifurcohaptor spp. (Monogenoidea: Dactylogyridae) reported from India using molecular methods with inclusion of insilico study: a brief report on its host-specificity, Trop. Biomed. 36 (2019) 726–741.
[39] B.L. Ramaekers, M. Pijls-Johannesma, M.A. Joore, P. van den Ende, J.A. Langendijk, P. Lambin, A.G. Kessels, J.P. Grutters, Systematic review and meta-analysis of radiotherapy in various head and neck cancers: comparing photons, carbon-ions and protons, Cancer Treat. Rev. 37 (2011) 185–201.
[40] N. Rani, R. Singh, Molecular modelling studies of 1,4-diaryl-2-mercaptoimidazole derivatives for antimicrobial potency, Curr. Comput. Aided Drug Des. 15 (2019) 409–420.
[41] M.M.V. Rao, T.P.N. Hariprasad, In silico analysis of a potential antidiabetic phytochemical erythrin against therapeutic targets of diabetes, In silico Pharmacol. 9 (2021) 5.
[42] S. Raza, G. Abbas, S.S. Azam, Screening pipeline for Flavivirus based inhibitors for Zika virus NS1, IEEE/ACM Trans. Comput. Biol. Bioinform. 17 (2020) 1751–1761.

[43] D. Roy, O. Mazumder, A. Sinha, S. Khandelwal, Multimodal cardiovascular model for hemodynamic analysis: simulation study on mitral valve disorders, PLoS One 16 (2021), e0247921.

[44] H. Roy, S. Nandi, In-silico modeling in drug metabolism and interaction: current strategies of lead discovery, Curr. Pharm. Des. 25 (2019) 3292–3305.

[45] H. Roy, B.S. Nayak, S. Nandi, Chitosan anchored nanoparticles in current drug development utilizing computer-aided pharmacokinetic modeling: case studies for target specific cancer treatment and future prospective, Curr. Pharm. Des. 26 (2020) 1666–1675.

[46] J. Roy, U.C. Kumar, P.K. Machiraju, R.K. Muttineni, B.V.S.S. Kumar, R. Gundla, R. Dayam, J.A. Sarma, Insilico studies on anthrax lethal factor inhibitors: pharmacophore modeling and virtual screening approaches towards designing of novel inhibitors for a killer, J. Mol. Graph. Model. 29 (2010) 256–265.

[47] P.N. Samanta, S. Kar, J. Leszczynski, Recent advances of in-silico modeling of potent antagonists for the adenosine receptors, Curr. Pharm. Des. 25 (2019) 750–773.

[48] R. Sankhe, E. Rathi, S. Manandhar, A. Kumar, S.R.K. Pai, S.G. Kini, A. Kishore, Repurposing of existing FDA approved drugs for Neprilysin inhibition: an in-silico study, J. Mol. Struct. 1224 (2021), 129073.

[49] G. Saravanan, T. Panneerselvam, V. Alagarsamy, S. Kunjiappan, P. Parasuraman, I. Murugan, P. Dinesh Kumar, Design, graph theoretical analysis, density functionality theories, insilico modeling, synthesis, characterization and biological activities of novel thiazole fused quinazolinone derivatives, Drug Dev. Res. 79 (2018) 260–274.

[50] A. Sarma, H. Phukan, N. Halder, M.G. Madanan, An in-silico approach to study the possible interactions of miRNA between human and SARS-CoV2, Comput. Biol. Chem. 88 (2020), 107352.

[51] M.W. Sarwar, I.B. Saleem, A. Ali, F. Abbas, Insilico characterization and homology modeling of arabitol dehydrogenase (ArDH) from candida albican, Bioinformation 9 (2013) 952–957.

[52] P. Selzer, H.J. Roth, P. Ertl, A. Schuffenhauer, Complex molecules: do they add value? Curr. Opin. Chem. Biol. 9 (2005) 310–316.

[53] Y. Setty, In-silico models of stem cell and developmental systems, Theor. Biol. Med. Model. 11 (2014) 1.

[54] A. Shah, V. Patel, B. Parmar, Discovery of Some Antiviral Natural products to fight against Novel Corona virus (SARS-CoV-2) using insilico approach, Comb. Chem. High Throughput Screen. (2020).

[55] A. Shanker, K.R. Pardasani, Insilico model for prediction of lateral gene transfer in Rhodopseudomonas paulistris, Interdiscip. Sci. Comput. Life Sci. 6 (2014) 323–330.

[56] T. Shanmugam, M. Selvaraj, S. Poomalai, Corrigendum to "Epigallocatechin gallate potentially abrogates fluoride induced lung oxidative stress, inflammation via Nrf2/Keap1 signaling pathway in rats: an in-vivo and in-silico study" [Int. Immunopharmacol. 39 (2016) 128-139], Int. Immunopharmacol. 80 (2020), 106203.

[57] J. Shim, M. Hwang, J.S. Song, B. Lim, T.H. Kim, B. Joung, S.H. Kim, Y.S. Oh, G.B. Nam, Y.K. On, S. Oh, Y.H. Kim, H.N. Pak, Virtual in-silico modeling guided catheter ablation predicts effective linear ablation lesion set for longstanding persistent Atrial Fibrillation: multicenter prospective randomized study, Front. Physiol. 8 (2017) 792.

[58] V. Shunmuga Priya, D. Pradiba, M. Aarthy, S.K. Singh, A. Achary, M. Vasanthi, In-silico strategies for identification of potent inhibitor for MMP-1 to prevent metastasis of breast cancer, J. Biomol. Struct. Dyn. 39 (2021) 7274–7293.

[59] V. Shyni, D.R. Leenaraj, R. Ittyachan, L. Joseph, D. Sajan, Spectroscopic, density functional theoretical study, molecular docking, and in vitro studies based on anticancer activity studies against A(549) lung cancer cell line of diphenylhydantoin adsorbed on AuNPs surface, J. Mol. Recognit. 34 (2021), e2916.

[60] J.S. Song, Y.S. Lee, M. Hwang, J.K. Lee, C. Li, B. Joung, M.H. Lee, E.B. Shim, H.N. Pak, Spatial reproducibility of complex fractionated atrial electrogram depending on the direction and configuration of bipolar electrodes: an in-silico modeling study, Korean J. Physiol. Pharmacol. 20 (2016) 507–514.
[61] N. Sood, S. Chaudhary, T. Pardeshi, S. Mujawar, K.B. Deshmukh, S.A. Sheikh, P. Sharma, In-silico study of small cell lung cancer based on protein structure and function: a new approach to mimic biological system, J. Adv. Pharm. Technol. Res. 6 (2015) 125–129.
[62] A. Sridhar, S. Saremy, B. Bhattacharjee, Elucidation of molecular targets of bioactive principles of black cumin relevant to its anti-tumour functionality—an Insilico target fishing approach, Bioinformation 10 (2014) 684–688.
[63] P. Srivastava, A. Tiwari, A new insight of herbal promises against ocular disorders: an occuloinformatics approach, Curr. Top. Med. Chem. 16 (2016) 634–654.
[64] S. Subramaniyam, R. Mathiyalagan, I. Jun Gyo, L. Bum-Soo, L. Sungyoung, Y. Deok Chun, Transcriptome profiling and insilico analysis of gynostemma pentaphyllum using a next generation sequencer, Plant Cell Rep. 30 (2011) 2075–2083.
[65] S. Suganya, B. Nandagopal, A. Anbarasu, Natural inhibitors of HMG-CoA reductase-an insilico approach through molecular docking and simulation studies, J. Cell. Biochem. 118 (2017) 52–57.
[66] S. Sundar, L. Thangamani, S. Piramanayagam, J. Natarajan, Discovering mycobacterial lectins as potential drug targets and vaccine candidates for tuberculosis treatment: a theoretical approach, J. Proteins Proteom. (2021) 1–12.
[67] A. Swargiary, M. Daimari, Identification of major compounds and α-amylase and α-glucosidase inhibitory activity of rhizome of Musa balbisiana Colla: an in-vitro and in-silico study, Comb. Chem. High Throughput Screen. 25 (2020).
[68] S. Tagore, N. Chowdhury, R.K. De, Analyzing methods for path mining with applications in metabolomics, Gene 534 (2014) 125–138.
[69] P. Theivendren, A. Subramanian, I. Murugan, S.D. Joshi, U.A. More, Graph theoretical analysis, insilico modeling, design, and synthesis of compounds containing benzimidazole skeleton as antidepressant agents, Chem. Biol. Drug Des. 89 (2017) 714–722.
[70] G. Thirumoorthy, S.P. Tarachand, P. Nagella, V.V. Lakshmaiah, Identification of potential ZIKV NS2B-NS3 protease inhibitors from Andrographis paniculata: an insilico approach, J. Biomol. Struct. Dyn. (2021) 1–13.
[71] S. Tulsyan, G. Agarwal, P. Lal, S. Agrawal, R.D. Mittal, B. Mittal, CD44 gene polymorphisms in breast cancer risk and prognosis: a study in North Indian population, PLoS One 8 (2013), e71073.
[72] K. Vasodavan, V.K. Neela, Twitching motility of Stenotrophomonas maltophilia under iron limitation: in-silico, phenotypic and proteomic approaches, Virulence 11 (2020) 104–112.
[73] S.B. Varthya, P. Sarma, A. Bhatia, N. Shekhar, M. Prajapat, H. Kaur, P. Thangaraju, S. Kumar, R. Singh, A. Siingh, A. Prakash, B. Medhi, Efficacy of green tea, its polyphenols and nanoformulation in experimental colitis and the role of non-canonical and canonical nuclear factor kappa beta (NF-kB) pathway: a preclinical in-vivo and in-silico exploratory study, J. Biomol. Struct. Dyn. 39 (2021) 5314–5326.
[74] H. Veith, F. Wiechert, C. Luebbert, G. Sadowski, Combining crystalline and polymeric excipients in API solid dispersions—opportunity or risk? Eur. J. Pharm. Biopharm. 158 (2021) 323–335.
[75] B.J. Wilson, Meta-analysis of SUMO1, BMC Res. Notes 1 (2008) 60.
[76] G. Yang, M. Mozzicafreddo, P. Ballarini, S. Pucciarelli, C. Miceli, An in-silico comparative study of lipases from the Antarctic Psychrophilic Ciliate Euplotes focardii and the mesophilic congeneric species Euplotes crassus: insight into molecular cold-adaptation, Mar. Drugs 19 (2021).

[77] N. Ye, Survey of in-silico prediction of anticancer peptides, Curr. Top. Med. Chem. 21 (2021) 1310–1318.
[78] M. Zahoor, I. Khan, A. Zeb, M.U.K. Sahibzada, S. Naz, W.U. Bari, A.W. Kamran, Pharmacological evaluation and in-silico modeling study of compounds isolated from Ziziphus oxyphylla, Heliyon 7 (2021), e06367.
[79] B. Zainab, Z. Ayaz, M.S. Alwahibi, S. Khan, H. Rizwana, D.W. Soliman, A. Alawaad, A. Mehmood Abbasi, In-silico elucidation of Moringa oleifera phytochemicals against diabetes mellitus, Saudi, Aust. J. Biol. Sci. 27 (2020) 2299–2307.
[80] G. Agarwal, K. Kv, S.B. Prasad, A. Bhaduri, G. Jayaraman, Biosynthesis of hyaluronic acid polymer: dissecting the role of sub structural elements of hyaluronan synthase, Sci. Rep. 9 (2019) 12510.
[81] D.G. Amoako, A.M. Somboro, A.L.K. Abia, M. Allam, A. Ismail, L.A. Bester, S.Y. Essack, Genome mining and comparative pathogenomic analysis of an endemic methicillin-resistant staphylococcus aureus (MRSA) clone, ST612-CC8-t1257-SCCmec_IVd(2B), Isolated in South Africa, Pathogens 8 (2019) 166.
[82] R. Aparnaa, N. Mahalakshmi, A. Harini, P.J. Jeyaprita, G. Anugraha, N.P. Amdare, V.K. Khatri, M.V. Reddy, P. Kaliraj, Wuchereria bancrofti 20/22 a homologue of abundant larval transcript L3 stage filarial antigen: molecular and immunological characterization, Parasite Immunol. 36 (2014) 475–484.
[83] L. Artigas, M. Coma, P. Matos-Filipe, J. Aguirre-Plans, J. Farrés, R. Valls, N. Fernandez-Fuentes, J. de la Haba-Rodriguez, A. Olvera, J. Barbera, R. Morales, B. Oliva, J.M. Mas, In-silico drug repurposing study predicts the combination of pirfenidone and melatonin as a promising candidate therapy to reduce SARS-CoV-2 infection progression and respiratory distress caused by cytokine storm, PLoS One 15 (2020), e0240149.
[84] S.M. Baliban, M. Yang, G. Ramachandran, B. Curtis, S. Shridhar, R.S. Laufer, J.Y. Wang, J. Van Druff, E.E. Higginson, N. Hegerle, K.M. Varney, J.E. Galen, S.M. Tennant, A. Lees, A.D. MacKerell Jr., M.M. Levine, R. Simon, Development of a glycoconjugate vaccine to prevent invasive Salmonella Typhimurium infections in sub-Saharan Africa, PLoS Negl. Trop. Dis. 11 (2017), e0005493.
[85] S. Borse, M. Joshi, A. Saggam, V. Bhat, S. Walia, A. Marathe, S. Sagar, P. Chavan-Gautam, A. Girme, L. Hingorani, G. Tillu, Ayurveda botanicals in COVID-19 management: an in silico multi-target approach, PLoS One 16 (2021), e0248479.
[86] M.K. Chaurasia, G. Ravichandran, F. Nizam, M.V. Arasu, N.A. Al-Dhabi, A. Arshad, R. Harikrishnan, J. Arockiaraj, In-silico analysis and mRNA modulation of detoxification enzymes GST delta and kappa against various biotic and abiotic oxidative stressors, Fish Shellfish Immunol. 54 (2016) 353–363.
[87] P. Chemmugil, P.T.V. Lakshmi, A. Annamalai, Exploring Morin as an anti-quorum sensing agent (anti-QSA) against resistant strains of Staphylococcus aureus, Microb. Pathog. 127 (2019) 304–315.
[88] H. Chen, X. Xu, C. Hua, H. Zhang, J. Jian, T. Ge, J. Xie, Z. Yu, Polymorphisms of matrix metalloproteinases affect the susceptibility of esophageal cancer: evidence from 20412 subjects, systematic review and updated meta-analysis, Medicine 100 (2021), e27229.
[89] D. Devang Divakar, S.A.S. Alanazi, M.Y.A. Assiri, S. Mohammed Halawani, S. Zaid Alshehri, S.A.S. Al-Amri, M. Mustafa, Association between ENAM polymorphisms and dental caries in children, Saudi J. Biol. Sci. 26 (2019) 730–735.
[90] K. Domb, D. Keidar-Friedman, K. Kashkush, A novel miniature transposon-like element discovered in the coding sequence of a gene that encodes for 5-formyltetrahydrofolate in wheat, BMC Plant Biol. 19 (2019) 461.
[91] S. Fan, J. Meng, L. Zhang, X. Zhang, C. Liang, CAV1 polymorphisms rs1049334, rs1049337, rs7804372 might be the potential risk in tumorigenicity of urinary cancer: a systematic review and meta-analysis, Pathol. Res. Pract. 215 (2019) 151–158.

[92] V. Fernandes, D. Sharma, K. Kalia, V. Tiwari, Neuroprotective effects of silibinin: an in silico and in vitro study, Int. J. Neurosci. 128 (2018) 935–945.
[93] S.B. Ganorkar, Y. Vander Heyden, A.A. Shirkhedkar, D.K. Lokwani, D.M. Dhumal, P.S. Bobade, Pharmaceutical analysis combined with in-silico therapeutic and toxicological profiling on zileuton and its impurities to assist in modern drug discovery, J. Pharm. Biomed. Anal. 179 (2020), 112982.
[94] V. Gopu, C.K. Meena, P.H. Shetty, Quercetin influences quorum sensing in food borne bacteria: in-vitro and in-silico evidence, PLoS One 10 (2015), e0134684.
[95] M. Goske, V.R.V. Ramachander, P.L. Komaravalli, P.F. Rahman, C. Rao, P. Jahan, CTLA-4 genetic variants (rs11571317 and rs3087243): role in susceptibility and progression of breast cancer, World J. Oncol. 8 (2017) 162–170.
[96] B. Guillen-Guio, J.M. Lorenzo-Salazar, S.F. Ma, P.C. Hou, T. Hernandez-Beeftink, A. Corrales, M.I. García-Laorden, J. Jou, E. Espinosa, A. Muriel, D. Domínguez, L. Lorente, M.M. Martín, C. Rodríguez-Gallego, J. Solé-Violán, A. Ambrós, D. Carriedo, J. Blanco, J.M. Añón, J.P. Reilly, T.K. Jones, C.A. Ittner, R. Feng, F. Schöneweck, M. Kiehntopf, I. Noth, M. Scholz, F.M. Brunkhorst, A. Scherag, N.J. Meyer, J. Villar, C. Flores, Sepsis-associated acute respiratory distress syndrome in individuals of European ancestry: a genome-wide association study, Lancet Respir. Med. 8 (2020) 258–266.
[97] N. Gupta, A. Kumar, Designing an efficient multi-epitope vaccine against Campylobacter Jejuni using immunoinformatics and reverse vaccinology approach, Microb. Pathog. 147 (2020), 104398.
[98] A. Iqubal, S. Sharma, A.K. Najmi, M.A. Syed, J. Ali, M.M. Alam, S.E. Haque, Nerolidol ameliorates cyclophosphamide-induced oxidative stress, neuroinflammation and cognitive dysfunction: plausible role of Nrf2 and NF-κB, Life Sci. 236 (2019), 116867.
[99] K. Johnson George, O. Rosana Babu, I.P. Vijesh Kumar, J. Santhosh Eapen, M. Anandaraj, Interplay of genes in plant-pathogen interactions: in planta expression and docking studies of a beta 1,3 glucanase gene from Piper colubrinum and a glucanase inhibitor gene from Phytophthora capsici, Physiol. Mol. Biol. Plants 22 (2016) 567–573.
[100] P. Kalaiarasan, B. Kumar, R. Chopra, V. Gupta, N. Subbarao, R.N. Bamezai, In silico screening, genotyping, molecular dynamics simulation and activity studies of SNPs in pyruvate kinase M2, PLoS One 10 (2015), e0120469.
[101] R. Kataria, A. Khatkar, In-silico design, synthesis, ADMET studies and biological evaluation of novel derivatives of Chlorogenic acid against urease protein and H Pylori bacterium, BMC Chem. 13 (2019) 41.
[102] D. Kaur, S. Patiyal, C. Arora, R. Singh, G. Lodhi, G.P.S. Raghava, In-silico tool for predicting, scanning, and designing defensins, Front. Immunol. 12 (2021), 780610.
[103] S. Khan, A. Khan, A.U. Rehman, I. Ahmad, S. Ullah, A.A. Khan, S.S. Ali, S.G. Afridi, D.Q. Wei, Immunoinformatics and structural vaccinology driven prediction of multi-epitope vaccine against Mayaro virus and validation through in-silico expression, Infect. Genet. Evol. 73 (2019) 390–400.
[104] S. Kumar, A.P. Reddy, X. Yin, P.H. Reddy, Novel MicroRNA-455-3p and its protective effects against abnormal APP processing and amyloid beta toxicity in Alzheimer's disease, Biochim. Biophys. Acta Mol. basis Dis. 2019 (1865) 2428–2440.
[105] Y.L. Kung, C.Y. Lu, K.F. Badrealam, W.W. Kuo, M.A. Shibu, C.H. Day, R.J. Chen, S.Y. Lu, V.V. Padma, C.Y. Huang, Cardioprotective potential of amygdalin against angiotensin II induced cardiac hypertrophy, oxidative stress and inflammatory responses through modulation of Nrf2 and NF-κB activation, Environ. Toxicol. 36 (2021) 926–934.

[106] M. Laskowski, V.R. Duvvuri, D.L. Buckeridge, G. Wu, J. Wu, S.M. Moghadas, Influenza H3N2 variant viruses with pandemic potential: preventing catastrophe in remote and isolated Canadian communities, Prev. Med. 57 (2013) 910–913.
[107] S. Liang, Z. Chen, H. Li, Z. Cang, K. Yin, M. Wu, S. Luo, Neuroprotective effect of Umbelliferone against cerebral ischemia/reperfusion induced neurological deficits: in-vivo and in-silico studies, J. Biomol. Struct. Dyn. 39 (2021) 4715–4725.
[108] A. Mahboob, S.M. Farhat, G. Iqbal, M.M. Babar, N.U. Zaidi, S.M. Nabavi, T. Ahmed, Alpha-lipoic acid-mediated activation of muscarinic receptors improves hippocampus- and amygdala-dependent memory, Brain Res. Bull. 122 (2016) 19–28.
[109] A. Marathe, V. Krishnan, T. Vinutha, A. Dahuja, M. Jolly, A. Sachdev, Exploring the role of inositol 1,3,4-trisphosphate 5/6 kinase-2 (GmITPK2) as a dehydration and salinity stress regulator in glycine max (L.) Merr. Through heterologous expression in E. coli, Plant Physiol. Biochem. 123 (2018) 331–341.
[110] J.A. Mazumder, E. Khan, M. Perwez, M. Gupta, S. Kumar, K. Raza, M. Sardar, Exposure of biosynthesized nanoscale ZnO to Brassica juncea crop plant: morphological, biochemical and molecular aspects, Sci. Rep. 10 (2020) 8531.
[111] S. Mhatre, S. Naik, V. Patravale, A molecular docking study of EGCG and theaflavin digallate with the druggable targets of SARS-CoV-2, Comput. Biol. Med. 129 (2021), 104137.
[112] R. Mohamed, S. Tarannum, M. Yariswamy, H.K. Vivek, J.M. Siddesha, N. Angaswamy, B.S. Vishwanath, Ascorbic acid 6-palmitate: a potent inhibitor of human and soybean lipoxygenase-dependent lipid peroxidation, J. Pharm. Pharmacol. 66 (2014) 769–778.
[113] M.A. Nawaz, F. Azeem, A.M. Zakharenko, X. Lin, R.M. Atif, F.S. Baloch, T.F. Chan, G. Chung, J. Ham, S. Sun, K.S. Golokhvast, In-silico exploration of channel type and efflux silicon transporters and silicification proteins in 80 sequenced viridiplantae genomes, Plants (Basel, Switzerland) 9 (2020) 1612.
[114] S.S. Nerurkar, A.R. Olzinski, K.S. Frazier, R.C. Mirabile, S.P. O'Brien, J. Jing, D. Rajagopalan, T.L. Yue, R.N. Willette, P38 MAPK inhibitors suppress biomarkers of hypertension end-organ damage, osteopontin and plasminogen activator inhibitor-1, Biomarkers 12 (2007) 87–112.
[115] J.G. Owen, D.F. Ackerley, Characterization of pyoverdine and achromobactin in Pseudomonas syringae pv. phaseolicola 1448a, BMC Microbiol. 11 (2011) 218.
[116] A. Parvaiz, G. Mustafa, H. Khan, F.A. Joyia, A.K. Niazi, S. Anwar, M.S. Khan, Field evaluation ratified by transcript and computational analyses unveils myco-protective role of SUGARWIN proteins in sugarcane, 3Biotech 9 (2019) 377.
[117] F. Patel, K. Parwani, P. Rao, D. Patel, R. Rawal, P. Mandal, Prophylactic treatment of probiotic and metformin mitigates ethanol-induced intestinal barrier injury: in vitro, in vivo, and in silico approaches, Mediat. Inflamm. 2021 (2021) 5245197.
[118] A. Paul, S. Rao, S. Mathur, The α-crystallin domain containing genes: identification, phylogeny and expression profiling in abiotic stress, phytohormone response and development in tomato (Solanum lycopersicum), Front. Plant Sci. 7 (2016) 426.
[119] S. Piplani, V. Saini, R.R. Niraj, A. Pushp, A. Kumar, Homology modelling and molecular docking studies of human placental cadherin protein for its role in teratogenic effects of anti-epileptic drugs, Comput. Biol. Chem. 60 (2016) 1–8.
[120] R. Ponnulakshmi, B. Shyamaladevi, P. Vijayalakshmi, J. Selvaraj, In silico and in vivo analysis to identify the antidiabetic activity of beta sitosterol in adipose tissue of high fat diet and sucrose induced type-2 diabetic experimental rats, Toxicol. Mech. Methods 29 (2019) 276–290.
[121] A. Presbitero, E. Mancini, R. Brands, V.V. Krzhizhanovskaya, P.M.A. Sloot, Supplemented alkaline phosphatase supports the immune response in patients undergoing cardiac surgery: clinical and computational evidence, Front. Immunol. 9 (2018) 2342.

[122] S.O. Rahman, M. Kaundal, M. Salman, A. Shrivastava, S. Parvez, B.P. Panda, M. Akhter, M. Akhtar, A.K. Najmi, Alogliptin reversed hippocampal insulin resistance in an amyloid-beta fibrils induced animal model of Alzheimer's disease, Eur. J. Pharmacol. 889 (2020), 173522.
[123] K.K. Rai, N. Rai, M. Aamir, D. Tripathi, S.P. Rai, Interactive role of salicylic acid and nitric oxide on transcriptional reprogramming for high temperature tolerance in lablab purpureus L.: structural and functional insights using computational approaches, J. Biotechnol. 309 (2020) 113–130.
[124] S. Raj, S. Sasidharan, V.K. Dubey, P. Saudagar, Identification of lead molecules against potential drug target protein MAPK4 from L. donovani: an in-silico approach using docking, molecular dynamics and binding free energy calculation, PLoS One 14 (2019), e0221331.
[125] C.M.F. Rezende, J.B. Coitinho, M. Costa, M.R. Silva, M. Giusta, R. Oliveira-Prado, R. Corrêa-Oliveira, R. Nagem, A.M. Goes, Biochemical analysis and identification of linear B-cell epitopes from recombinant Sm21.7 antigen from Schistosoma mansoni, Mol. Immunol. 101 (2018) 29–37.
[126] J.J. Sahayarayan, K.S. Rajan, R. Vidhyavathi, M. Nachiappan, D. Prabhu, S. Alfarraj, S. Arokiyaraj, A.N. Daniel, In-silico protein-ligand docking studies against the estrogen protein of breast cancer using pharmacophore based virtual screening approaches, Saudi, Aust. J. Biol. Sci. 28 (2021) 400–407.
[127] S. Sarkar-Banerjee, S. Chowdhury, D. Sanyal, T. Mitra, S.S. Roy, K. Chattopadhyay, The role of intestinal fatty acid binding proteins in protecting cells from fatty acid induced impairment of mitochondrial dynamics and apoptosis, Cell. Physiol. Biochem. 51 (2018) 1658–1678.
[128] D. Scumaci, E. Olivo, C.V. Fiumara, M. La Chimia, M.T. De Angelis, S. Mauro, G. Costa, F.A. Ambrosio, S. Alcaro, V. Agosti, F.S. Costanzo, G. Cuda, DJ-1 proteoforms in breast cancer cells: the escape of metabolic epigenetic misregulation, Cell 9 (2020) 1968.
[129] P. Shah, V. Chavda, S. Patel, S. Bhadada, G.M. Ashraf, Promising anti-stroke signature of voglibose: investigation through in-silico molecular docking and virtual screening in in-vivo animal studies, Curr. Gene Ther. 20 (2020) 223–235.
[130] A. Shalmani, U. Ullah, I. Muhammad, D. Zhang, R. Sharif, P. Jia, N. Saleem, N. Gul, A. Rakhmanova, M.M. Tahir, K.M. Chen, N. An, The TAZ domain-containing proteins play important role in the heavy metals stress biology in plants, Environ. Res. 197 (2021), 111030.
[131] R.A. Shey, S.M. Ghogomu, C.M. Shintouo, F.N. Nkemngo, D.N. Nebangwa, K. Esoh, N.E. Yaah, M. Manka'aFri, J.E. Nguve, R.A. Ngwese, F.N. Njume, F.A. Bertha, L. Ayong, R. Njemini, L. Vanhamme, J. Souopgui, Computational design and preliminary serological analysis of a novel multi-epitope vaccine candidate against onchocerciasis and related filarial diseases, Plants (Basel, Switzerland) 10 (2021).
[132] G. Shi, Y. Cheng, Y. Zhang, R. Guo, S. Li, X. Hong, Long non-coding RNA LINC00511/miR-150/MMP13 axis promotes breast cancer proliferation, migration and invasion, Biochim. Biophys. Acta Mol. basis Dis. 1867 (2021), 165957.
[133] N. Shrivastava, A. Verma, P.K. Dash, Identification of functional epitopes of structural proteins and in-silico designing of dual acting multiepitope anti-tick vaccine against emerging Crimean-Congo hemorrhagic fever virus, Eur. J. Pharm. Sci. 151 (2020), 105396.
[134] C.L. Strope, K. Mansouri, H.J. Clewell 3rd, J.R. Rabinowitz, C. Stevens, J.F. Wambaugh, High-throughput in-silico prediction of ionization equilibria for pharmacokinetic modeling, Sci. Total Environ. 615 (2018) 150–160.
[135] M.K. Sundaram, M.Z. Ansari, A. Al Mutery, M. Ashraf, R. Nasab, S. Rai, N. Rais, A. Hussain, Genistein induces alterations of epigenetic modulatory signatures in human cervical cancer cells, Anti Cancer Agents Med. Chem. 18 (2018) 412–421.

[136] Y. Swarnalatha, I.S. Jerrine Joseph, T. Jayakrishna, Rosmarinic acid plays a protective role in the embryogenesis of zebrafish exposed to food colours through its influence on aurora kinase A level, Biomed. Pharmacother. 89 (2017) 1166–1171.
[137] B. Tilocca, A. Soggiu, M. Sanguinetti, V. Musella, D. Britti, L. Bonizzi, A. Urbani, P. Roncada, Comparative computational analysis of SARS-CoV-2 nucleocapsid protein epitopes in taxonomically related coronaviruses, Microbes Infect. 22 (2020) 188–194.
[138] P. Žuvela, J. David, X. Yang, D. Huang, M.W. Wong, Non-linear quantitative structure-activity relationships modelling, mechanistic study and in-silico design of flavonoids as potent antioxidants, Int. J. Mol. Sci. 20 (2019) 2328.

CHAPTER 2

Computational approaches in drug discovery and design

Priyanka Sharma[a], Kalicharan Sharma[b], and Mukesh Nandave[a]
[a]Department of Pharmacology, Delhi Pharmaceutical Sciences and Research University, New Delhi, India
[b]Department of Pharmaceutical Chemistry, Delhi Pharmaceutical Sciences and Research University, New Delhi, India

1. Drug discovery and computer-aided drug design

Computer-aided drug design (CADD) assists scientists in reducing the amount of time and money spent on chemical and therapeutic testing by focusing solely on the most probable chemicals. It not only explains the molecular mechanism of biological effects but it also forecasts potential derivatives that could improve it. CADD entails.

(1) The usage of computing power has sped up the drug development and establishment process.
(2) Experts use physiochemical and biological knowledge about sites and/or receptors to identify and optimize innovative therapies.
(3) ADMET, poor activity, and poor absorption, distribution, metabolism, excretion, and toxicity are the features of undesired compounds, which could be removed by the in silico filter, which would result in the selection of the most promising candidate.

2. Introduction to CADD

New medication development is a laborious and costly process. As individual compounds progress through the preclinical and clinical stages of development, they are rigorously tested for efficacy, pharmokinetic (PK), and side effects [1]. Medicinal chemistry, automation, and high-throughput screening (HTS) have sped up the screening of hundreds to millions of compounds against specific therapeutic targets over the past two decades [2,3]. For example, the projected pharmaceutical research cost of fexinidazole, which was licensed for treatment of sleeping sickness, an ignored condition, was €55 million, is much lesser than the cost of developing no orphan drugs, which is anticipated to be more than USD2 billion [4] As per Brandish

Computational Approaches in Drug Discovery, Development and Systems Pharmacology
https://doi.org/10.1016/B978-0-323-99137-7.00009-5

et al., >1 million chemicals library analysis took 12 weeks to evaluate their capacity to cross the cell membrane and inhibit D-amino acid oxidase by implementing cell-based HTS in 2006 [5]. To put it another way, current drug design relies not just on accessible molecular knowledge on suggested molecular targets but also antitarget information. Alteration of a recognized potent scaffold (molecular optimization) or linking of known effective scaffolds is the most prevalent method of drug design. However, de novo drug creation (i.e., from scratch) is also conceivable (e.g., fragment growing approximations).

In any instance, to build up or optimize the active ingredient, a starting point or seed is required [6]. Computer-assisted methods have become more important in both stages of current drug discovery: identifying potential beginning points and making sensible decisions about which chemical alterations to adopt.

In addition to HTS and other testing methodologies, the completion of the Human Genome Project (HGP) has paved the way for huge improvements in the new design of drugs, notably customized medicines and disease goals [7,8] (Figs. 1 and 2)

This chapter will go through the computational techniques that can be utilized to uncover new potent chemotypes and inform future chemical improvement. Aspects of rational drug development are shown in Fig. 3.

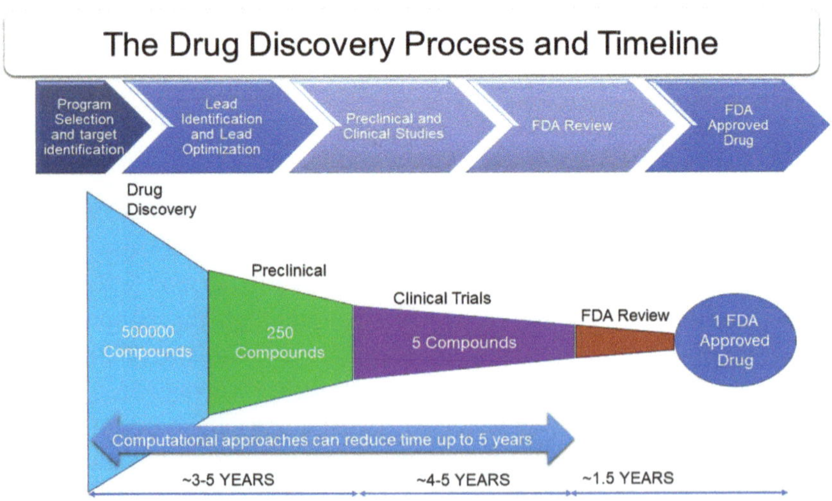

Fig. 1 The drug discovery process is depicted in a diagram.

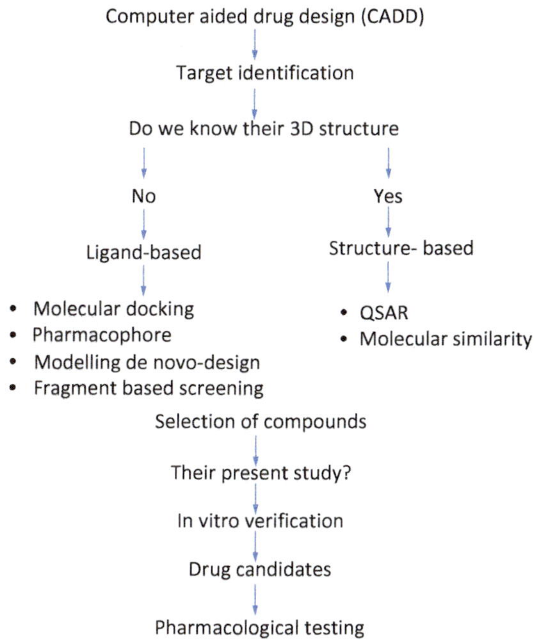

Fig. 2 A diagram depicting a typical computer-aided drug design process.

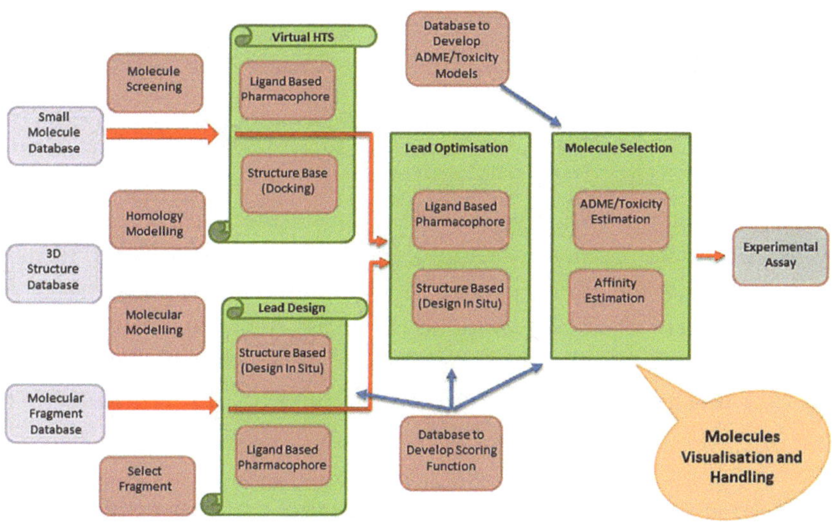

Fig. 3 Complete overview of drug design pipeline.

The CADD technique greatly reduces the cost of drug discovery while also speeding it up [9]. CADD employs two different methodologies: ligand-based and structure-based methods [10]. The structure-based method examines the structure of potential sites and pinpoints the critical locations for biological processes. The computer will be the advanced tool in the production of compounds that interact also with the target to change its physiological functioning [11,12]. However, the ligand-based strategies examine the physicochemical characteristic and properties of the targeted ligand. Then they give the several development of novel molecules with the desirable properties [13].

3. Current approaches used in drug designing by using CADD

CADD incorporates a variety of methodologies to address biological-pharmaceutical-related concerns. Structure-based, ligand-based, and hybrid approaches are the three major classes of CADD methods.

3.1 Structure-based drug discovery

Structure-based approaches rely on the molecular target's 3D information. Docking and molecular dynamics (MD) are two prominent examples of these approaches [14]. Structure-based techniques have been used to characterize binding sites, explain the mode of action of bioactive components at the atomic level, and analyze the dynamics and thermodynamics associated with ligand-target identification. Table 1 summarizes some techniques for structure-based drug design.

3.2 Ligand-based drug designing

The information regarding the structures of molecules and a set of ligands, as well as the known therapeutic activity, is used in these procedures. Its main goal is to evaluate the most potent molecule or improve the properties of the active molecules [19]. This technique eliminates the need for prior knowledge of active ligands, which is a huge benefit. New ligands could be created to elicit a therapeutic effect from 3D structures [20]. Table 2 summarizes some techniques to ligand-based drug design.

3.3 Hybrid methods and methods based on end-points

When both the structure of the active molecules and the structure of the target are known, hybrid or combined approaches, i.e. of structure-based

Table 1 Approaches of structure-based drug design.

S.No.	Approaches	Action	Advantages
1	Virtual high-throughput screening structure-based	To identify putative hits from the known structure	It is possible to screen a large number of compounds in a small number of conformational samples of proteins and ligands [15]
2	Structure-based virtual screening	To identify potential drug candidates to bind to a drug target	To estimate the binding affinity of the drug to the protein targets [16]
3	Fragment-based LEAD discovery	Based on NMR-derived structure-activity correlations,	Effective binding, good aqueous solubility [17,18]
4	Structure-based LEAD optimization: In silico	To raise the optimization of LEAD by delineating the prediction	Experimental time decrease in vitro and in vivo
5	Modeling ADMET	To predict absorption, distribution, metabolism, excretion, and toxicology (ADMET) of drugs/compounds	Cost and time effective

and ligand-based combination technologies, can be used. The specific pharmacophore modeling process provides an example. Another example is using in silico techniques to estimate therapeutic dependencies on the morphological profile of chemical compounds. (Fig. 4).

3.4 The fragment-based drug design

It can contemplate the molecular innovation of the 2000s, and this chapter will explore the standards behind FBDD and to what degree it ended up implanted in drug designing of the long run. Before diving into the details of FBDD, it is important to understand the key principles and obstacles that this method of drug discovery entails [25].

There are a few concepts toward fragment-based drug designing as listed below in Table 3.

Biophysical approaches are used to screen roughly 1000 fragments in FBDD. The fragments will be 150 to 250 MW in size, and a broad nonspecific

Table 2 Approaches of ligand-based drug design.

S.No.	Approaches	Action	Advantages
1	Ligand-based virtual screening (LBVS)	Isofunctional molecular structures have been identified	Helpful in drug repurposing [21]
2	Molecular descriptors	On the basis of physicochemical features, reference molecules are compared to a large library of low-cost chemicals	For successful task execution, use symbolic representation [22]
3	Quantitative structure-activity relationship models (QSAR)	QSAR can as well be employed for linking compounds to their biological functions	The ability to come up with the right mathematical relationship [23]
4	Pharmacophore modeling	With a large enough number of ligands, a pharmacophore model of the receptor site can be created	Improved stability and bioavailability [24]

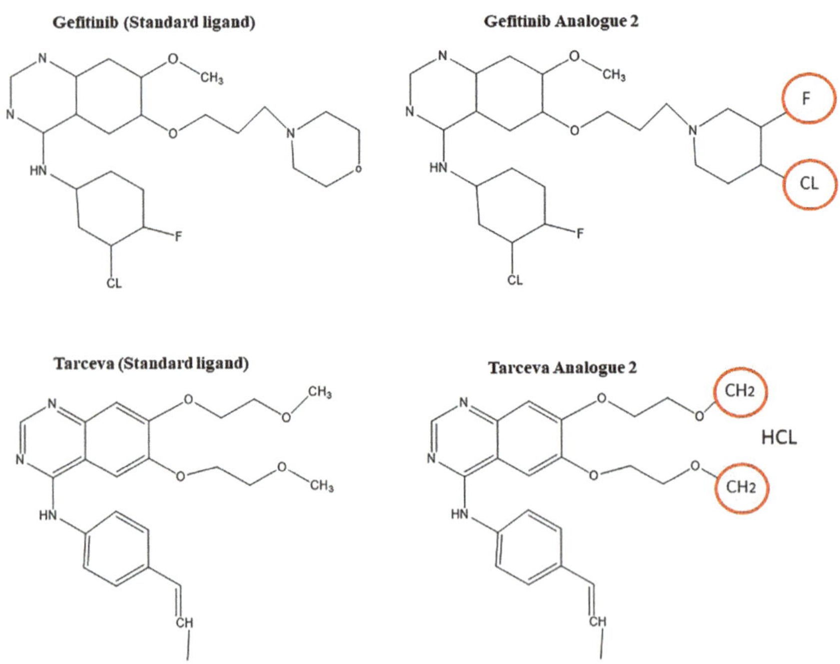

Fig. 4 Gefitinib and Tarceva structures with their analogues.

Table 3 The concept on fragment-based drug designing.

Approaches	Description	Advantages
Concept 1	Small-molecule medications suffer from a lot of attrition due to physical qualities that aren't right	With a large enough number of ligands, a pharmacophore model of the receptor site can be created
Concept 2	Despite their low power, fragments from high-quality interactions	It highlights how fragments must provide high-quality interactions and can be used to construct larger, more effective drugs
Concept 3	The term "ligand efficiency" refers to how well different-sized molecules can be optimized	To assist in determining the variations in physicochemical properties between a fragment lead and the final medication entity
Concept 4	To sample chemical space, only a limited number of fragment libraries are necessary	Multiple hits with high ligand efficiency should be found more easily with chemical sampling

component database will be chosen to cover a diverse range of chemical scaffolds and functionalities that have previously been exploited in drug development. Some examples of typical fragments are shown below [26]

(A) In most cases, the experimental binding mechanism of fragment hits is determined in the protein of interest. Structure-based drug design is used to develop fragments to form novel interactions.

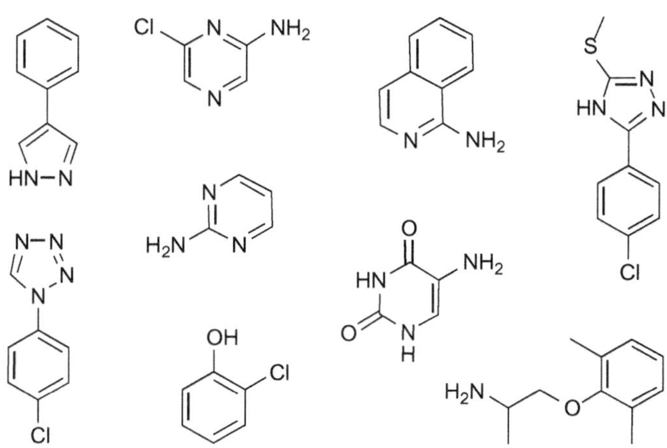

(B) If distinct fragments are detected to bind to proximal locations in the protein, fragment linking can be used. Because of their tiny size, first fragment hits have modest potency, but they create high-quality interactions and can be easily refined into potent lead compounds.

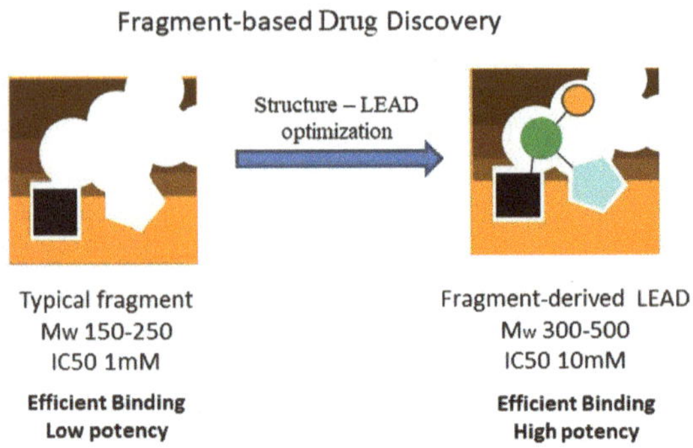

4. CADD concepts and technologies

The environment of drug research and discovery is continually shifting. We hope to give a succinct but comprehensive snapshot of overall trends and developing concepts in CADD. This part is discussed in Table 3.

4.1 Big data

The phrase "bigdata" refers to massive amounts of data that are difficult to store, analyze, and visualize using typical computational methods due to their enormous, varied, and complicated data structures [39] (Fig. 5). Here we are writing some features of big data that are

- Volume: Data size.
- Velocity: The new data of generation speed.
- Variety: Formats of various data.
- Veracity: Quality of data.
- Validity: Authenticity of data.
- Vocabulary: Terminology of data.
- Venue: A platform for data generation.
- Visualization: Data view.
- Volatility: Usefulness of data duration.
- Value: Data has the potent to lower the cost of medication research and development.

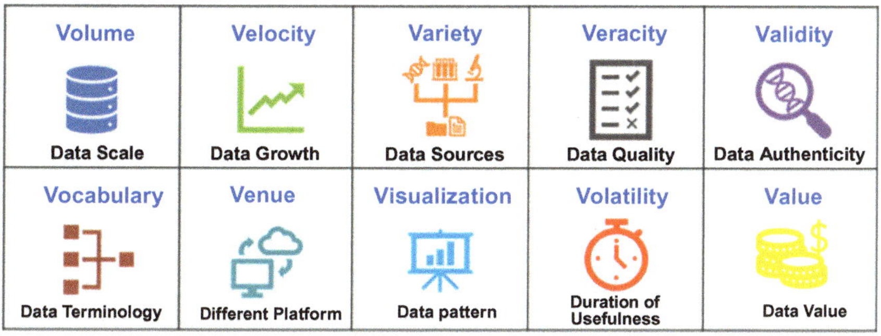

Fig. 5 The Big data can help in drug research and discovery.

4.2 Web servers

As per Chen et al., information was created in response to the demand for chemical data management using informatics. It serves as a stepping stone or doorway to virtual screening in the drug discovery process. As a result, it is critical to be aware of the resources accessible to assist such endeavors. As a result, it is critical to be aware of the resources accessible to assist such endeavors. Table 4 shows the virtual screening of a few web-based systems and their potential uses [40].

4.3 Workflows

Let's take a look at a typical scenario including virtual screening for lead discovery and/or optimization. The initial stage in a procedure is usually to obtain relevant data from libraries or in-house databases [41] Molecular area or similarity metrics, such as the Tanimoto index, can be used to filter data. Finally, molecular docking would be used in in silico testing to pick lead candidates [42]. The sample workflow could be completed with a variety of tools, such as commercial software suites like Schrodinger or Molecular Operating Environment, which strive to be full drug discovery toolboxes. Academic suites or programs exist as well, albeit their effectiveness is sometimes restricted by the methodologies or descriptors provided.

4.4 Machine learning

What exactly does it mean to learn? Learning, from a physiological standpoint, entails a variety of cognitive processes that all contribute to the memory of certain actions or amount of knowledge for a specific reason. To a degree, machines and algorithms can imitate this process [43]. Consider the junk mail that finds its way into the junk folder. To do so, the server

Table 4 Computer-aided drug design: selected trending concepts and technologies.

S.No.	Concept	Information
1	Big data	Refers to a vast or complex volume of data that is either in place or available in the public domain [27–31]
2	Web servers	Databases or web-based apps that could be used during a virtual screening campaign [32]
3	Workflows	In a virtual screening campaign, an ordered set of algorithms and steps [33]
4	Machine learning	Self-feeding algorithms and models aimed at data optimization and improvement [34]
5	Deep learning	Machine learning implementation using artificial neural networks and nonlinear processing units [35,36]
6	Artificial intelligence	Refers to a computer or program capable of simulating cognitive functions without the need for human supervision or input [37]
7	Molecular dynamics	Molecular mechanics and force fields are used to simulate and model molecules (typically proteins) [38]

runs a query based on the originator and/or effective delivery, and then decides on a message's fate based on a history of user actions. However, as the reader is likely aware, this approach is flawed, as wanted mail frequently winds up in the spam folder. Table 5 shows instances of machine learning approaches used in drug development from the literature.

4.5 Deep learning

Deep learning is a method of scaling machine learning by employing multilayered neural networks to try to abstract massive data models [51]. Deep learning, like machine learning, was inspired by a cognitive process. Deep learning is used in this case to extract features from numerous observations via neural connections, replicating the perceptual process [52]. To put it another way, deep learning recognizes patterns in data by using neural networks with various topologies that have been trained to identify characteristics according to a complexity scale [35,36]. Iteratively altering the weight values of artificial neural networks (ANN) teaches them to self-optimize. These techniques were created in the 1980s and have since expanded to include support for vector machines and random forests [53]. Deep learning methods' dependence on data organization is a significant restriction to their

Table 5 Examples of molecular docking, chemoinformatics, drug discovery, and/or lead optimization web servers.

S.No.	Name	Type	Description
1	*E*-Babel	File Format Converters	OpenbBabel's online version. The Virtual Computational Chemistry Laboratory is in charge of its upkeep
2	Corina online demo	File format Converters	CORINA is available as a demo online. SMILES are converted into 3D coordinates
3	Binding Database	Database	A public database comprising 1.1 million reports of protein-ligand complex binding affinity
4	BRENDA	Database	Enzymatic data from 82,568 proteins was manually curated
5	PUMA	Chemoinformatic tool	Several analyses on chemical space and specific molecular variation are being implemented on a server
6	USR-VS	Virtual screening tool	Virtual screening server with rapid form recognition algorithms. The queries are compared to about 94,000 ZINC conformers.
7	SwissModel	Homology modeling tool	Server for homology modeling
8	Hex Server	Protein-protein docking	Protein-protein docking server depend on target shape and electrostatics
9	ProBuilder	File format Converters	From 1D to 3D protein/ peptide builder
10	PROPKA	Molecular modeling	Calculate the pK_a of protein titratable functions using a web server
11	metaPocket	Binding site prediction	To predict ligand-binding sites, a meta server is used to locate pockets on protein surfaces
12	PASS	Binding site prediction	A program for estimating drug interaction pockets based on protein structure

efficiency. Beyond pattern identification, an important distinction among knowledge and true vision is that ANNs cannot employ their "logic" to judgment.

4.6 Artificial intelligence

Artificial intelligence (AI) is a branch of computer science concerned with the introduction of intelligence into automated machinery and computer [54]. Apple's Siri, Amazon's Alexa, and Microsoft's Cortana are all examples of AI in technology today. They are all digital helpers that can supply info and schedules. Is medical research a viable alternative? For intensive care and operative planning, AI has made inroads into medical settings [55]. As a result of the efficacy of these approaches and the advent of data-driven paradigms, AI has now been used to patients with medical treatment [56]. Significant breakthroughs in scanning processing and identification have been revealed, leading to the claim that, while AI is now in the development, it may soon overtake clinicians. However, whether that is a real separation among deep learning and AI approaches (at least for the time being) is debatable [57,58]. Finally, machine learning and its derivatives have the potential to significantly improve medication research and discovery. After all, the pharmaceutical business had invested more than $400 million on AI research and development as of 2017. Nonetheless, as with any other method, it is vital to maintain a healthy level of skepticism about AI's genuine merits.

4.7 Molecular dynamics

MD has been recognized as the successor to molecular docking in drug discovery. It has mostly been employed in the modeling of potential allosteric sites and research of binding modes [59]. MD scalability has recently enabled novel ways to handle problems that go beyond protein flexibility [60]. Consider free potential fluctuations, which allow you to determine the energy involved in ligand binding as well as various derivatives [61]. pH-REMD, an upgraded sampling method for assessing the environment of active sites and correcting pK_a on sidechains, and QM/MM, a hybrid methodology for modeling electronic changes based on ab initio and physical changes produced by molecular mechanics, are two further methods [62]. This approach can be used to investigate enzymatic mechanisms like covalent inhibition.

Since the 1970s, MD has evolved slowly but consistently. A cursory scan of academic repositories reveals the subject's exponential surge in popularity

[63]. There is various MD simulation software, which is available for both free and commercial purposes.

5. Prediction of protein structures through CADD

Proteins with drug-binding sites are inherently dynamic systems that can demonstrate extensive structural and functional flexibility. A single structural model, whether experimental or anticipated, consists of only a static snapshot and hence cannot always represent all of a protein's relevant features, as illustrated in Table 6. In a nutshell, there can be no such thing as "the" sequence of amino acids, and this holds true even for experimental structures that must deal with issues like protein mobility, experimental circumstances, and structural mistakes, among other things. The importance of

Table 6 Examples of machine learning applications in drug discovery.

S.No.	Applications	Results
1	Virtual screening	Lead structures for a novel TB target have been discovered. In addition, hit molecules can be repurposed into new drugs [44].
2	High throughput screening	Fingerprints were created using image data. These allowed for the linkage of biological tests with the prediction of activity [45]
3	Protein-ligand interactions	Although the chemical variety is not large enough to provide a thorough assessment of binding and nonbinding molecules, machine learning algorithms are effective for recognizing interactions [46]
4	Estimation on adverse effect	K-Seeds, a new clustering algorithm, was created. It performed better than other methods in terms of enrichment [47]
5	Neoplastic and mutagenic Classification	The models and experimental knowledge were found to be in agreement. Descriptors for multicells were developed with a 70% accuracy rate [48]
6	Molecular docking accuracy	The DUD set was used to create effective models of protein-ligand interactions [49]
7	Binding affinity prediction	Molecular dynamics data can help machine learning models a lot. This, in turn, can help molecular dynamics by improving force fields [50]

target and binding site flexibility in CADD cannot be overstated, and failing to do so can jeopardize its success [64].

In the pharmaceutical sector, computational approaches for predicting 3D protein models are widely employed, and significant effort has gone into increasing model accuracy and broadening the breadth of these methods.

The following steps can be performed until a satisfactory model is obtained in a homology modeling pipeline:

(i) Template selection to find the most appropriate experimentally measured components.
(ii) Alignment of the target and template sequences;
(iii) Constructed of 3D models of structures;
(iv) Refinement of the model; and
(v) Estimation of model quality.

Model refinement usually means removing conflicts and regularizing bond angles and length geometrically, but it can also entail more complicated structural alterations. As a general rule, focus on steps I (ii), (iii), and (v), rather than global model refinement (iv), which often yields a poor return on investment [73]. Expert expertise and time-consuming manual intervention are frequently required in techniques, necessitating the creation of completely automated homology modeling procedures few soft wares used in as shown in Table 7.

Table 7 MD simulation software for both free and commercial purposes.

Name of Software	Availability	Description	URL
CHARMM	Commercial	Source code and demos are included in this package of molecular simulation applications	https://www.charmm.org//
GROMACS	Free/open	Molecular dynamics simulation package	http://www.gromacs.org/
NAMD	Free/open	Free parallel molecular dynamics code designed for high-performance simulation of large biomolecular systems	http://www.ks.uiuc.edu/Research/namd/

Table 7 MD simulation software for both free and commercial purposes—cont'd

Name of Software	Availability	Description	URL
OPENMD	Free/open	Using atom types with orientational degrees of freedom, molecular dynamics can be used to mimic liquids, proteins, nanoparticles, surfaces, and other complicated systems	https://openmd.net/
CHARMm	Commercial	Multiple graphical front ends	https://www.3ds.com/products-services/biovia/products/discovery-studio/simulations.html?wockw=products%20services%20OR%20biovia%20OR%20products%20OR%20discovery%20studio%20OR%20simulations.html
MacroModel	Commercial	Distributed by Schrodinger	https://www.schrodinger.com/
PrimaDORAC	Free/open	Tiny molecules' bound properties for use in molecular mechanics or molecular dynamics calculations	http://www1.chim.unifi.it/orac/primadorac/
ORAC	Free/open	Molecular dynamics simulations program	http://www1.chim.unifi.it/orac/

It is envisaged that, with the advancement of NGS, such models would eventually be able to predict individual and species-specific treatment reactions, encouraging personalized therapy and minimizing animal sacrifice. We believe that a combination of newly solved X-ray crystal structures, an ever-increasing number of sequences, gotten better modeling approaches, and product evaluation techniques will result in strong homology modeling methods that will aid in the advancement of intricate obstacles in drug development.

6. Illumination of phytopharmacology of natural products through CADD

Drug research and development projects have frequently looked to plant sources for hit/lead chemical identification [75–79]. This is due to the fact that nature provides a vast array of structurally different chemical scaffolds from which pharmaceuticals can be extracted and/or manufactured [80,81]. Furthermore, natural products (NPs) differ from synthetic chemicals and pharmaceuticals in that they will be typically high in chiral carbon centers and occupy a molecular area that most synthetic compounds and treatments do not [82].

Computer-assisted technologies such as ligand docking, pharmacophore searching, neural networking, and binding free energy estimates of prospective medicines toward a target receptor are all used in modern drug development. The goal of these in silico technologies has been to use 3D computer models to mimic the interaction between a putative therapeutic molecule and its receptor or binding site (typically the drug target) [83]. As indicated in Table 8, the chemical structure of the most promising phytochemical elements derived from these plant species has been used traditionally to treat a variety of life-threatening diseases, including many targeted diseases.

PASS prediction: Using the PASS program, the identified main chemicals were subjected to an analysis of putative biological effects. This program predicts the biological features of a compound (up to 4000 types) based on its chemical structure analysis, such as potential activity and probable inactivity, where the standard values of Pa and Pi vary from 0.000 to 1.000. When Pa Pi, a chemical is considered physiologically active. Pa 0.7 indicates high pharmacological activity, Pa 0.5 indicates moderate pharmacological potentiality, and Pa 0.5 indicates poor pharmacological potentiality [95].

Table 8 Protein structure homology modeling servers and tools.

S.No.	Resources	URL
1	Protein Model Portal	http://www.proteinmodelportal.org HHpred [65]
2	HHpred	http://toolkit.tuebingen.mpg.de/hhpred ICM [66]
3	ICM	http://www.molsoft.com/ IntFOLD [67]
4	IntFOLD	http://www.reading.ac.uk/bioinf/IntFOLD [68]
5	Modeler, ModWeb	http://salilab.org/modeller/ Phyre2 [69]
6	Phyre2	http://www.sbg.bio.ic.ac.uk/phyre2/ Robetta [70]
7	Robetta	http://robetta.bakerlab.org/ SWISS-MODEL [71]
8	SWISS-MODEL	http://swissmodel.expasy.org [72]

The most important example of using CADD is herbal management and treatment of COVID. The continuing Coronavirus disease (COVID-19) pandemic is caused by the SARS-CoV-2 virus. SARS-CoV-2 has a higher infectivity than the SARS-CoV virus that was first detected in 2003, and there is no known therapy. The virus's rapid spread over such a brief span of time has resulted in a large number of individuals (over 2 million) becoming infected worldwide, posing a serious challenge to healthcare systems. COVID-19 exhibits an age-related distribution curve of sickness and a total mortality [96], despite the fact that the data are moving as the disease advances.

The Ayurvedic philosophy recommends administering "a set of phytoconstituents" that have the potential to have adaptogenic, immunomodulatory, and drug-targeting effects [97–99]. Chromatographic techniques were used to identify phytochemicals in Shatavari, also known as *Asparagus racemosus* (AR), Guduchi, also known as *Tinospora cordifolia* (TC), and *Withania somnifera* (WS). To better understand the immunomodulatory effects of phytochemicals, a network pharmacology model was created to find and depict the links between phytochemicals and pharmacological targets in innate immunity. The phytoconstituents were also docked to three SARS-CoV-2 molecular targets to see if they have antiviral action. Predictive methods were also employed to evaluate the possibility for interactions between phytoconstituents and regularly prescribed medications as shown in Table 9.

Table 9 Frequently used servers and tools for protein prediction of binding site.

S.No.	Software	Description	URL
1	MED-SuMo	Surface similarity detecting program for macromolecules. Similar binding surfaces are found in 3D databases, and 3D superpositions are generated based on shared surface chemical characteristics and similar form	http://medit-pharma.com/index.php
2	CAVER	Channels and Tunnels in protein structures are analyzed and visualized using software	https://www.caver.cz/
3	GHECOM	Using mathematical morphology, a program for identifying multiscale pockets on protein surfaces has been developed	http://strcomp.protein.osaka-u.ac.jp/ghecom/download_src.html
4	SURFNET	Surfaces and empty zones between surfaces are generated using coordinate data from a PDB file	https://www.ebi.ac.uk/thornton-srv/software/SURFNET/
5	Phosfinder	Phosphate-binding sites in protein structures can be predicted using this method	http://phosfinder.bio.uniroma2.it/overview.html
6	VOIDOO	Cavity detection and volume analysis software	http://xray.bmc.uu.se/usf/voidoo.html
7	POVME	Binding-pocket volume measurement software that is free and open source	http://rocce-vm0.ucsd.edu/data/sw/hosted/POVME/
8	POCASA	Roll is an algorithm that can predict binding sites by recognizing pockets and cavities in proteins with known 3D structures. It is implemented as an automatic web service	http://g6altair.sci.hokudai.ac.jp/g6/service/pocasa/
9	FunFOLDQA	Based on 3D models of proteins, this program evaluates the validity of ligand binding site residue predictions	http://www.reading.ac.uk/bioinf/downloads/

Table 9 Frequently used servers and tools for protein prediction of binding site—cont'd

S.No.	Software	Description	URL
10	LISE	Ligand Binding Site Prediction is a free and open-source application. Protein Triangles with Ligand Interacting and Binding Sites	https://sourceforge.net/projects/msdock/files/
Frequently used servers and tools for protein target prediction [74]			
11	PatchSearch	PatchSearch uses a limited amount of flexibility to search for homologous binding sites on protein surfaces. To express all possible matches between two structures, it uses product graphs	
12	IXCHEL	Ixchel is a program that predicts biological activity based on proteins. A database of over 9000 protein cavities is used to dock the input molecule (in SDF or SMILE)	
13	CABRAKAN	Abrakan is a ligand-based virtual profiling program that works in two dimensions. It compares chemicals and predicts their biological activity using their 2D fingerprints	
14	HURAKAN	It analyzes molecules without superimposition based on their interactions with their surroundings to produce compounds with diverse structures but similar bioactivity anticipated	
15	MolScore-Antivirals	Antiviral medication candidates are identified and prioritized using an expert system	
16	MolScore-Antibiotics	Antibacterial medication candidates are identified and prioritized using an expert system	

Finally, due to their ability to prevent SARS-CoV-2 replication, our research identified promising bioactive ingredients for medical evaluation of Rasayana herbs in prophylactic [100] (Table 10).

7. CADD in illustration of phytopharmacology

Pharmacophore modeling is a CADD technology that has the potential to be one of the most promising candidates for experimental efforts in current

Table 10 List of herbs and their potent chemicals used against various diseases.

Botanical source	Active parts	Chemical constituents	Disease
Abroma Augusta	Root, bark, leaves	Fredeline, choline, betaine	Antidiabetic, anti-inflammatory [84]
Abelmoschus moschatus	Root, leaves and seeds	Myricetin, farnesol	Anti-diabetic, antistroke, antimicrobial activity and anti-inflammatory [85]
Acacia nilotica	Gum, leaves, root and stem	Polyphenol, tannins, gallic acid	Cardiovascular disease, antidiabetic [86]
Acacia polyacantha	Seed	Tryptamines, B-carbolines	Antidiabetic, antifungal and antimalaria [87]
Aconitum palmatum	Root	Alkaloids flavanoids	Antidiabetic [88]
Aegle marmelos	Leaves, root, fruits and seed	Lupeol, cineole, citral	Antidiabetic [89]
Agrimonia eupatoria	Whole plant, leaves	Volatile oil, apigenin, luteolin, glycosides	Antidiabetic, antibacterial [90]
Allium sativum	Bulb	Allicin peptides, steroids, flavonoids, phenols	Antidiabetic, antiallergic, antiatherosclerotic [91]
Asparagus racemosus	Stems, leaves and seed	Essential oil, asparagine, flavonoid	Antibacterial and antidiabetic [92]
Azadirahta indica	Root, leaves bark	Azadirachtin, nimbadiol, nimbinene	Antidiabetic [93]
Bacopa monnieri	Aerial part	Nicotinine, alkaloid	Alzheimer's disease [94]

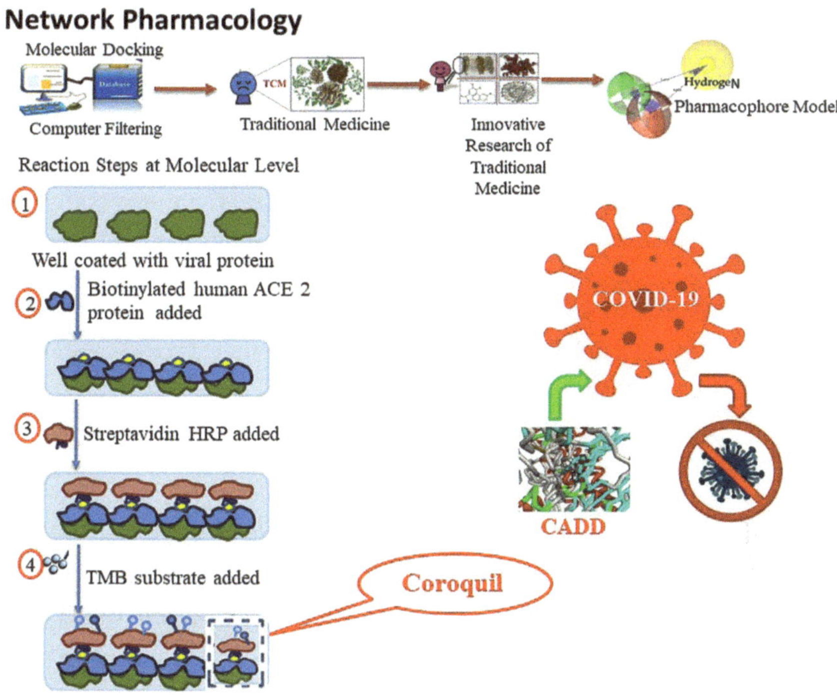

Fig. 6 CADD in illustration in development of antiviral drug.

medicinal chemistry. Powerful molecular modeling tools have been useful in designing lead targets in the search for high affinity antiviral medication against Covid-19 (Fig. 6).

A novel strategy for understanding herbal formulations has been proposed through network pharmacology by following below points.

7.1 Active compound identification and screening

The Traditional Chinese Medicine Systems Pharmacology Database and Analysis Platform was used to certify all molecules of the 14 Chinese medicinal plants in HSBDF. We screened HSBDF molecules using the absorption, distribution, metabolism, and excretion (ADME) processes, which are important in drug research and discovery.

7.2 Identification of protein targets

The TCMSP database, which contained information on 6511 drug entities and 3987 targets along interactions between them, was used to find protein targets linked with active compounds.

7.3 Component-target gene network construction

Based on the aforementioned data sets, a visual component-target network was created in Cytoscape 3.7.2 to show the complicated interactions between potent chemicals and their active site. The active components and targets that have been screened are represented by the nodes in the network, while the interaction among the nodes indicate the therapeutic analysis relationships.

7.4 The targets of COVID-19 prediction

The knowledge on COVID-19-associated target genes was gathered using the Gene Cards database and the Therapeutic Target Database (TTD). Gene Cards is a collection of functions for proteomics, genomics, and transcriptomics.

7.5 Protein-protein interactions (PPI) network construction

STRING (to develop the PPI network interaction) was used put the HSBDF core targets. The PPI network was built and visualized using Cytoscape V3.7.2. For topological study of PPI networks, CytoNCA, a network topology analysis plug-in in Cytoscape, was utilized.

7.6 Molecular docking of components and targets

The ligand coordinate in the target protein complex defined the active site of molecular docking. The ligand was designed to be flexible, while the receptor was designed to be rigid. Small compounds were docked with the ACE2 protein and the SARS-CoV-2 3CL protein, respectively, using Autodock Vina 1.1.2.

8. CADD in the treatment of diseases

Traditional medicine (TM), a system that has been practiced for over 2000 years, utilized by about one-fifth of the globe's population and is centered globally [101]. Modernization of the TM is both a theoretical and a technological breakthrough. On the one hand, component-based medicine was originally presented in 1999, thanks to the current use of cutting-edge technology in chemical analysis and medicine [102]. Component-based medicine, on the one hand, was initially offered in 1999 as a result of the recent use of cutting-edge technology in chemical analysis and medicine. It is distinguished by reasonably obvious pharmacodynamics ingredients, methods of action, codes and standards, and consistent manufacturing procedures. A range of modern synthetic and computational biology technologies were used extensively in the research of TM.

A growing number of severe disorders are being investigated by merging multiomics methods with data science in order to successfully record the unified biological reaction [103]. These findings showed that network pharmacology is a relatively young field that focuses on "network-targeted, multicomponent therapies." It offered a new medical strategy for TCM's holistic approach [104].

9. Assessment of early stage drug toxicity through CADD

The most important consideration while producing a pharmaceutical is safety, which includes a wide range of toxicities and adverse pharmacological effects that must be assessed during the preclinical and clinical trial phases. In vitro and in vivo assays are commonly used to study medication safety, which includes a wide range of toxicities and adverse pharmacological effects. In recent years, some efforts have been made to produce in vitro models, such as "organ on a chip," in order to cut costs [114]. Those methods, however, are still expensive and lengthy. When compared to experimental procedures, technical process has demonstrated to have significant advantages because they are environmentally friendly, quick, inexpensive, and precise, and most significantly, they may be performed before a molecule is manufactured [115].

In this chapter, we will examine the evolution of in silico chemical toxicity prediction over the last 5 years, covering machine learning and structural alerting approaches, as well as significant toxicity endpoints in drug research and discovery.

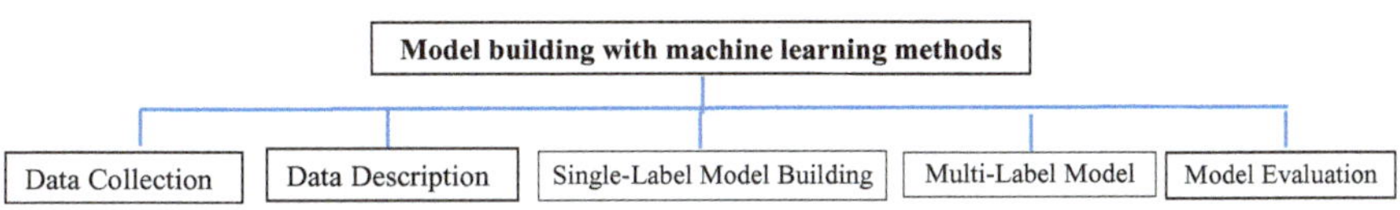

Data collection, data description, model development, and model evaluation are the four processes in the typical procedure for constructing a predictive model. Each stage has its own set of requirements to ensure that the models are reliable and accurate. Table 11 shows some commonly used databases (Tables 12–14).

PROGRESS IN THE PREDICTION OF TOXICITY: For medication safety assessment, many computer models have been created, which can

Table 11 Pharmacokinetics of phytoconstituents from *AR*, *TC*, and *WS* in silico.

Herbs	Phytoconstituents	Expected oral bioavailability[a]	Predicted drug-likeness[b]	Pharmacokinetics				
				CYP[c]	P-gp substrate	BBB permeability	GI absorption	Log K_p (cm/s)
Asparagus racemosus	Muzanzagenin	Orally bioavailable	Yes	No	Yes	Yes	High	−6.94
	Asparanin A	Not orally bioavailable because polarity, solubility, and size axes lie outside the pink region	No	No	Yes	No	Low	−8.48
	Asparagamine A	Orally bioavailable	Yes	No	No	Yes	High	−6.95
	Isoagatharesinol	Due to saturation parameter does not lie inside the pink area, it is not orally bioavailable	Yes	CYP2D6, CYP3A4 only	No	No	High	−6.43

	Rutin	Due to its increased molecular weight and polarity, it is not orally accessible	No	No	Yes	No	Low	−10.26
	Shatavarin I	Due to its greater polarity, molecular weight, and flexibility, it is not orally accessible	No	No	Yes	No	Low	−13.47
	Shatavarin IV	Due to its increased molecular weight and polarity, it is not orally accessible	No	No	Yes	No	Low	−10.53
	Shatavarin VI	Due to its increased molecular weight and polarity, it is not orally accessible	No	No	Yes	No	Low	−10.53

Continued

Table 11 Pharmacokinetics of phytoconstituents from *AR, TC,* and *WS* in silico—cont'd

Herbs	Phytoconstituents	Expected oral bioavailability	Predicted drug-likeness	Pharmacokinetics				
				CYP	P-gp substrate	BBB permeability	GI absorption	Log K_p (cm/s)
	Shatavarin VII	Due to its increased molecular weight and polarity, it is not orally accessible	No	No	Yes	No	Low	−10.97
	Shatavarin IX	Due to its increased molecular weight and polarity, it is not orally accessible	No	No	Yes	No	Low	−10.99
	Shatavarin X	Due to its greater polarity, molecular weight, and flexibility, it is not orally accessible	No	No	Yes	No	Low	−11.23

Tinospora cordifolia	Berberine	Orally bioavailable	Yes	CYP1A2, CYP2D6, CYP3A4 only	Yes	Yes	High	−5.78
	Columbamine	Orally bioavailable	Yes		Yes	Yes	High	−5.94
	Menisperine	Orally bioavailable	Yes		Yes	Yes	High	−6.30
	Magnoflorine	Orally bioavailable	Yes	CYP1A2, CYP3A4 only	Yes	Yes	High	−6.44
	Tinopsoraside	Because of its increased molecular weight and polarity, it is not orally accessible	No	No	Yes	No	Low	−9.13
	Tinosporide	Orally bioavailable	Yes	CYP2D6 only	Yes	No	High	−7.64
	Tinocordiside	Orally bioavailable	Yes	No	Yes	No	High	−8.56
	Syringin	Orally bioavailable	Yes	No	N	No	Low	−9.50
	Columbin	Orally bioavailable	Yes	No	Yes	No	High	−6.95
	20-β-Hydroxy Ecdysone	Orally bioavailable	No	No	Yes	No	High	−8.91

Continued

Table 11 Pharmacokinetics of phytoconstituents from *AR, TC,* and *WS* in silico—cont'd

Herbs	Phytoconstituents	Expected oral bioavailability	Predicted drug-likeness	Pharmacokinetics				
				CYP	P-gp substrate	BBB permeability	GI absorption	Log K_p (cm/s)
Withania somnifera	Withacoagin	Orally bioavailable	Yes	CYP2C9 only	Yes	No	High	−6.29
	Withanolide B	Orally bioavailable	Yes		Yes	No	High	−5.76
	Withastramonolide-12-Deoxy	Orally bioavailable	Yes		Yes	No	High	−6.35
	Withanoside IV	Because of its increased molecular weight and polarity, it is not orally accessible	No	No	Yes	No	Low	−10.37
	Withanolide A	Orally bioavailable	Yes	No	Yes	No	High	−6.86

[a]Predicted oral bioavailability from RADAR graph (Supplementary Material).
[b]Predicted CYP inhibition for CYP1A2, CYP2C9, CYP2C19, CYP2D6, and CYP3A4.
[c]Predicted Drug-likeness (Results of Lipinski, Ghose, Veber, Egan and Muegge rules).

Note: The phase-I drug-metabolizing enzymes CYP-Cytochrome P450 are responsible for >95% of xenobiotic metabolism; P-gp-P-glycoprotein is a critical efflux drug transporter; the BBB—blood-brain barrier plays an important role in preventing drug transport into the brain; and K_p-skin permeability coefficient all explain skin permeability coefficient. Lipophilicity and molecule size are linearly related to K_p. The lower the log K_p (in cm/s), the less permeant the molecule is to the skin.

Table 12 CADD steps for designing a medicinal drugs.

Method	URL
Active compound identification and screening	http://tcmspw.com/
Identification of protein targets	http://lsp.nwsuaf.edu.cn/tcmsp.php
Component-target gene network construction	http://www.cytoscape.org/
Predicting the targets of COVID-19	https://www.genecards.org/
Protein-protein interactions (PPI) network construction	https://string-db.org/cgi/input.pl
Molecular docking of components and targets	https://www.rcsb.org/
The information sharing platform's target system structure	http://ncovtarget.qnlm.ac/web/mg/hm
PubChem database	https://pubchem.ncbi.nlm.nih.gov/

Table 13 A few diseases can be treated using their herbal preparation by using CADD.

S.No.	Diseases	Herbal formulation	Reference
1	Cardiocerebrovascular diseases (CCVDs)	Hawthorn Berry Vasguard	[105]
2	Diabetes mellitus (DM)	Di Dang Decoction	[106]
3	Chronic obstructive pulmonary disease (COPD)	Ginsenoside extract	[107]
4	Chronic bronchitis	Radix Bupleuri powder	[36]
5	Bronchial asthma	Scutellariae Radix tablets	[108]
6	Lung cancer	Rheum palmatum powder	[109]
7	Chronic gastritis	Moluodan	[110]
8	Hyperlipidemia	Xuezhiqing	[111]
9	Rheumatoid arthritis	Kangen-karyu	[112]
10	Liver disease	Qing Gan Zi Shen Tang	[113]

be classified into three categories: qualitative classification, quantitative regression, and read-across. Most of the prediction database online and web server as shown in Table 15.

To improve the accuracy of predictive models, more computational approaches should be created. For example, read-across has recently gotten a lot of interest since it can fill in the gaps left by missing data. Many programs

Table 14 Some of the most widely used databases for chemical toxicity prediction.

Database name	URL
TOXNET	https://toxnet.nlm.nih.gov/
ToxBank Data Warehouse	http://www.toxbank.net/data-warehouse
admetSAR	http://lmmd.ecust.edu.cn/admetsar1/
Pharmaco Kinetics Knowledge Base (PKKB)	http://cadd.zju.edu.cn/pkkb/
ToxCas	https://www.epa.gov/chemical-research/toxicity-forecasting
Tox21	https://tripod.nih.gov/tox21
CTD (Comparative Toxicogenomics Database)	http://ctdbase.org/
ECOTOX	https://cfpub.epa.gov/ecotox/
SuperToxic	http://bioinformatics.charite.de/supertoxic/
DSSTox	https://www.epa.gov/chemical-research/distributed-structure-searchable-toxicity-dsstox-database
ACToR	https://actor.epa.gov/actor/home.xhtml
T3DB	http://www.t3db.ca
eChemPortal	https://www.echemportal.org/echemportal/index.action
PubChem	http://pubchem.ncbi.nlm.nih.gov/
ChEMBLdb	https://www.ebi.ac.uk/chembldb/
BindingDB	http://www.bindingdb.org/bind/index.jsp
ChemProt	http://potentia.cbs.dtu.dk/ChemProt/
STITCH	http://stitch.embl.de/
DrugBank	http://www.drugbank.ca/
TTD	http://bidd.nus.edu.sg/group/cjttd/
IntAct	http://www.ebi.ac.uk/intact/
SIDER	http://sideeffects.embl.de/
MetaADEDB	http://lmmd.ecust.edu.cn/online_services/metaadedb/
OFFSIDES	http://www.pharmgkb.org
Chemical Effects in Biological Systems (CEBS)	http://tools.niehs.nih.gov/cebs3/ui/
IntSide	http://intside.irbbarcelona.org
Reactome	Pathway http://www.reactome.org/
Pathway Commons	Pathway http://www.pathwaycommons.org/
KEGG	Pathway http://www.kanehisa.jp/
PharmGKB	Pathway https://www.pharmgkb.org/

Table 15 Most of the prediction database online and web server.

Categories	Models	Online server	URL
Carcinogenicity and Mutagenicity	Naïve Bayes, kNN, probabilistic neural network, and SVM	CarcinoPred-EL [116]	https://www.compudrug.com/?q=node/35
Acute Oral Toxicity	MACCS-SVMOAO, SubFP-SVMOAO, MACCS-kNN	DLAOThome [117]	https://www.simulations-plus.com/software/admetpredictor/
Cardiotoxicity	LCFP_8 fingerprints	ADMEWORKS Predictor [118]	https://www.fqs.pl/en/products
Hepatotoxicity	Cruz-Monteagudo ID 4, Leave-one-out (LOO)	Metabolizer [119].	https://chemaxon.com/products
Respiratory Toxicity	Workplace Exposure Limit (WEL), lymph node assay	IMPACT-F. [120]	http://www.pharmainformatic.com/html/impact-f.html

Table 16 Some software commonly used to predict toxicity.

Software	Activity	Type
ADMET Predictor, Leadscope and Lhasa Derek	Drug design	Commercial tool
OCED Toolbox	QSTR is used for toxicity prediction and modeling	Commercial tool
Lazar	With a user interface that involves drawing chemical compounds, it is possible to predict numerous toxicity outcomes	Web server
ToxTree	Using a decision tree approach, assess the toxic danger	Web server
ChemSAR	Molecular descriptors	Web server

and web servers can now forecast chemical toxicity prior to synthesis. Few of them are mentioned in Table 16.

10. Challenges and problems in CADD- based drug design and discovery

CADD continues to encounter numerous obstacles, including but not limited to: (1) Increasing the volume and quality of computing resources available online; (2) the field of computational chemo genomics is being developed further; (3) enhancing medication design with various molecular targets in mind; and (4) enhancing the ability of toxicity models and side effects to forecast, enhancing collaboration with other fields in order to improve the hunt for bioactive compounds for disease therapy and/or prevention. The writers' perspectives on some of the areas in CADD that need to be improved are presented in the below schematic section (Fig. 7).

10.1 Combination with other methodologies

CADD could be viewed as a component of a multidisciplinary effort rather than a stand-alone strategy for bringing pharmaceuticals to market [121]. CADD is utilized in concert with other methodologies such as HTS and/or combinatorial chemistry in most practical applications. However, because some research organizations are still unwilling to use computational tools to guide their investigations, there is still room for progress. Here are a few examples of how computational approaches have been combined with other technologies:

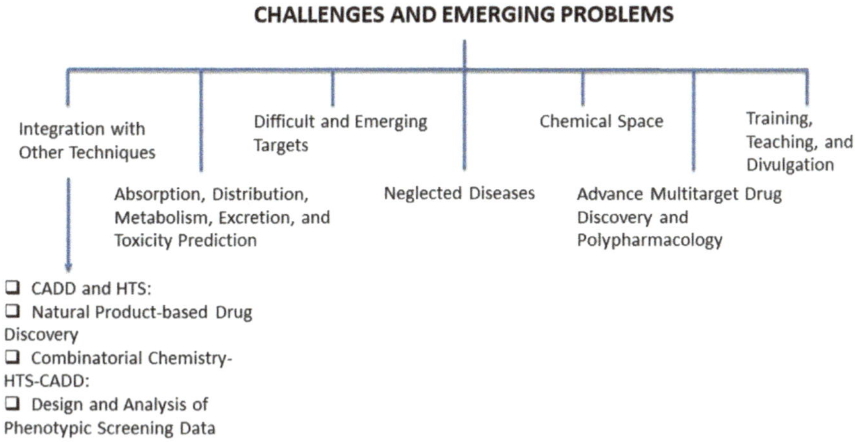

Fig. 7 Schematic representation for challenges and emerging problems of CADD.

10.2 Absorption, distribution, metabolism, and excretion, and toxicity prediction

Bit of the bottlenecks in drug design is ADME. Computational approaches are helping to predict potential ADME and toxicity issues, as well as minimizing the amount of animal testing experiments. However, due to the intricacy of numerous toxicity mechanisms, precisely estimating toxicity is a difficult endeavor. A recent review of in silico chemical toxicity prediction was released. As a result, more progress in the field of informatics toxicology is expected [125] (Tables 17 and 18).

Table 17 Various computational methods used in drug discovery and development.

Computational methods	Description
CADD and HTS	The topics covered include computer-assisted screening library selection (including informatic filtering of frequent hitters), informatic analysis of screening data, the construction of structure-activity correlations, data visualization, and the organizing, storing, and administration of output data [122]
Natural product-based drug discovery	Natural product databases, as well as target fishing and structural elucidation, are being constructed, organized, and mined [32]
Combinatorial chemistry-HTS-CADD:	Target fishing and structural elucidation are underway, as well as the creation, organization, and mining of natural product databases [123]
Deconvolution	Data from phenotypic screening were designed and analyzed [124]

Table 18 A recent trends in drug discovery to address polypharmacology.

Activity	Method	References
Chemogenomics	Virtual screening	[11]
Toxicity of molecules-targets-cell/based data	Deconvolution of phenotypic screening	[39]
Poly molecules interaction	Drugs with dual and multiple targets are being developed	
Quantitative structural relationship	Structure multiple-activity relationships (SmARTs)	[122]
Drug repurposing	Pull-down of Chemical Similarity Network Analysis	

10.3 Difficult and novel objectives

CADD is a promising technique for tackling tough topics, such as protein-protein interactions (PPI), which are currently regarded problematic [126]. Because of the nonclassical drug-like features of PPI inhibitors, rational design and optimization pose significant hurdles. Similarly, CADD approaches may open up new paths for addressing orphan, neglected, or developing targets with clinical potential, such as epigenetic targets [127].

10.4 Neglected diseases

There is considerable research being conducted to address neglected diseases. When it comes to detecting new hits and/or enhancing their activity, computational methods have a lower total cost than traditional experimental procedures [128].

10.5 Chemical space

It is still difficult to define and explore the medicinally relevant chemical space effectively. This is true for both investigating the molecular area of compound sites (e.g., epigenetic targets) and studying the molecular area from the perspective of commercially available and/or regularly utilized chemicals in HTS campaigns, such as dark chemical matter [129].

10.6 Polypharmacology and multitarget drug discovery

A recent trend in drug discovery is the development of multitarget drugs. CADD can also address polypharmacology and related concerns in this regard [130].

10.7 Training, teaching, and divulgation

Strengthening undergraduate and graduate education, as well as ensuring to support the development of data and methodologies to enhance CADD, is critical. Learning is currently done on the fly (in response to individual needs), but the creation of CADD-focused textbooks could make training much easier. Attending one of the many CADD conferences currently accessible can enhance formal training [126].

11. Conclusion

One of the most complex and challenging processes in the pharmaceutical industry is the creation of novel medications with potential therapeutic applications. The search for new medicinal agents consumes millions of dollars and labor hours. Since many variables, like bioavailability, toxicity, and metabolism, affect a medication's function, rational drug design has long been considered an ideal. Recent significant technological advancements in the fields of computer science, molecular biology, and structural characterization of biomacromolecules have made rational medication design possible. CADD is no longer just a cutting-edge method. It is a sensible and effective method to support the medicinal chemist. It is unlikely to result in pharmacological novelties on its own, but it has developed into an important tool that serves as a thinking help and a manual for synthesis. However, medications that are created and tested using computational methods might give a clear molecular justification and, more importantly, can spark the imagination.

Appendix: Supplementary material

Supplementary material related to this chapter can be found on the accompanying CD or online at https://doi.org/10.1016/B978-0-323-99137-7.00009-5.

References

[1] L. Zhao, L. Heather, C.M. Lauren, A. HaoZhu, Advancing computer-aided drug discovery (CADD) by big data and data-driven machine learning modelling, Drug Discov. Today 25 (9) (2020) 1624–1638.
[2] X.T. Zheng, et al., On-chip investigation of cell-drug interactions, Adv. Drug Deliv. Rev. 65 (2013) 1556–1574.
[3] J.P. Hughes, et al., Principles of early drug discovery, Br. J. Pharmacol. 162 (2011) 1239–1249.

[4] N. Berdigaliyev, M. Aljofan, An overview of drug discovery and development, Future Med. Chem. 10 (2020) 4155. fmc-2019-0307.
[5] P.E. Brandish, et al., A cell-based ultra-high-throughput screening assay for identifying inhibitors of D-amino acid oxidase, J. Biomol. Screen. 11 (2006) 481–487.
[6] M.A. Hamburg, F.S. Collins, The path to personalized medicine, N. Engl. J. Med. 363 (2010) 301–304.
[7] C.A. Nicolaou, N. Brown, Multiobjective optimization methods in drug design, Drug Discov. Today Technol. 10 (2013) e427–e435.
[8] A. Talevi, Tailored multi-target agents. Applications and design considerations, Curr. Pharm. Des. 22 (2016) 3164–3170.
[9] G. Sliwoski, S. Kothiwale, J. Meiler, E.W. Lowe, Computational methods in drug discovery, Pharmacol. Rev. 66 (1) (2014) 334–395.
[10] A. Abdolmaleki, J.B. Ghasemi, F. Ghasemi, Computer aided drug design for multi-target drug design: SAR/QSAR, molecular docking and pharmacophore methods, Curr. Drug Targets 18 (5) (2017) 556–575.
[11] J. Bajorath, Computational chemistry and computer-aided drug discovery: part II, Future Med. Chem. 8 (15) (2016) 1799–1800.
[12] J.C. Faver, M.N. Ucisik, W. Yang, K.M. Merz, Computer-aided drug design: using numbers to your advantage, ACS Med. Chem. Lett. 4 (9) (2013) 812–814.
[13] T.I. Oprea, J.P. Overington, Computational and practical aspects of drug repositioning, Assay Drug Dev. Technol. 13 (6) (2015) 299–306.
[14] P. Sledz, A. Caflisch, Protein structure-based drug design: from docking to molecular dynamics, Curr. Opin. Struct. Biol. 48 (2018) 93–103.
[15] O.M. Becker, D.S. Dhanoa, Y. Marantz, et al., An integrated in silico 3D model-driven discovery of a novel, potent, and selective amidosulfonamide 5-HT1A agonist (PRX-00023) for the treatment of anxiety and depression, J. Med. Chem. 49 (2006) 3116–3135.
[16] T. Cheng, Q. Li, Z. Zhou, Y. Wang, S.H. Bryant, Structure-based virtual screening for drug discovery: a problem-centric review, AAPS J. 14 (2012) 133–141.
[17] J.R. Bienstock, Overview: fragment-based drug design, ACS Symp. Ser. 1076 (2011) 1–26. Molecular modeling merges with combinatorial chemistry. Curr. Opin. Chem. Biol. 4, 283–286.
[18] M. Congreve, R. Carr, C. Murray, H. Jhoti, A 'rule of three' for fragment based lead discovery? Drug Discov. Today 8 (2003) 876–877.
[19] E.N. Siju, G.R. Rajalakshmi, A.P. Paulose, F.T. Dhanya, N. Hariraj, K. Rahul, CADD: pharmacological approaches in drug design and drug discovery, World J. Pharm. Pharm. Sci. 6 (2017) 892–908.
[20] P. Kolb, R.S. Ferreira, J.J. Irwin, B.K. Shoichet, Docking and chemoinformatic screens for new ligands and targets, Curr. Opin. Biotechnol. 20 (2009) 429–436.
[21] T. Kalliokoki, Accelerating Three Dimensional Virtual Screening, 2010. Dissertations in Health Sciences.
[22] D. Prada-Graciaa, S. Huerta-Yépezb, L.M. Moreno-Vargasb, Application of computational methods for anticancer drug discovery, design, and optimization, Bol. Med. Hosp. Infant. Mex. 73 (6) (2016) 411–423.
[23] H. Kubinyi, in: M.E. Wolff (Ed.), Burger's Medicinal Chemistry, vol. 1, John Wiley & Sons, 1995, pp. 497–571.
[24] K.J. Nielsen, D. Adarns, L. Thomas, et al., Structure-activity relationships of omega-conotoxins MVIIA, MVIIC and 14 loop splice hybrids at N and P/Q-type calcium channels, J. Mol. Biol. 289 (5) (1999) 1405–1421.
[25] C.W. Murray, D.C. Rees, The rise of fragment-based drug discovery, Nat. Chem. 1 (3) (2009) 187–192.
[26] D. Fattori, Molecular recognition: the fragment approach in lead generation, Drug Discov. Today 9 (2004) 229–238.

[27] S. Sagiroglu, D. Sinanc, Big data: a review, in: Proc. 2013 Int. Conf. Collab. Technol. Syst, vol. 2013, 2013, pp. 42–47.
[28] E.E. Schadt, et al., Cloud and heterogeneous computing solutions exist today for the emerging big data problems in biology, Nat. Rev. Genet. 12 (2011) 224.
[29] V. Marx, Biology: the big challenges of big data, Nature 498 (2013) 255–260.
[30] (a) Swarup V. and Geschwind D.H. (2013) Alzheimer's disease: from big data to mechanism. Nature 500, 34–35. (b) Wu, X.D. et al. (2014) Data mining with big data. IEEE Trans. Knowledge Data Eng. 26, 97–107.
[31] N. Brown, J. Cambruzzi, P.J. Cox, M. Davies, J. Dunbar, D. Plumbley, D.W. Sheppard, Big data in drug discovery, Prog. Med. Chem. 57 (2018) 277–356.
[32] M. Gonza'lez-Medina, J.J. Naveja, N. Sa'nchez-Cruz, J.L. Medina-Franco, Open chemoinformatic resources to explore the structure, properties and chemical space of molecules, RSC Adv. 7 (2017) 54153–54163.
[33] A. Cereto-Massague, M.J. Ojeda, C. Valls, M. Mulero, G. Pujadas, S. Garcia-Vallve, Tools for in silico target fishing, Methods 71 (2015) 98–103.
[34] M.A. Khamis, W. Gomaa, W.F. Ahmed, Machine learning in computational docking, Artif. Intell. Med. 63 (2015) 135–152.
[35] L. Zhang, J. Tan, D. Ha, H. Zhu, From machine learning to deep learning: progress in machine intelligence for rational drug discovery, Drug Discov. Today 22 (2017) 1680–1685.
[36] Q. Zhang, H. Yu, J. Qi, D. Tang, X. Chen, J.B. Wan, P. Li, H. Hu, Y.T. Wang, Y. Hu, Natural formulas and the nature of formulas: exploring potential therapeutic targets based on traditional Chinese herbal formulas, PLoS One 12 (2) (2017), e0171628.
[37] W. Duch, K. Swaminathan, J. Meller, Artificial intelligence approaches for rational drug design and discovery, Curr. Pharm. Des. 13 (2007) 1497–1508.
[38] M. De Vivo, M. Masetti, G. Bottegoni, A. Cavalli, Role of molecular dynamics and related methods in drug discovery, J. Med. Chem. 59 (2016) 4035–4061.
[39] F.D. Prieto-Martı'nez, J.L. Medina-Franco, Molecular docking: current advances and challenges, Tip Rev. Espec. Cienc. Quím.-Biol. 21 (2018) 65–87.
[40] K. Dhananjayan, Molecular docking study characterization of rare flavonoids at the Nac-binding site of the first Bromodomain of BRD4 (BRD4 BD1), J. Cancer Res. 2015 (2015) 1–15.
[41] J.P. Ebejer, S. Fulle, G.M. Morris, P.W. Finn, The emerging role of cloud computing in molecular modelling, J. Mol. Graph. Model. 44 (2013) 177–187.
[42] C. Grosan, A. Abraham (Eds.), Machine learning, in: Intelligent Systems, Springer, 2011, pp. 261–268.
[43] S. Shalev-Schwartz, S. Ben-David, Understanding Machine Learning: From Theory to Algorithms, Cambridge University Press, New York, 2014.
[44] S. Ekins, A.A. Godbole, G. Keri, L. Orfi, J. Pato, R.S. Bhat, Machine learning and docking models for *Mycobacterium tuberculosis* topoisomerase I, Tuberculosis (Edinb.) 103 (2017) 52–60.
[45] J. Simm, G. Klambauer, A. Arany, M. Steijaert, J.K. Wegner, E. Gustin, H. Ceulemans, Repurposing highthroughput image assays enables biological activity prediction for drug discovery, Cell Chem. Biol. 25 (2018) 611–618.e3.
[46] L.J. Colwell, Statistical and machine learning approaches to predicting protein–ligand interactions, Curr. Opin. Struct. Biol. 49 (2018) 123–128.
[47] G.M. Dimitri, P. Lió, DrugClust: a machine learning approach for drugs side effects prediction, Comput. Biol. Chem. 68 (2017) 204–210.
[48] N.H.N. Moorthy, S. Kumar, V. Poongavanam, Classification of carcinogenic and mutagenic properties using machine learning method, Comput. Toxicol. 3 (2017) 33–43.
[49] J.C. Pereira, E.R. Caffarena, C.N. Dos Santos, Boosting docking-based virtual screening with deep learning, J. Chem. Inf. Model. 56 (2016) 2495–2506.

[50] A. Perez, G. Martı'nez-Rosell, G. De Fabritiis, Simulations meet machine learning in structural biology, Curr. Opin. Struct. Biol. 49 (2018) 139–144.
[51] C. Cao, F. Liu, H. Tan, D. Song, W. Shu, W. Li, Z. Xie, Deep learning and its applications in biomedicine, Genomics Proteomics Bioinformatics 16 (2018) 17–32.
[52] M. Riesenhuber, T. Poggio, Hierarchical models of object recognition in cortex, Nat. Neurosci. 2 (1999) 1019–1025.
[53] H. Chen, O. Engkvist, Y. Wang, M. Olivecrona, T. Blaschke, The rise of deep learning in drug discovery, Drug Discov. Today 23 (2018) 1241–1250.
[54] P.P. Groumpos, Deep learning vs. wise learning: a critical and challenging overview, IFAC-PapersOnLine 49 (2016) 180–189.
[55] S.G. Tzafestas, Artificial Intelligence, Springer, Cham, 2016, pp. 25–33.
[56] S.A. Bini, Artificial intelligence, machine learning, deep learning, and cognitive computing: what do these terms mean and how will they impact health care? J. Arthroplasty 33 (2018) 2358–2361.
[57] V.L. Patel, E.H. Shortliffe, M. Stefanelli, P. Szolovits, M.R. Berthold, R. Bellazzi, A. Abu-Hanna, The coming of age of artificial intelligence in medicine, Artif. Intell. Med. 46 (2009) 5–17.
[58] C. Krittanawong, The rise of artificial intelligence and the uncertain future for physicians, Eur. J. Intern. Med. 48 (2018) e13–e14.
[59] E. Papaleo, G. Saladino, M. Lambrughi, K. Lindorff-Larsen, F.L. Gervasio, R. Nussinov, The role of protein loops and linkers in conformational dynamics and allostery, Chem. Rev. 116 (2016) 6391–6423.
[60] J.P. Arcon, L.A. Defelipe, C.P. Modenutti, E.D. Lo'pez, D. Alvarez-Garcia, X. Barril, M.A. Martı, Molecular dynamics in mixed solvents reveals protein-ligand interactions, improves docking, and allows accurate binding free energy predictions, J. Chem. Inf. Model. 57 (2017) 846–863.
[61] J. Mortier, C. Rakers, M. Bermudez, M.S. Murgueitio, S. Riniker, G. Wolber, The impact of molecular dynamics on drug design: applications for the characterization of ligand-macromolecule complexes, Drug Discov. Today 20 (2015) 686–702.
[62] M. Aldeghi, A. Heifetz, M.J. Bodkin, S. Knapp, P.C. Biggin, Accurate calculation of the absolute free energy of binding for drug molecules, Chem. Sci. 7 (1) (2016) 207–218.
[63] D.E. Shaw, J.C. Chao, M.P. Eastwood, J. Gagliardo, J.P. Grossman, C.R. Ho, K.J. Bowers, Anton, a special-purpose machine for molecular dynamics simulation, Commun. ACM 51 (2008) 91.
[64] A. Bergner, et al., Use of Relibase for retrieving complex three-dimensional interaction patterns including crystallographic packing effects, Biopolymers 61 (2001) 99–110.
[65] K. Arnold, et al., The protein model portal, J. Struct. Funct. Genomics 10 (2009) 1–8.
[66] A. Hildebrand, et al., Fast and accurate automatic structure prediction with HHpred, Proteins 77 (Suppl. 9) (2009) 128–132.
[67] R.A. Abagyan, et al., ICM—a new method for protein modeling and design. Applications to docking and structure prediction from the distorted native conformation, J. Comput. Chem. 15 (1994) 488–506.
[68] L.J. McGuffin, D.B. Roche, Automated tertiary structure prediction with accurate local model quality assessment using the IntFOLD-TS method, Proteins 79 (Suppl. 10) (2011) 137–146.
[69] N. Eswar, et al., Comparative protein structure modeling using modeller, Curr. Protein Pept. Sci. 9 (2007) (Chapter 2, Unit 2).
[70] L.A. Kelley, M.J. Sternberg, Protein structure prediction on the web: a case study using the Phyre server, Nat. Protoc. 4 (2009) 363–371.
[71] S. Raman, et al., Structure prediction for CASP8 with all-atom refinement using Rosetta, Proteins 77 (Suppl. 9) (2009) 89–99.

[72] L. Bordoli, et al., Protein structure homology modeling using SWISS-MODEL workspace, Nat. Protoc. 4 (2009) 1–13.
[73] J.L. MacCallum, et al., Assessment of protein structure refinement in CASP9, Proteins 79 (Suppl. 10) (2011) 74–90.
[74] N. Guex, et al., Automated comparative protein structure modeling with SWISS-MODEL and Swiss-PdbViewer: a historical perspective, Electrophoresis 30 (Suppl. 1) (2009) 162–173.
[75] O. Akerele, In summary of WHO guidelines for the assessment of herbal medicine, HerbalGram 28 (1993) 13–19.
[76] O. Potterat, M. Hamburger, Drug discovery and development with plant-derived compounds, in: F. Petersen, R. Amstutz (Eds.), Progress in Drug Research: Natural Compounds as Drugs, Verlag AG, Birhäusser, 2008, pp. 45–118.
[77] Y.W. Chin, M.J. Balunas, H.B. Chai, A.D. Kinghorn, Drug discovery from natural sources, AAPS J. 8 (2) (2006) E239–E253.
[78] J.W.H. Li, J.C. Vederas, Drug discovery and natural products: end of an era or an endless frontier? Science 325 (2009) 161–165.
[79] R.J. Quinn, A.R. Carroll, M.B. Pham, P. Baron, M.E. Palframan, et al., Developing a drug-like natural product library, J. Nat. Prod. 71 (2008) 464–468.
[80] S.M.N. Efange, Natural products: a continuing source of inspiration for the medicinal chemist, in: M.M. Iwu, J.C. Wootton (Eds.), Advances in Phytomedicine, Elsevier Science, Amsterdam, 2002, pp. 61–69.
[81] K. Grabowski, K.H. Baringhaus, G. Schneider, Scaffold diversity of natural products: inspiration for combinatorial library design, Nat. Prod. Rep. 25 (2008) 892–904.
[82] H.D. Höltje, W. Sippl, D. Rognan, G. Folkers, Molecular Modeling: Basic Principles and Applications, WILEY-VCH Verlag GmbH & Co. KGaA, Weinheim, 2008, pp. 181–258.
[83] R. Khanra, S. Dewanjee, T. K Dua, et al., *Abroma augusta* L. (Malvaceae) leaf extract attenuates diabetes induced nephropathy and cardiomyopathy via inhibition of oxidative stress and inflammatory response, J. Transl. Med. 13 (2015) 6.
[84] M.Z. Gul, L.M. Bhakshu, F. Ahmad, et al., Evaluation of *Abelmoschus moschatus* extracts for antioxidant, free radical scavenging, antimicrobial and antiproliferative activities using *in vitro* assays, BMC Complement. Altern. Med. 11 (2011) 64.
[85] K. Bargali, S.S. Bargali, Acacia nilotica: a multipurpose leguminous plant, Nat. Sci. 7 (4) (2009). 1545–0740.
[86] M.C. Gessler, M.H.H. Nkunya, L.B. Mwasumbi, M. Heinrich, M. Tanner, Screening Tanzanian medicinal plants for antimalarial activity, Acta Trop. 56 (1) (1994) 65–77.
[87] Y. Li, L. Yx, Z. Mj, et al., The effects of *Rheum palmatum* L. on the pharmacokinetic of major diterpene alkaloids of *Aconitum carmichaelii* Debx. in rats, Eur. J. Drug Metab. Pharmacokinet. 42 (2017) 441–451.
[88] T. Narender, S. Shweta, P. Tiwari, K. Papi Reddy, T. Khaliq, P. Prathipati, A. Puri, A.K. Srivastava, R. Chander, S.C. Agarwal, K. Raj, Antihyperglycemic and antidyslipidemic agent from *Aegle marmelos*, Bioorg. Med. Chem. Lett. 17 (6) (2007) 1808–1811.
[89] A. Copland, L. Nahar, C.T. Tomlinson, V. Hamilton, M. Middleton, Y. Kumarasamy, S.D. Sarker, Antibacterial and free radical scavenging activity of the seeds of *Agrimonia eupatoria*, Fitoterapia 74 (1-2) (2003) 133–135.
[90] J. Koscielny, D. Klüssendorf, R. Latza, R. Schmitt, H. Radtke, G. Siegel, H. Kiesewetter, The antiatherosclerotic effect of *Allium sativum*, Atherosclerosis 144 (1) (1999) 237–249.
[91] S.C. Mandal, A. Nandy, M. Pal, B.P. Saha, Evaluation of antibacterial activity of Asparagus racemosus willd. root, Phytother. Res. 14 (2) (2000) 118–119.
[92] H. Schmutterer, Properties and potential of natural pesticides from the neem tree, *Azadirachta indica*, Annu. Rev. Entomol. 35 (1990) 271–297.

[93] N. Uabundit, J. Wattanathorn, S. Mucimapura, K. Ingkaninan, Cognitive enhancement and neuroprotective effects of *Bacopa monnieri* in Alzheimer's disease model, J. Ethnopharmacol. 127 (1) (2010) 26–31.
[94] M. Mojumdar, M. Kabir, M. Hasan, T. Ahmed, M.R. Rahman, Y. Akter, M.M. Rahman, Molecular docking and pass prediction for analgesic activity of some isolated compounds from *Acalypha indica* L. and ADME/T property analysis of the compounds, World J. Pharm. Res. 5 (2016) 1761–1770.
[95] R.K. Goel, D. Singh, A. Lagunin, V. Poroikov, PASS-assisted exploration of new therapeutic potential of natural products, Med. Chem. Res. 20 (2011) 1509–1514.
[96] Z. Wu, J.M. McGoogan, Characteristics of and important lessons from the coronavirus disease 2019 (COVID-19) outbreak in China: summary of a report of 72 314 cases from the Chinese Center for Disease Control and Prevention, JAMA 323 (2020) 1239–1242.
[97] A. Roy, B. Patwardhan, R. Chaguturu, Reigniting pharmaceutical innovation through holistic drug targeting, Drug Discov. World 17 (2016) 45–55.
[98] R.C. Bhushan Patwardhan, Innovative Approaches in Drug Discovery: Ethnopharmacology, Systems. Biology and Holistic Targeting, Academic Press, 2016.
[99] B. Patwardhan, A.D.B. Vaidya, Natural products drug discovery: accelerating the clinical candidate development using reverse pharmacology approaches, Indian J. Exp. Biol. (2010) 220–227.
[100] S. Borse, M. Joshi, A. Saggam, V. Bhat, S. Walia, A. Marathe, S. Sagar, P. Chavan-Gautam, A. Girme, L. Hingorani, G. Tillu, Ayurveda botanicals in COVID-19 management: an in silico multi-target approach, PLoS One 16 (6) (2021), e0248479.
[101] D. Cyranoski, China is promoting coronavirus treatments based on unproven traditional medicines, Nature 10 (2020).
[102] Z. Liu, Y. Liu, G. Zeng, B. Shao, M. Chen, Z. Li, Y. Jiang, Y. Liu, Y. Zhang, H. Zhong, Application of molecular docking for the degradation of organic pollutants in the environmental remediation: a review, Chemosphere 203 (2018) 139–150.
[103] J.H. Zhang, Y. Zhu, X.H. Fan, B.L. Zhang, Efficacy-oriented compatibility for component-based chinese medicine, Acta Pharmacol. Sin. 36 (2015) 654–658.
[104] M. Hong, Y. Zhang, S. Li, H.Y. Tan, N. Wang, S. Mu, X. Hao, Y. Feng, A network pharmacology-based study on the hepatoprotective effect of fructus schisandrae, Molecules 22 (2017) 1617.
[105] R. Guo, M.H. Pittler, E. Ernst, Hawthorn extract for treating chronic heart failure, Cochrane Database Syst. Rev. 1 (2008), CD005312.
[106] B. Pang, M. Li, J. Song, et al., Luo Tong formula attenuates retinal inflammation in diabetic rats via inhibition of the p38MAPK/NF-κB pathway, Chin. Med. 15 (2020) 5.
[107] S. Guan, W. Xu, F. Han, W. Gu, L. Song, W. Ye, Q. Liu, X. Guo, Ginsenoside Rg1 attenuates cigarette smoke-induced pulmonary epithelial-mesenchymal transition via inhibition of the TGF-β1/Smad pathway, Biomed. Res. Int. 2017 (2017) 7171404.
[108] X. Xuan, Z. Sun, C. Yu, J. Chen, M. Chen, Q. Wang, L. Li, Network pharmacology-based study of the protective mechanism of conciliatory anti-allergic decoction on asthma, Allergol. Immunopathol. (Madr). 48 (5) (2020) 441–449.
[109] Y. Chen, J. Zhu, W. Zhang, Antitumor effect of traditional Chinese herbal medicines against lung cancer, Anticancer Drugs 25 (9) (2014) 983–991.
[110] S. Dwivedi, D. Chopra, B. Bhandari, Role of *Terminalia arjuna* Wight and Arn. in the treatment of chronic coronary artery disease from pharmacovigilance point of view, Ayu 40 (2) (2019) 104–108.
[111] X.B. Dou, X.D. Wo, C.L. Fan, Progress of research in treatment of hyperlipidemia by monomer or compound recipe of Chinese herbal medicine, Chin. J. Integr. Med. 14 (1) (2008) 71–75.

[112] T. Makino, H. Wakushima, T. Okamoto, et al., Effects of Kangen-karyu on coagulation system and platelet aggregation in mice, Biol. Pharm. Bull. 25 (2002) 523–525.
[113] Z.Y. Jiang, C.Y. Xu, X.X. Chang, et al., Fatty liver index correlates with non-alcoholic fatty liver disease, but not with newly diagnosed coronary artery atherosclerotic disease in Chinese patients, BMC Gastroenterol. 13 (2013) 110.
[114] D. Huh, B.D. Matthews, A. Mammoto, M. Montoya-Zavala, H.Y. Hsin, D.E. Ingber, Reconstituting organ-level lung functions on a chip, Science 328 (2010) 1662–1668.
[115] M.D. Segall, C. Barber, Addressing toxicity risk when designing and selecting compounds in early drug discovery, Drug Discov. Today 19 (2014) 688–693.
[116] H. Zhang, Z. Cao, M. Li, Y. Li, C. Peng, Novel naive Bayes classification models for predicting the carcinogenicity of chemicals, Food Chem. Toxicol. 97 (2016) 141–149.
[117] X. Li, L. Chen, F. Cheng, Z. Wu, H. Bian, C. Xu, et al., In silico prediction of chemical acute oral toxicity using multi-classification methods, J. Chem. Inf. Model. 54 (2014) 1061–1069.
[118] S. Wang, H. Sun, H. Liu, D. Li, Y. Li, T. Hou, ADMET evaluation in drug discovery. 16. Predicting hERG blockers by combining multiple pharmacophores and machine learning approaches, Mol. Pharm. 13 (2016) 2855–2866.
[119] M. Hewitt, K. Przybylak, In silico models for hepatotoxicity, Methods Mol. Biol. 1425 (2016) 201–236.
[120] J. Jarvis, M.J. Seed, S.J. Stocks, R.M. Agius, A refined QSAR model for prediction of chemical asthma hazard, Occup. Med. (Lond.) 65 (2015) 659–666.
[121] F.I. Saldı'var-Gonza'lez, F.D. Prieto-Martı'nez, J.L. Medina-Franco, Descubrimiento y desarrollo de fa'rmacos: un enfoque computacional, Educ. Quim. 28 (2017) 51–58.
[122] J.L. Medina-Franco, M.A. Giulianotti, G.S. Welmaker, R.A. Houghten, Shifting from the single to the multitarget paradigm in drug discovery, Drug Discov. Today 18 (2013) 495–501.
[123] F. Lopez-Vallejo, T. Caulfield, K.A. Martinez-Mayorga, M. Giulianotti, A. Nefzi, R. Houghten, J. MedinaFranco, Integrating virtual screening and combinatorial chemistry for accelerated drug discovery, Comb. Chem. High Throughput Screen. 14 (2011) 475–487.
[124] J.G. Moffat, F. Vincent, J.A. Lee, J. Eder, M. Prunotto, Opportunities and challenges in phenotypic drug discovery: an industry perspective, Nat. Rev. Drug Discov. 16 (2017) 531–543.
[125] H. Yang, L. Sun, W. Li, G. Liu, Y. Tang, In silico prediction of chemical toxicity for drug design using machine learning methods and structural alerts, Front. Chem. 6 (2018) 30.
[126] B.I. Díaz-Eufracio, J.J. Naveja, J.L. Medina-Franco, Protein–protein interaction modulators for epigenetic therapies, Adv. Protein Chem. Struct. Biol. 110 (2018) 65–84.
[127] T.I. Oprea, C.G. Bologa, S. Brunak, A. Campbell, G.N. Gan, A. Gaulton, Zahor-a'nszky-Kohalmi G., Unexplored therapeutic opportunities in the human genome, Nat. Rev. Drug Discov. 17 (2018) 317–332.
[128] C.H. Andrade, B.J. Neves, C.C. Melo-Filho, J. Rodrigues, D.C. Silva, R.C. Braga, P.V.L. Cravo, In silico chemogenomics drug repositioning strategies for neglected tropical diseases, Curr. Med. Chem. 26 (2018) 4355–4379.
[129] A.M. Wassermann, E. Lounkine, D. Hoepfner, G. Le Goff, F.J. King, C. Studer, M. Glick, Dark chemical matter as a promising starting point for drug lead discovery, Nat. Chem. Biol. 11 (2015) 958–966.
[130] T. Walker, C.M. Grulke, D. Pozefsky, A. Tropsha, Chembench: a cheminformatics workbench, Bioinformatics 26 (2010) 3000–3001.

CHAPTER 3

Alternative biological screening methods

Shikha Joon[a,b,*], Rajeev K. Singla[a,b,*], Enty Tjoa[c,†], Ketan C. Parmar[d,†], and Bairong Shen[a]
[a]Institutes for Systems Genetics, Frontiers Science Center for Disease-Related Molecular Network, West China Hospital, Sichuan University, Chengdu, China
[b]iGlobal Research and Publishing Foundation, New Delhi, India
[c]Department of Microbiology, School of Medicine and Health Sciences, Atma Jaya Catholic, University of Indonesia, Jakarta, Indonesia
[d]Department of Chemistry, Sir P.T. Sarvajanik College of Science, Veer Narmad South Gujarat University, Surat, India

1. Introduction

Efforts have been undertaken in recent decades to speed up the process of discovering new drugs for clinical use, but no major progress has been made. Further, the rise of deadly diseases and health problems that necessitate the development of novel drug discovery and screening methods has aggravated this issue. Novel drug development and screening methodologies demand a thorough understanding of the underlying molecular mechanisms involved in disease metabolism and control, as well as an in-depth understanding of disease-causing microorganism genomes. To speed up the drug development process, realistic disease models are required along with improved and integrated biological (assay platforms) and computational screening techniques. The next step is identifying potential targets whose chemical modification could result in a therapeutic effect. Further, potential molecules with the required pharmacological activity are identified among the preliminary hits. During the hit-to-lead discovery phase, these molecules are then modified to achieve side-effect minimizations, potency, and physicochemical characteristics improvisation [1,2]. Several elements of various biological screening technologies, as well as their advantages and drawbacks, have been examined in depth in this chapter. The careful selection and

* These authors have contributed equally to this work and share the first authorship.
† These authors have contributed equally to this work and share the second authorship.

Computational Approaches in Drug Discovery, Development and Systems Pharmacology
https://doi.org/10.1016/B978-0-323-99137-7.00011-3

application of various strategies and approaches, either separately or in combination, have the potential to speed up the drug discovery and development process.

2. High-throughput screening methods

2.1 High-throughput screening: Definitions and concepts

HTS is a drug discovery approach that allows for the automated testing of a large number of molecules (chemical and/or biological) against a specific biological target. In the pharmaceutical sector, HTS technologies are widely used to quickly assess the biological or biochemical activity of a large number of compounds, mainly pharmaceuticals, using robotics, and automation. They speed up target analysis by allowing large-scale compound libraries to be screened rapidly and economically. HTS can be used to evaluate pharmacological targets, as well as pharmacologically characterize agonists and antagonists for various enzymes and receptors. As HTS methods allow for the rapid identification of antibodies, active compounds, and/or specific-biomolecule pathway modulating genes, these provide a foundation for drug designing [3–12].

2.2 Basic steps involved in the HTS

In general, HTS consists of the four steps listed below.

- Samples and compound library preparation (preparation of an assay plate)
- Development of a suitable method for laboratory automation
- Setting up a robotic workstation and its configuration
- Data collection and handling

2.2.1 Samples and compound library preparation (preparation of an assay plate)

Depending on the assay, there are typically cellular or biochemical samples. These samples must be prepared in an array for HTS. The microplate is thus the primary platform or the sample carrier or key lab wares used. It is a disposable small testing vessel comprising a grid of wells for sample inoculation. In general, these come in a format of either 96-, 192-, 384, 1536-, 3456-, or 6144-well plates. The selection of the microplate format may be influenced by the sample type (its nature) and the assay for its detection. "Stock plates" are used by screening facilities to store their compound library collections.

These do not have a direct experimental use; however, compounds are copied to an assay plate via pipetting [3–12].

2.2.2 Development of a suitable method for laboratory automation

Automation is a crucial component of HTS because it imposes specific constraints on the practical design of the assay. Miniaturization must be adopted for an HTS assay, wherein, it should ideally be carried out in a single well with minimal use of reagents. Also, a little or no manipulation other than the sample (intended for testing) was injected. As a result, automation issues must be a priority over the assay and the optimal detection mode selection. For setting up an automated screen, stringent assay and quality control methods are of significant concern. The more distinct the negative and positive controls are, the more likely it is to achieve high-quality data. This generates negligible false negatives or false positives [3–12].

2.2.3 Setting up a robotic workstation and its configuration

A robotic platform's purpose is to simultaneously manage numerous plates autonomously. This accelerates the data collection considerably. HTS robot platforms vary from basic automated liquid handling machines to multidimensional workstations that can execute several tasks. Mechanical arms are used to achieve this. A robotic system transports the microplates from one station to another to accomplish the addition of reagents, their mixing, incubation, and detection [8].

2.2.4 Data collection and handling

An optical measurement that quantifies the light that passes through the sample is exploited to acquire the HTS data. These can be in the form of various readouts including luminescent or fluorescent detection, turbidity (light scatter), or colorimetric. The detection modes comprise time-resolved fluorescence (examples, LANCE, HTRF), FRET (fluorescence resonance energy transfer), fluorescence intensity and polarization, nonradioactive amplified luminescent proximity homogeneous assay (example, AlphaScreen), and luminescence (example, NanoBRET) [3–12].

2.3 Quantitative high-throughput screening (qHTS)

qHTS employs an HTS platform to evaluate multiple concentrations of test compounds. Post-screening, the concentration-response curves for the tested compounds are obtained. In recent times, qHTS is widely used in the field of toxicology because it provides a complete biological characterization of the tested compounds along with diminished chances of false negatives or false positives [6].

2.4 HTS and drug discovery

The main objective of HTS is the identification of candidates that influence the target in the preferred, also known as "hits" or "leads," through compound library screenings. This is typically accomplished through the use of detectors such as plate readers, robotics, liquid handling devices, and instrument control and data processing software. Notably, HTS methods sometimes fail to identify potential drug molecules. This could be because the compound library screening cannot assess numerous attributes essential to drug development. For example, HTS cannot evaluate bioavailability and toxicity. Instead, HTS assays are essentially involved in the identification of "leads" and their optimization strategies. Therefore, the HTS assay results serve as an initial point in the drug discovery process and unravel the role and interaction of a specific biochemical process. As a result, HTS should be viewed as a quick scan of biological processes in which compounds with negligible or no effect can be eliminated quickly from the drug discovery process [10].

2.5 High-throughput virtual screening (HTVS)

It is a process of validating a target, wherein a database of interest is searched for bioactive molecules. These are desired to match the structure of the given query. Specifically, it HTVS tests the binding activity of the compounds against the given target. Therefore, HTVS is used for the discovery of enzymes, ion channels, pharmacophore targets, or receptors. To study biomolecules' functions, a variety of bioactive has been used [13–15]. Chemical probes are needed to identify the target proteins for the given bioactive. This, in turn, helps to decipher their mechanism of action. Although there exist different approaches for discovering the lead compounds and deciphering their mechanism of action or biological function, HTVS exploits small molecular probes to unravel the functional attributes of the given bioactive. For this, a variety of efficient HTVS tools have been developed for drug discovery and development [16]. Lead molecules with high quality are discovered using HTVS, which, in turn, selects promising drug candidates for further in vitro and in vivo testing. This reduces the economic

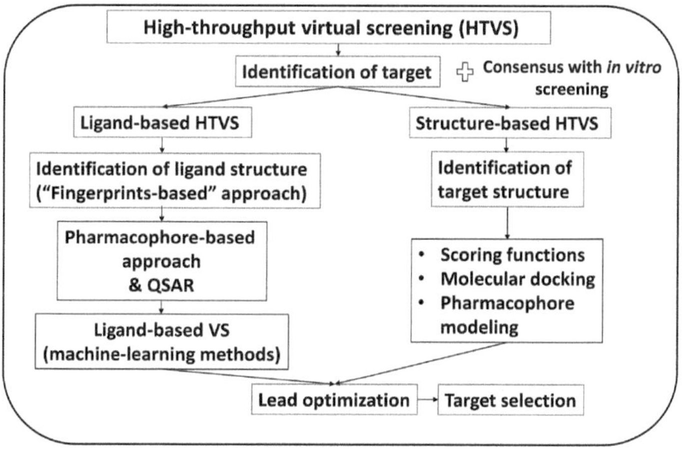

Fig. 1 An illustration of the HTVS methodology.

burden incurred in the synthesis of a range of bioactive and their testing. Fig. 1 illustrates the HTVS methodology.

3. Docking as an alternative to biological screening

Molecular docking or docking is the most popular structure-based drug design (SBDD) method for lead identification, which is used in conjunction with HTS [17]. Accordingly, the binding mode of a ligand is predicted for the specific binding site on the intended target. It is assumed that the ligand is flexible, while the intended target's three-dimensional (3D) structure is known to bear a ligand-specific rigid binding site. Also, scoring functions are used to measure the affinity of the target-ligand binding. Various databases are searched for promising compounds for the intended target. The ranking is then carried out for these compounds to derive a subset of compounds with improved target-specificity. Later, biological assays are commenced to ascertain their candidature as drugs [18–20]. Fortunately, ligand placement and their scoring (scoring functions, SF) can be carried out using advanced docking tools having inbuilt algorithms [21]. These are outlined in Table 1, for example, Surflex [22], FlexX [23], GLIDE [24], FRED [26], GOLD [27], DOCK [25], AutoDock [28], and LigandFit [29]. Molecular docking is widely applied for virtual screening (structure-based) as documented in various studies [30–37]. This indeed has geared up the discovery of drugs and their development [38]. Ligand placement can be relied upon when target-ligand binding possibilities are to be assessed.

Table 1 Molecular docking tools for virtual screening.

Tool	Strategy used	References	Websites/URLs
Surflex	Surface-based molecular similarity	[22]	http://www.biopharmics.com/downloads.Html
FlexX	Incremental reconstruction and ligand fragmentation	[23]	https://www.biosolveit.de/flexx/index.html?ct51
GLIDE	Systematic search algorithms	[24]	https://www.schrodinger.com/productpage/14/5/
FRED DOCK	Molecular shape	[25,26]	http://www.eyesopen.com/oedocking http://dock.compbio.ucsf.edu
GOLD AutoDock	Genetic algorithms	[27,28]	https://www.ccdc.cam.ac.uk/solutions/csd-discovery/components/gold/ http://autodock.scripps.edu
LigandFit	Monte Carlo optimization	[29]	http://accelrys.com

This considers their geometries as well. SF, on the other hand, cannot be depended upon for all of the targets. This could be owing to its inability to accurately predict entropy effects [39]. This could be avoided by creating manual and customized (empirical) SF for certain applications. For lead optimization (rational), it is amongst the best approach since it enables the visualization of possible docking (target-ligand binding). And although basic energy calculations are involved, it provides quick access to compounds from multiple libraries [40,41]. As a result, the in vitro experiments are now easier to perform with a reduced number of false positives [20]. A schematic representation of molecular docking methodology is shown in Fig. 2. Fig. 3 illustrates the applications of molecular docking in drug discovery.

4. De novo drug design

This strategy is built on the concept of "from the beginning." Accordingly, the active site of a prospective pharmacological target is structurally defined.

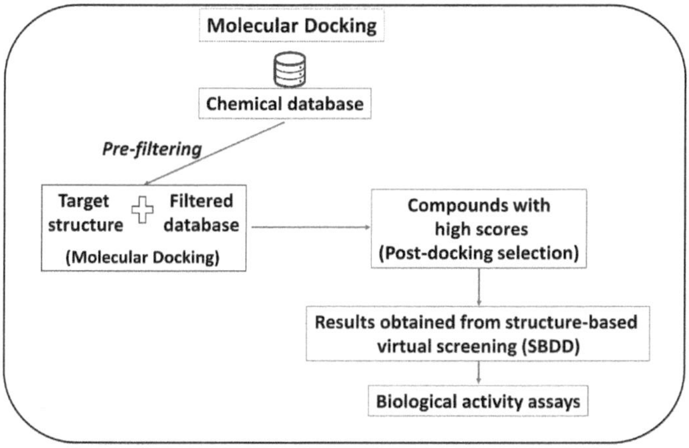

Fig. 2 A schematic representation of molecular docking methodology.

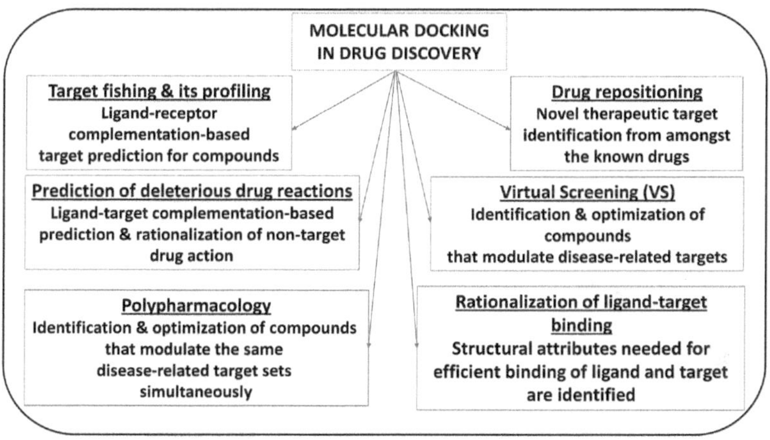

Fig. 3 Applications of molecular docking in drug discovery.

For this, the amino acid sequences (forming the active site of the target of interest) and their orientation (which determines the target binding site and ligand specificity) are identified. This is indispensable for ligand designing and obtaining ligands that bind to their therapeutic targets with precision. The structural data for the target protein's active site can be obtained, and several computational approaches can be used to analyze it. It is carried out using computational tools, which are collectively called computer-aided ligand designing (CALD) methods [42]. As reported, random connection methods, fragment location methods, fragment connection methods, site point connection methods, whole molecule methods, and

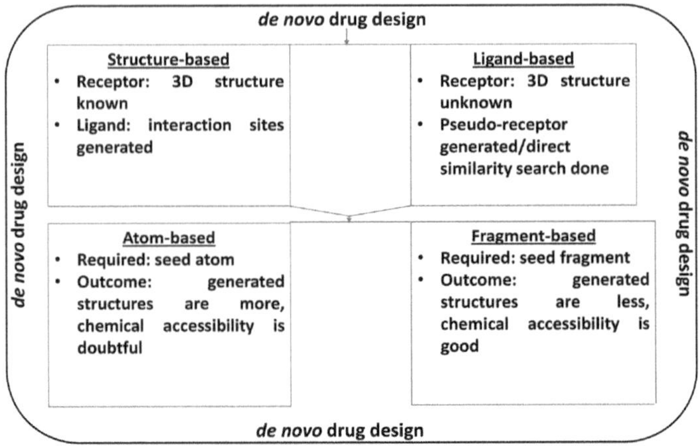

Fig. 4 Methodology for de novo drug design.

sequential build-up methods are said to be the six primary groups of CALD methods [42]. These are outlined in Table 2. Fig. 4 illustrates the methodology for de novo drug design.

5. In silico pharmacological drug screening

Virtual screening (VS) is the most popular approach for SBDD for lead identification (3D), which is used in conjunction with HTS. This includes

Table 2 Classification of CALD methods.

Method	Description
Random connection methods	Combines fragment connection and sequential build-up methods with the introduction of randomness via bond disconnection strategy
Fragment location methods	Determines the location of intended small fragment(s) in the active site
Fragment connection methods	Positions and connects the fragments via the "scaffolds" or "linkers" to attain intended orientation of the positioned fragments
Site-point connection methods	Determination of site or location points and placement of fragment in the active site to place atoms in these determined location points
Whole molecule methods	Compounds are placed in the active site of the target using distinct conformations to allow assessment of complementarity between the target and the ligand with reference to their electrostatic force and shape
Sequential build-up methods	Construction of ligand via atom to atom/fragment to fragment

mainly molecular docking and scoring functions. The search for likely target binding molecules/compounds in the database is done here. The ranking for these compounds is then carried out to have a target-specific subset of compounds. Next, biological assays are commenced for further validation [18–20]. As mentioned in the previous section, this can be carried out using docking tools having inbuilt algorithms as outlined in Table 1 [22]. For example, Surflex [22], FlexX [23], GLIDE [24], FRED [26], GOLD [27], DOCK [25], AutoDock [28], and LigandFit [29]. As evidenced by numerous research, molecular docking is commonly used for virtual screening (structure-based) [30–33,35–37,43]. Structure-based VS has boosted the efficiency of the drug research and development process [38]. Ligand placement is a good way to test several possibilities for ligand binding to the target of interest (also their geometries). The scoring functions, on the other hand, cannot be depended upon for all of the targets. This could be owing to its inability to accurately predict entropy effects [39]. This could be avoided by creating manual and customized (empirical) scoring functions for certain applications. This is a potential approach for rational lead optimization since it enables the visualization of possible target-ligand binding (docking). Even though the basic energy calculations are needed if makes the compounds readily available from large libraries. Consequently, in vitro experiments are easier to perform accompanied by a reduced number of false positives [20].

6. Pharmacophore modeling as an alternative approach

6.1 Definitions and concepts

Paul Ehrlich introduced the term "pharmacophore". It is a combination of "phoros" and "pharmacon". "Phoros" means "carrier," while "pharmacon" refers to the "drug" [44]. Appropriately, a pharmacophore is a structural characteristic or attribute of a molecular framework. A drug's biological or pharmacological qualities, such as receptor recognition and binding, are conferred by it [44,45]. It aspires (a) to identify the characteristics that are required to confer a given biological activity, (b) to identify the desired molecular or bioactive conformation, and (c) to make a rule for compound series' alignment or superposition. A stepwise computational approach is used to accomplish the above. Accordingly, this includes selecting a suitable drug target, preparing a database, creating a pharmacophore model, and finally carrying out 3D screening [46–50]. Fortunately, automated pharmacophore modeling programs have been developed for this. For example,

Table 3 Pharmacophore modeling tools.

Tools	Strategy used	References
LigandScout	It obtains the pharmacophore from protein-ligand complexes, the ligand geometries are interpreted, assigns accurate hybridization states, and classifies plausible interactions occurring between the ligand and the protein via application of preset rules	[57–59]
GASP, Catalyst, MOE, Phase	The n-point pharmacophore fingerprint (cascading) is used to superposition the pharmacophore molecule	[47,51,53–56]

GASP [51], DISCO [52], Catalyst [47,53], Phase [54], MOE [55,56], and LigandScout [57–59]. These are outlined in Table 3. Interaction site recognition is carried out by these automated programs. Precisely, these are hydrogen bond donor (D), hydrogen bond acceptor (A), hydrophobic (H), aromatic rings (R), ionizable/positive ionic (P), and ionizable/negative ionic (N). The pharmacophore models are developed using the attributed "activity" that segregates the nonactives and the actives. Those models of pharmacophores that show inactivity are not considered for further evaluation. The pharmacophore-based VS has recently become an important method for identifying hits in drug discovery research. This is particularly useful when the 3D information on the structure of the target is unavailable. In addition to this, it allows for quick screening of a large library of compounds to find potential compounds. Furthermore, the models so generated are transparent and descriptive, which are accessible to modifications. The results obtained are easily interpretable. The major drawback is that the drug's biophysical interactions are not completely addressed here [60–65].

6.2 Pharmacophore fingerprint and pharmacophore query in computer-aided drug design (CADD)

Pharmacophore modeling is a popular and important tool in CADD. A molecule possesses certain atoms and groups, each of these displays specific characteristics concerning molecular recognition. These can be conveniently simplified to a pharmacophore attribute. Accordingly, the molecular patterns are labeled as hydrophobic, anionic, cationic, aromatic, hydrogen bond donors or acceptors, or any plausible combinations [60–65]. A comparison can be made for various molecules at the pharmacophore level known as "pharmacophore fingerprints." A pharmacophore is referred to as a "query" when only a few pharmacophore properties are taken into account in a 3D model.

6.3 VS-based pharmacophore modeling

The most common application of pharmacophore modeling to VS is to find compounds that trigger the intended biological effect. Researchers do this by creating a query or a pharmacophore model that encodes the correct 3D organization of the desired interaction pattern. Various options for constructing such a query are available; however, this depends on the data availability for the specific target (usually a protein). Four scenarios can be considered or are encountered while carrying out the VS-based pharmacophore search. These are (a) when the structural information for both the protein and ligand is absent, and in vitro screening is the only alternative available [66–69], (b) the structural information for the protein is absent, but active ligands are present, and ligand-based VS can be performed using the pharmacophores [70–72], (c) the structural information for both the protein and ligand is present and is the best scenario [59,73,74], and (d) the only available information is that of protein's structure, and hence, is the most challenging of all the above-mentioned scenarios [75–80].

When several active ligands or their inactive derivatives are known, the ligand data must be divided into training and evaluation sets, respectively. This is critical for validating the pharmacophore query so generated. The resulting pharmacophore query is usually treated as the "positive filters" for compound identification. However, to avoid side-effects, these may be utilized as "negative filters" too [81,82].

6.4 Pharmacophore modeling in docking simulations: Methodology

As mentioned in the preceding section, pharmacophore models make excellent queries for VS of databases. Nonetheless, a so-called hierarchical strategy in VS, in which several technologies are merged sequentially, is one of the most prevalent options, and is known as the "funnel principle."

Here, the compounds with a lesser chance of being active are eliminated consecutively at each step and the potential compounds are then proceeded for VS [83]. Here, the pharmacophore models are used as filters for compound identification. This relies on the fulfillment of the requirements concerning the query's geometric and chemical functionality. Usually, this is undertaken before more sophisticated approaches, for example, molecular docking. Docking-based VS and pharmacophore-based VS can be combined using a variety of options as follows:

(a) A pharmacophore query can be used to prefilter the database of ligands. This can be done using docking simulations before evaluation [83].

(b) A pharmacophore query can be used to post-filter the docking simulations. This eliminates those compounds that do not bind as per the pharmacophore query [84].

(c) During the docking simulations, ligand placement can be guided using the pharmacophore alignment [85,86]. Accordingly, for ligand placement, the pharmacophore model can be exploited, which is similar to a molecule fitting into the query. Further, a constraint can be used for guiding the ligand placement when distinct docking poses are scored. This query can be an automated receptor-based or a user-defined query [87].

(d) The results obtained for the active compounds having top scores can be enriched using the pharmacophore models as was done in the SAMPL4 VS challenge. Here, a set of compounds were ranked for HIV-integrase (target). The activities of these compounds were not known while performing the task. The hierarchical approach was exploited to obtain the top scores. The docking results were subjected to both the pharmacophore prefiltering and post-filtering [72,88].

6.5 Pharmacophore modeling and its applications

6.5.1 ADME/T and pharmacophores

The main reason for the nonsuccessful drug development and clinical trials is poor ADME/T (absorption, distribution, metabolism, excretion, and toxicity) [89–92]. It is, therefore, advisable to profile ADME/T early during the process of drug development. This can be done using various pharmacophore modeling approaches [93]. The plausible enzyme-(specifically those that metabolize drugs) drug interactions can be identified using the pharmacophore models. Here, the test molecules' equivalent chemical groups are matched to those of ADME/T-profiled drug molecules [94]. In particular, the cytochrome (CYP) P450s are involved in drug metabolism initiation and are of particular interest for ADME/T profiling of the candidate drug [95]. Accordingly, the receptor-based pharmacophore models for CYP P450s and known drug interactions have already been generated. These are capable of predicting CYP P450s and drug-like compound's binding interactions along with a plausible enzyme metabolism assessment of the intended compound [96–99]. Likewise, the uridine 5′-diphosphate-glucuronosyltransferases' (UGT) ADME/T pharmacophore models are available [100–102].

6.5.2 Identification of the drug target using pharmacophore guiding

There are times when we know the drug molecules; however, their activity mechanisms remain elusive. Usually, these drug molecules are either procured from drugs that were developed phenotypically or herbal medicines. In this situation, CADD can aid in target identification. For instance, compounds with known activity mechanisms can be identified using similarity tools that are based on cheminformatics fingerprint [100,103]. Alternately, the most appropriate pharmacophore models can be identified (manual construction or automated via protein databank, PDB) that fits into the "query" using the pharmacophore modeling approach. Here, the "query" is the molecule itself [76]. The target (or targets) for any compound whose activity mechanisms are unknown can also be identified using the pharmacophore modeling approach [104]. Investigations for myriad plant metabolites were done via LigandScout followed by their drug target identification. These findings were validated by experimental testing. With the developments in drug repositioning and polypharmacology, pharmacophore models have become crucial for drug development [81,103,105]. Finally, off-targets or plausible side-effects can be predicted using pharmacophore modeling, which generated target-specific compounds or drugs [82]. Fig. 5 illustrates pharmacological modeling and its applications.

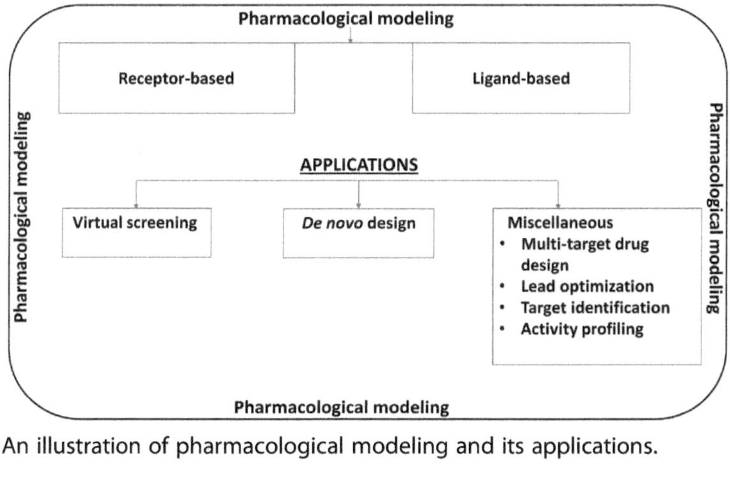

Fig. 5 An illustration of pharmacological modeling and its applications.

6.6 Pharmacophore modeling and its limitations

Even though pharmacophore modeling is integral to drug design, it has various limitations as follows:

(a) First, the lack of good scoring metrics is a fundamental constraint of pharmacophore-based VS. A general and reliable scoring metric is absent in pharmacophore queries. In general, the root means square deviation (RMSD) between the query's attributes and molecule's atoms is used to express the quality of ligand fitting into a pharmacophore query. Unfortunately, RMSD does not consider any similarity with the inhibitory molecules already known and fails to predict the overall ligand-receptor protein compatibility. As a result, the molecules that respond to or "hit" a pharmacophore query may differ significantly from other inhibitors. These might possess noncomplementary functional groups to the binding site of the receptor. Despite being a "hit," this could render these molecules inactive [81].

(b) Secondly pharmacophore-based VS relies upon a precomputed conformation database. Unfortunately, there are only a few low-energy conformations for every molecule in these databases. Quite possibly, this can lead to the nonidentification of an active molecule owing to the missing confirmation. In particular, this is true for the small molecular functional groups that possess various rotatable bond conformations, for example, the hydroxyl groups. As such, it is difficult to distinguish these different rotations, while the generation of the conformations using the differences in the RMSD. This leads to poor sampling. During the process of fitting, various tools for the pharmacophore search can rotate these bonds. This is done to obtain correctly oriented conformations on small, functional groups that are polar and flexible [106,107].

(c) Finally, the precise methodology for constructing a pharmacophore query is lacking. Although the molecules are retrieved by the pharmacophore models most of the time, the possibility of the occurrence of various other promising molecules cannot be denied. In a study, a little different pharmacophore was built for a similar target. Even though a similar data set was screened, the identified molecules were different [108,109]. Another example is that of the kinase inhibitors. The kinome has distinct activity profiles, but similarity occurs among the kinase inhibitors. Even though the molecules similar to the kinase inhibitors can be identified by the pharmacophore approaches, their target kinase-inhibitory activity is dubious [110].

It will, therefore, be appropriate to state here that the applications of pharmacophore modeling, that is, identification of the target, side-effects prediction, profiling of ADME-tox, are still undermined by its applicability to newer classes of molecules with missing links [111].

7. Chemogenomics approaches in drug screening

Chemogenomics, also known as chemical genomics, involves screening small-molecule chemical libraries against specific drug target families systematically. Here, the common drug target families include proteases, kinases, nuclear receptors, and G protein-coupled receptors (GPCRs), etc. for discovering novel drugs and their targets [112]. This also comprises members with unknown ligands and functions. Accordingly, hits that are capable of modulating the lesser characterized target family members' activities can be identified via chemogenomics screening approaches. This, in turn, enables the functional elucidation of the novel targets. Chemogenomics, therefore, aims to investigate how all possible drug-target interactions occur [112]. Table 4 outlines some common chemogenomics libraries.

7.1 Basic strategy and approaches for chemogenomics

Here, the drug and target discovery is integrated via active compounds. These active compounds are either probes or ligands employed for the functional characterization of the proteome. Phenotype is induced via the protein and small compound interaction. Post-characterization of the induced phenotype, associations between a molecular event and a protein can be drawn. The function of a protein, and not a gene, can be modified using chemogenomics. Also, real-time reversals and interactions can be observed using chemogenomics. For instance, a phenotype modification is brought by the addition of a specific compound and the same can be reversed by its removal from the medium. At present, the chemogenomics approaches can be classified as classical or forward chemogenomics and reverse chemogenomics [113]. Fig. 6 depicts chemogenomics strategies for drug screening.

7.1.1 Forward chemogenomics

Forward chemogenomics aims at the identification of the drug targets. For this, the molecules responsible for a particular phenotype are searched. Here, a specific phenotype is investigated, followed by the identification of small compounds or compounds that interact with it. The identified modulators are exploited as tools to study proteins causing the particular phenotype.

Table 4 Chemogenomics libraries and their description.

Chemogenomics libraries	Description
GlaxoSmithKline Biologically Diverse Compound Set	Comprises targets of G-protein-coupled receptors (GPCR) & kinase with varied mechanisms
$LOPAC_{1280}$: Sigma Library of Pharmacologically Active Compounds	Commercial, serves the purpose for screens having a known biology for GPCR in association with the phenotypic effects
Pfizer Chemogenomic library	Target-specific pharmacological probe-based selection of compounds, majorly comprise ion channels, GPCRs, and kinases, broad biological and chemical diversity
Prestwick Chemical Library	Target diversity, bioavailability, & safety-based preselected approved drugs by EMA, FDA, and other agencies
Molecular Libraries Program Probes (NIH)	Specifically it does not fulfil the criteria of a screening library, provides open-access biological assay data, and broadly covers the proteins that bind to the nucleic acids
Protein Kinase Inhibitor Set (GlaxoSmithKline)	GlaxoSmithKline kinase chemical probes (probes are publishes already) based set of kinase (open-source), and amenable to collaborations with more than 250 collaborators
Mechanism Interrogation PlatE 3.0 (NCATS)	Focused on the oncology, Kinase inhibitors dominated, and serves well for screens specific to the anticancer phenotypes

Following the identification of compounds that cause a particular phenotype (target phenotype), the subsequent step should be to discover the gene and protein targets The most difficult aspect of this strategy is to design the phenotypic assays that go straight from screening to target identification [113].

7.1.2 Reverse chemogenomics

Reverse chemogenomics aims at the validation of phenotypes. For this, small molecules that interact with a particular protein are searched. Here, small compounds that cause functional alterations in an enzyme (in terms of in vitro) will be identified. Following the identification of modulators,

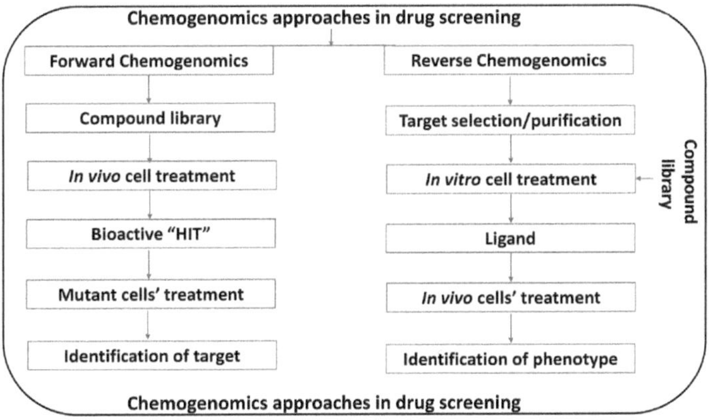

Fig. 6 Chemogenomics strategies for drug screening.

the small molecule-induced phenotype is investigated in vitro or in vivo. Hence, the biological functions of an enzyme are confirmed using this approach. This approach is similar to target-based drug discovery. Parallel screening and the ability to execute lead optimization on several targets belonging to the same family have improved this method [113].

7.2 Applications of chemogenomics

7.2.1 Drug discovery and identification of novel drug targets

Chemogenomics has also been employed as an efficient approach for drug discovery [114]. For this, genomics and chemistry have now been integrated for profiling, optimizing, monitoring the drug candidates and drug treatment [114]. Novel drug targets can be identified using chemogenomics profiling [115]. For example, chemogenomics was used to screen known ligands of the murD protein family (that partakes in the peptidoglycan biosynthesis pathway) from the murD ligand library (preexisting). This revealed two inhibitorsfor murC and murF, respectively. This provided the basis for the development of efficient peptidoglycan biosynthesis pathway-targeting antileptospirosis drug. These inhibitors were speculated to belong to the category of broad-spectrum drugs and mandate further in vitro and in vivo experimentation [115].

7.2.2 Investigation of the mechanism of action of anticancer drugs

The mechanism of action of anticancer drugs can be examined using comparative chemogenomics [116]. For instance, the action mechanism of

DNA-targeted platinum-acridine anticancer agents was investigated using a comparative chemogenomics approach [115]. For this, a library comprising platinum-acridine hybrid agents (nonclassical) was generated. Next, a genome-wide screening (a validated approach) was used to investigate their action mechanisms in *Saccharomyces cerevisiae* and *Schizosaccharomyces pombe*. Depending on the type of DNA repair modules needed, the platinum-acridine anticancer agents cause DNA damage that differed from cisplatin (an effective antitumor agent) as revealed by their chemogenomics profiles from the above two organisms. Apart from the anticancer drugs, chemogenomics approaches have also rationalized the mode of action of the Ayurvedic and Traditional Chinese Medicines (TCM) [117].

7.3 Advantages and limitations of chemogenomics

The main advantage of chemogenomics is its prediction using enormous biological data. The information on drugs' and targets' nucleotide sequences and chemical structures is available on public databases and, in turn, is used for the prediction of drug-target interactions (DTIs) [118]. The need for a meticulous integration of the information obtained from cheminformatics and bioinformatics, a rational technique for hit selection from vast virtual possibilities, and construction of information-specific catalogs are some of the limitations of chemogenomics [112].

8. Genomics and proteomics in drug discovery and designing

8.1 Genomics and proteomics: Definitions and concepts

The combined study of the structure, function, and evolution of genomes along with their mapping is termed "genomics," while that of proteomes (an entire set of proteins) is "proteomics" [119,120]. In recent times, the highly sophisticated and advanced genomics and proteomics technologies can perform a collateral gene (in a genome) and protein (in a proteome) analysis, respectively. As a result, it becomes possible to provide detailed information on the molecular mechanisms globally. Further, these are capable of reconstructing the metabolic pathways, signaling cascades, and regulatory networks in combination with various biochemical approaches post-drug administration [121–123]. An overview of the techniques used in proteomics is given in Fig. 7. Fig. 8 illustrates a general methodology employed in proteomics.

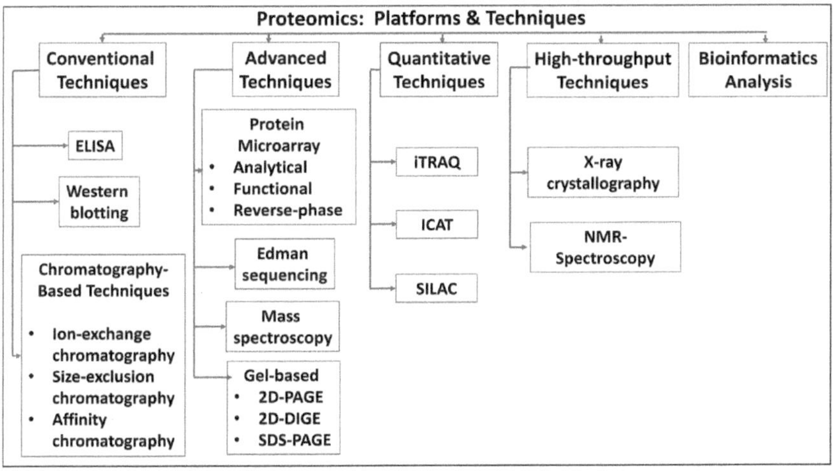

Fig. 7 An overview of the techniques used in proteomics.

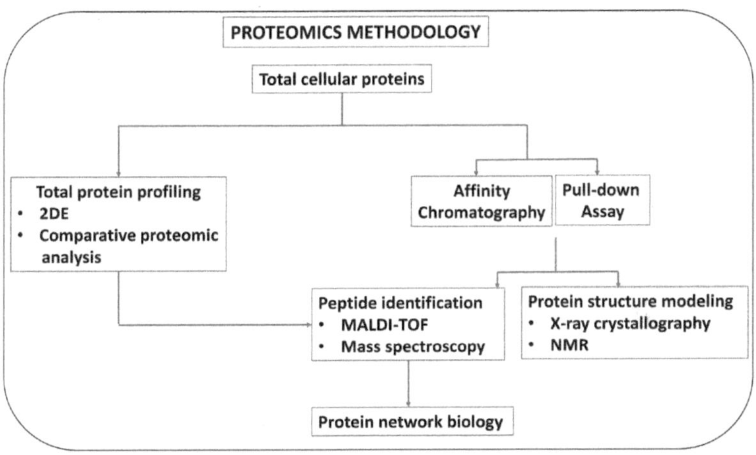

Fig. 8 An illustration of a general methodology employed in proteomics.

8.2 Genomics and proteomics: Subdisciplines

8.2.1 Computational proteomics

This involves the generation of information on the three-dimensional (3D) structure of a protein and its analysis on a large scale. It is pivotal to accurately predict the contact maps of the intended protein. Here, the current state of knowledge on the structures of proteins and nucleic acids is the most important resource, which is readily available at PDB (http//:www.rcsb.org/pdb/), 3D-GENOMICS (www.sbg.bio.ic.au.uk/3dgenomics/) and various other databases [124]. Table 5 outlines the proteomics databases, servers, and tools.

Table 5 Proteomics databases, tools, and servers.

Database, tools, and servers	Websites/URLs
BLASTP (BLAST)	http://blast.ncbi.nlm.nih.gov
BlockMakei (Motif based alignment server)	http://blocks.fhcrc.org/make_blocks.html
CASTp (Protein structure analysis server)	http://sts.bioe.uic.edu/castp/index.php
CATH (Protein structure databases)	http://www.biochem.ucl.ac.uk/bsm/cath/
ConSurf (Protein structure analysis server)	http://consurf.tau.ac.il/
CD server (Protein domain servers)	http://www.ncbi.nlm.nih.gov/Structure/cdd/cdd.shtml
DELTA-BLAST (Domain Enhanced Lookup Time Accelerated BLAST)	https://blast.ncbi.nlm.nih.gov
Dialign (Motif based alignment server)	http://bibiserv.techfak.uni-bielefeld.de/dialign/
EBI (Protein structure modeling server)	http://biotech.ebi.ac.uk:8400/
ESyPred3D (Protein structure modeling server)	http://www.fundp.ac.be/urbm/bioinfo/esypred
GenBank (database)	http://www.ncbi.nih.gov/entrez/query.fcgi?db=protein
Gibbs (Motif based alignment server)	http://bayesweb.wadsworth.org/gibbs/gibbs.html
InterProScan (Protein domain servers)	http://www.ebi.ac.uk/lnterProScan/
LigandProtein (Protein structure analysis server)	http://bip.weizmann.ac.il/oca-bin/lpccsu
Match Box (Motif based alignment server)	http://www.sciences.fundp.ac.be/biologie/bms/help.html
MEME (Motif based alignment server)	http://meme.sdsc.edu/meme/website/meme.html
MMDD (Protein structure databases)	http://www.ncbi.nlm.nih.gov/Structure/
ModBase (Protein structure databases)	http://alto.compbio.ucsf.edu/modbase-cgi/index.cgi
nr (database)	http://www.ncbi.nlm.nih.gov/BLAST/
O-GlycoBase (Protein structure analysis server)	http://www.cbs.dtu.dk/services/NetOGIyc/
OWL (database)	http://www.bioinf.man.ac.uk/dbbrowser/OWL/
PATTINPROT (Protein domain servers)	http://pbil.ibcp.fr/html/pbiljndex.html

Table 5 Proteomics databases, tools, and servers—cont'd

Database, tools, and servers	Websites/URLs
PDB (Protein structure databases)	http://www.rcsb.org/pdb/
PHI-BLAST (Pattern Hit Initiated BLAST)	https://blast.ncbi.nlm.nih.gov
PhosphoBase (Protein structure analysis server)	http://www.cbs.dtu.dk/services/NetPhos
PIR (database)	http://pir.georgetown.edu/
PSI-BLAST (Position Specific Iterated BLAST)	https://blast.ncbi.nlm.nih.gov
PredictProtein (Protein structure analysis server)	http://www.embl-heidelberg.de/predictprotein
ProtSkin (Protein structure analysis server)	http://www.mcgnmr.ca/ProtSkin/intro/
ProWleScan (Protein domain servers)	http://hits.isb-sib.ch/cgi-bin/PFSCAN
RefSeq (database)	https://www.ncbi.nlm.nih.gov/refseq/
ScanProsite (Protein domain servers)	http://us.expasy.org/tools/scanprosite/
SCOP (Protein structure databases)	http://scop.mrc-lmb.cam.ac.uk/scop/
SIRW (Protein domain servers)	http://sirw.embl.de/index.html
SwissModel (Protein structure databases)	http://swissmodel.expasy.org/repository/
SwissProt (database)	http://kr.expasy.org/sprot/
TBLASTN (BLAST)	https://blast.ncbi.nlm.nih.gov
TrEMBL (database)	http://kr.expasy.org/sprot/
UniParc (database)	http://www.pir.uniprot.org/database/archive.shtml
UniProt (database)	http://www.pir.uniprot.org/
UniRef (database)	http://www.pir.uniprot.org/database/nref.shtml
WhatIf (Protein structure modeling server)	http://www.cmbi.kun.nl/gv/servers/WIWWWI

8.2.2 Chemical proteomics

Here, the protein-modifying reagents or chemical probes are designed to study the functional attributes of various proteins that form a proteome. For this, biochemistry, cell biology, mass spectrometry (MS), and synthetic organic chemistry are used. Chemical probes are indispensable for chemical proteins as these are capable of targeting diverse families of enzymes. Essentially, these comprise a ligand, a linker, and target protein- or enzyme-specific tag, which allow target identification and its purification as well. Chemical proteomics utilize chemical probes, such as phenyl sulfonate, *S*-transferase, and serine hydrolase probes [125].

8.2.3 Structural genomics and proteomics

The structure of cellular proteins or those that occur in an organism is determined using structural genomics. The functional investigation of cellular proteins and rational drug design requires 3D structures. To a certain extent, cloning, expression, and purification of proteins encoded by a genome have been made possible by genome sequence databases. However, unraveling the functional attributes of all the cellular proteins and molecular protein-protein interactions (PPIs) require 3D structure determination of all these proteins (and their variants). This indeed is quite challenging but is overcome by structural genomics. The relationship amongst specific cell organellar proteins and/or their complexes is determined and established at the proteome-wide level using structural proteomics. The effective drugs can therefore be designed using structural proteomics that rely on combined structural biology, medicinal, and computational chemistry methods. Therefore, 3D protein structure determination is the key ideology of structural proteomics that allows for amino acid sequence similarity-based computational modeling of specific organelle proteins [126–129].

8.2.4 Topological proteomics

Here, whole protein networks occurring within a single cell are localized and characterized. This, in turn, disseminates information on their basic organization and paves way for novel drug target identification and lead selection. For example, the Multi-EpitopeLigan Kartographie (MELK) analyzes proteins occurring within a single cell. At the same time, protein patterns (subcellular and large scale) are also sketched out using this ultrasensitive technology. As a result, protein hierarchies connected to certain cellular functions or dysfunctions are revealed. Further, protein interaction networks can be analyzed using TopNet (a web-based automated tool, http://networks.gersteinlab.org/) [130].

8.3 Genomics and proteomics: Common platforms

8.3.1 Microarrays

These are genome analysis tools used for detecting the expression of myriad genes simultaneously. These are also referred to as DNA chips that are based on the binding specificity of complementary single-stranded nucleic acids. A global RNA expression profile is provided by chip microarrays. The gene expression patterns are analyzed using cDNA and oligonucleotide arrays. A schematic representation of complementary DNA (cDNA) microarray is shown in Fig. 9. The cDNA arrays comprise the polymerase chain reaction (PCR)-synthesized sequences of double-stranded cDNA that profile the expression patterns of myriad genes simultaneously. On the other hand, silicon wafer-or quartz-synthesized oligonucleotides are used for the preparation of oligonucleotide microarrays [131,132].

The fluorescent dyes are used to label the target cell or tissue-isolated mRNAs (experimental) and the controls. A quantitative binding then occurs between these fluorescent-labeled mRNAs and their complementary nucleic acid sequences present on the microarrays (hybridization). The fluorescence intensities of the sequences in the test and control samples are then compared to estimate their relative expression fold of difference [132–134].

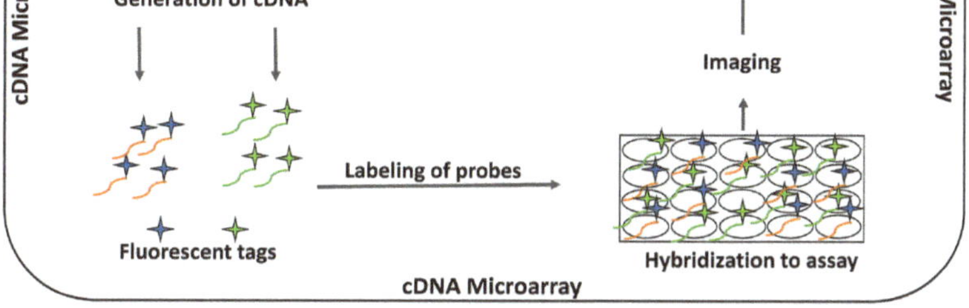

Fig. 9 A schematic representation of complementary DNA (cDNA) microarray.

8.3.2 Quantitative real-time PCR (qRT-PCR)

The qRT-PCR can be used to investigate differentially expressed genes in test and control groups in greater depth and across a greater sample size. In comparison to microarrays, it can perform quantitative evaluation of myriad genes. When compared to control groups, the qRT-PCR results disseminate vital information on gene expression alterations in a period in the treated test groups during treatment [135]. A schematic representation of qRT-PCR is shown in Fig. 10.

8.3.3 Two-dimensional electrophoresis (2DE) and high-performance liquid chromatography (HPLC): Proteomics separation methods

2DE is used to perform isoelectric point- and molecular weight-based separation of myriad proteins. A schematic representation of 2DE is shown in Fig. 11 [136,137]. It is therefore a vital proteomics platform that allows for the cell, tissue, and serum proteome analysis and detection of post-translationally modified proteins. Unfortunately, the less abundant proteins are not separated using this method. Prefractionation methods using isoelectric membranes-equipped multicompartment electrolyzers, affinity purification, subcellular fractionation, and protein-enrichment approaches, such as immobilized metal affinity chromatography (IMAC), can be employed [138–140].

HPLC is used to separate the complex protein mixture. However, it cannot separate the larger polypeptides. This can be overcome by 2D-HPLC that combines reversed-phase chromatography (RPC) and ion-exchange

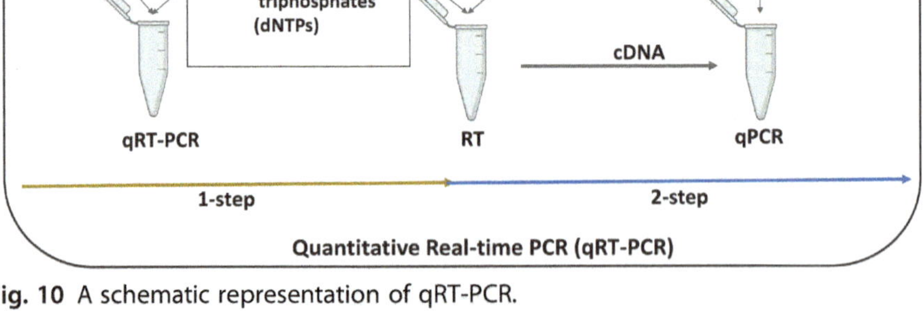

Fig. 10 A schematic representation of qRT-PCR.

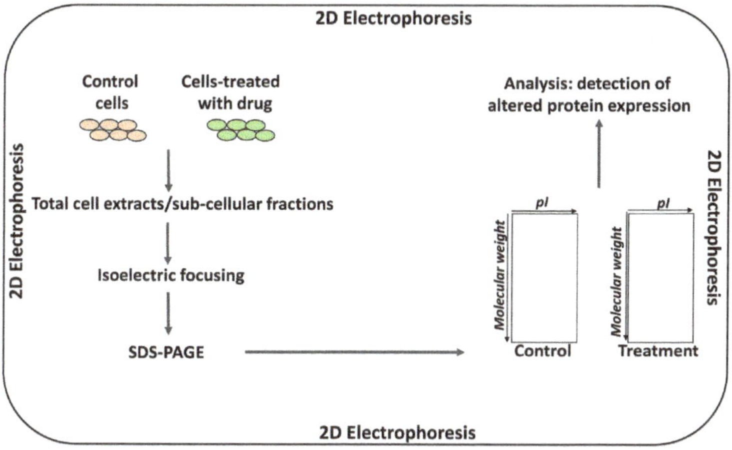

Fig. 11 A schematic representation of 2DE.

chromatography (IEC). In this, the IEC separates the peptides in the first dimension, while HPLC separates the obtained fractions in the second dimension. Finally, a complete peptide map is constituted (for the collected fragments) post-identification by the mass spectrometry (MS) [141–145].

8.3.4 Mass spectroscopy (MS), electrospray ionization (ESI), and surface-enhanced laser desorption/ionization-time of flight (SELDI-TOF)

In a matrix-assisted laser desorption/ionization-time of flight mass spectroscopy (MALDI-TOF MS), the proteins that are expressed differentially undergo protease-mediated digestion. This is done before performing a MALDI-TOF MS [146]. Peptides can be ionized with great sensitivity and minimal fragmentation using MALDI-TOF MS. It is performed in two steps. First, peptides are ionized using a time of the flight-coupled laser. Second, peptides are detected using a mass analyzer in the form of a mass-to-charge (m/z) ratio. Next, another MS analyzer is used for tandem mass spectrometry (MS/MS) to characterize these peptides. These are represented as a series of fragmented peptides (in the ionic form) in the generated MS/MS spectrum and an amino acid sequence (partial) can be constructed. Because it offers information about both peptide masses and peptide sequences, MS/MS-based protein identification is considered highly sensitive, robust, and accurate [146]. A schematic representation of MS/ESI is shown in Fig. 12.

In ESI MS, the dissolution of the samples to be analyzed (analyte) is done in a water/acetonitrile or a water/methanol mixture. This is then injected

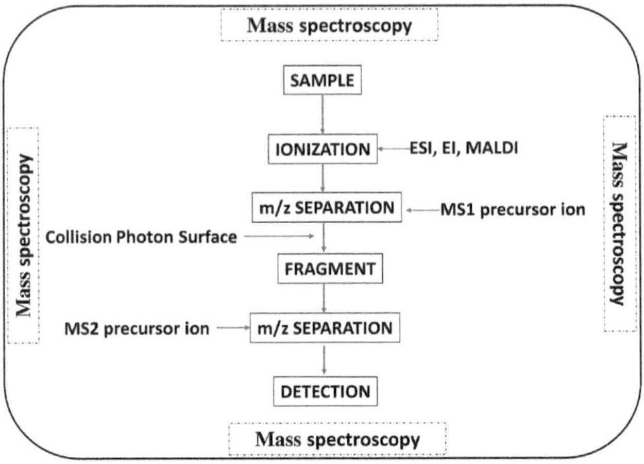

Fig. 12 A schematic representation of MS/ESI.

continuously using a nanoelectrospray (made of metal or metal-coated glass capillary) into an electric field. The flow rates are maintained at 1 to 5 mL/min (metal capillary) or nanoliters per minute (metal-coated glass capillary) depending upon the nanoelectrospray source used. The molecules of analytes are generated within the droplets (in the form of a mist) that are charged. These analyte molecules are then released from their respective solvents, as these droplets travel downward the pressure and potential gradients to the mass analyzer. ESI-coupled quadrupole or the triple quadrupole mass filters are used in tandem MS (MS/MS) [147–150].

MS analysis requires protein purification and separation before it is performed. This is overcome by surface-enhanced laser desorption/ionization-time of flight (SELDI-TOF) [151]. In this approach, the altered protein is identified by molecular weight and surface affinity using myriad selective chips (protein-chip array) [152]. This technique offers several other advantages over the above two techniques and ensures well-controlled experimental conditions. For instance, the binding activities are stringently adjusted using metal chelate surface, inhibitors (cation, anion, and hydrophobic exchangers), or cofactors in the binding assays. Moreover, proteins that are in relatively low abundance and the downstream enzyme (kinases, methyltransferases, phosphatases, and proteases) targets are also analyzed and identified using protein chip arrays. Altogether, it is a highly sensitive technique, in terms of low-molecular-weight protein (>6 kDa) detection and low abundant raw protein (purified protein samples not required) analysis [153,154].

8.4 Applications of genomics and proteomics: Current status in drug discovery and design

8.4.1 Identification and validation of drug targets

The discovery of the drug target is the foremost step in the pipeline of drug discovery. For this, the targets associated with the disease or diseases under study are to be identified and validated early. The altered gene or protein expression causes any particular disease. Therefore, the examination of this altered gene or protein expression profiles paves way for the detection of potential drug targets. Accordingly, the activities of these proteins can be modulated in a model system, and the effect on the concerned disease phenotype can then be evaluated. This, in turn, allows for the validation of the altered proteins (or target proteins) in the disease under study as potential drug candidates [155–157].

In the above scenario, global detection of alterations in the protein expressions in a particular disease and drug application can be carried out effectively using the genomics and proteomics approaches. Together, these allow for both the identification and validation of the target [155–157]. For example, the genomics- and proteomics-based approaches have been employed to identify transforming growth factor-β (TGF-β) in pancreatic carcinoma and lung epithelial cells [158], MIG2-like protein (MIG2B), and B-cell novel protein 1 (BCNP1) in chronic lymphocytic leukemia [159], tumor-invasion associated heat shock protein 90-alpha (HSP 90-α) [160,161], breast cancer-associated plasma membrane proteins [162], and methionine aminopeptidase inhibitors (bengamides) [163]. The cellular reaction- or signaling pathway-associated targets have also been identified using the proteomics approach [133,158]. Here, preprecipitation of proteins is performed before proceeding for the actual proteomics analysis. In an interesting study, the thioredoxin-targeted proteins were comprehensively analyzed in *Escherichia coli* via nanospray microcapillary tandem mass spectrometry, 2D-electrophoresis (2DE), and tandem affinity purification [164]. Further, thioredoxin-targeted proteins were also identified in *Chlamydomonas reinhardtii* via various proteomics tools. Further, protein kinase inhibitor (p38 MAPK inhibitor) targets have also been identified as potential inflammatory drugs using the proteomics approach [165].

Protein target validation for drugs with known or unknown mechanisms of action is another useful application of genomics and proteomics. Reportedly, HSP-70 and HSP-90 were validated as the farnesyl transferase inhibitor and antiallergic drug (amlexanox and disodium cromoglycate) targets in ovarian cancer cell lines using proteomics [160,166]. Interestingly, the PPIs can be mapped using functional proteomics for potential target identification [155]. It is well documented that receptor-ligand interaction or PPIs are important in myriad cellular processes and therefore provide valuable insights into these crucial cellular activities [167]. Alternatively, the PPIs can be studied using a combination of proteomics and other methods for drug target development. For example, a combination of proteomics with a dual-bait two-hybrid system efficiently detected peptides, proteins, and drugs with selective interaction for protein targets [168]. The kinetic regulation of PPIs was studied using combined proteomics and luciferase complementation imaging approaches. High-throughput proteomic analysis of PPIs was facilitated using a peptide array library (oriented) [169].

8.4.2 Actions of anticancer drugs

The rising understanding of the link between apoptosis and cancer has sparked a surge in research into apoptosis induction using chemotherapeutic drugs and small molecule inhibitors. The discovery of cellular proteins that induce apoptosis is a crucial step in the identification of therapeutic targets and the screening of new treatment candidates. Genomics and proteomics provide a comprehensive picture of gene and protein changes in entire cells and subcellular fractions. Efforts are now being channelized toward the use of genomics and proteomics for demonstrating the action mechanisms of candidate drugs [170]. For example, proteomics approach based on 2DE and MALDI-TOF MS was employed for the identification of altered cellular proteins and cellular responses in vitro posttreatment with the anticancer drug, gold(III) porphyrin 1a [171]. Further, alterations in Rho GDP-dissociation inhibitor alpha (RhoGDI alpha) and RNA-binding regulatory subunit/DJ-1 PARK7 (RS/DJ-1) were observed when profiled posttreatment with MAPK and paclitaxel in nonsmall lung carcinoma using a proteomics approach [172]. In another proteomics-based study, it was observed that apoptosis was counteracted by Raf-1 via mammalian sterile 20-like kinase (MST2) suppression. MST2 and Raf-1 depletion also thwarted apoptosis [173]. Furthermore, the proteomics approaches were employed for profiling the cellular targets of gefitinib, which is a well-known epidermal growth factor receptor (EGFR) kinase inhibitor. Also, its action mechanisms were deciphered. This, in turn, provided leads for developing potential inhibitors against various cellular protein kinases [174]. The dynamic changes in the proteome induced by activation of tyrosine kinase receptors (Trk)-receptors by their respective ligands [175], the chloride ion channel induction in the mitochondria directly by apoptosis by Myc [176], and initial modifications in the expression of the proteins via the inhibitors (Herceptin and Tarceva) of erbB [177] have all been identified using comparative proteomics studies.

Using proteomics approaches, the impacts of 5-fluorouracil- and diallyl trisulfide-induced apoptosis were also investigated in human cervical and gastric cancer cells, respectively [178,179]. Altogether, the proteomics-based identification of several intracellular pathway proteins, in particular, anticancer drug targets led to their classification as signaling transduction-related nuclear proteins, heat-shock proteins (HSPs), oxidative and endoplasmic reticulum (ER) stress proteins, and mitochondrial function-related proteins [180–184].

Combination approaches, such as a coupled 2D HPLC-MS/MS and amino acid-coded mass tagging (AACT) boosted proteomics quantification by MS-based methods [142]. This method was also used for investigating the anticancer effects caused by cyclin-dependent kinase (CDK) inhibition. The apoptosis induction in mouse liver was profiled using proteomics, transcriptomics, and a simulation technique [142]. In another study, protein expression changes were examined in breast epithelial cells during oxidative stress using a stable isotope-labeled proteome internal standard [185]. In the proteomic investigation of human O6-methylguanine-DNA methyltransferase (MGMT), affinity chromatography was coupled with MS/MS. When combined with other biochemical approaches, these investigations showed that proteomics can reveal protein expressions linked to the toxic and pharmacological consequences of an anticancer drug [186].

8.4.3 Drug resistance prediction

Drug resistance is a key issue that affects the results of cancer chemotherapies [170]. Acquired drug resistance implies that cancers are resistant not just to the medications that were previously used to treat them, but rather to other drugs with different modes of action [187]. Chemotherapy resistance can manifest itself in a variety of ways. This includes drug target alterations [188], apoptotic evasion [189], reduced drug influx, and enhanced drug efflux [188]. Given the genomics and proteomics biological system databases along with the advanced technology platforms, "fingerprints" are now available with functional proteomics. These provide information regarding therapeutic responses upon treatment [144]. The fundamental mechanisms for chemotherapeutic (e.g., vincristine [188], deoxycholate [189], vinblastine [188], and cisplatin [190]) resistance have been identified using genomics and proteomics. In vitro vinca resistance-associated alterations in the expression of cellular proteins were investigated via a differential proteomics approach [188].

8.4.4 Biomarkers for determining clinical effects

Biomarkers are genes and proteins whose expression has changed as a result of a disease. Clinical effects and drug efficacy can be determined using biomarkers as signatures. The identification of biomarkers in complex biological samples for correlating biological processes, and drug target validation, as well as response prediction is often a challenge in genomics and proteomics. However, these approaches can perform a direct identification of potential biomarkers in complex biological samples (such as tissues or blood) [191–193]. Reportedly, a global search for tumor-associated proteins in oral tongue carcinoma was performed using proteomics analysis. Here, alterations in the expression of several tumor-associated proteins were observed, which were identified as potential diagnostic and prognostic biomarkers for tongue carcinoma [194]. Similarly, proteomics analysis revealed potential diagnostic and prognostic biomarkers for buccal squamous cell carcinoma [180]. Recently, potential biomarkers (for example, vitronectin [195], ferritin light chain [196], cytokeratin 19 [197], and serum-associated fucosylated glycoproteins [198] were discovered for hepatocarcinoma via the proteomics analysis. This has also been extended to the identification of biomarkers for ovarian cancer [199,200], bladder cancer [191,201–203], and prostate cancer [201,204].

9. Conclusion

Conclusively, considerable technological strides have been achieved for precise and physiological disease models, which has boosted automation, throughput, and data management. However, the molecular mechanisms underlying the existing or emerging infections, novel targets, highly predictive in vitro models, and functional assay systems are indispensable to gain better clinical relevance of the discovered drugs.

References

[1] J.P. Hughes, S. Rees, S.B. Kalindjian, K.L. Philpott, Principles of early drug discovery, Br. J. Pharmacol. 162 (6) (2011) 1239–1249, https://doi.org/10.1111/j.1476-5381.2010.01127.x.

[2] R.C. Mohs, N.H. Greig, Drug discovery and development: role of basic biological research, Alzheimer's Dement. 3 (4) (2017) 651–657, https://doi.org/10.1016/j.trci.2017.10.005.
[3] C. Brideau, B. Gunter, B. Pikounis, A. Liaw, Improved statistical methods for hit selection in high-throughput screening, SLAS Discov. 8 (6) (2003) 634–647, https://doi.org/10.1177/1087057103258285.
[4] X. Douglas Zhang, X.C. Yang, N. Chung, A. Gates, E. Stec, P. Kunapuli, et al., Robust statistical methods for hit selection in RNA interference high-throughput screening experiments, Pharmacogenomics 7 (3) (2006) 299–309, https://doi.org/10.2217/14622416.7.3.299.
[5] M.M. Hann, T.I. Oprea, Pursuing the leadlikeness concept in pharmaceutical research, Curr. Opin. Chem. Biol. 8 (3) (2004) 255–263, https://doi.org/10.1016/j.cbpa.2004.04.003.
[6] J. Inglese, D.S. Auld, A. Jadhav, R.L. Johnson, A. Simeonov, A. Yasgar, et al., Quantitative high-throughput screening: a titration-based approach that efficiently identifies biological activities in large chemical libraries, Proc. Natl. Acad. Sci. 103 (31) (2006) 11473–11478, https://doi.org/10.1073/pnas.0604348103.
[7] R. Macarron, M.N. Banks, D. Bojanic, D.J. Burns, D.A. Cirovic, T. Garyantes, et al., Impact of high-throughput screening in biomedical research, Nat. Rev. Drug Discov. 10 (3) (2011) 188–195, https://doi.org/10.1038/nrd3368.
[8] S. Michael, D. Auld, C. Klumpp, A. Jadhav, W. Zheng, N. Thorne, et al., A robotic platform for quantitative high-throughput screening, ASSAY Drug Devel. Technol. 6 (5) (2008) 637–657, https://doi.org/10.1089/adt.2008.150.
[9] E. Schonbrun, A.R. Abate, P.E. Steinvurzel, D.A. Weitz, K.B. Crozier, High-throughput fluorescence detection using an integrated zone-plate array, Lab Chip 10 (7) (2010), https://doi.org/10.1039/b923554j.
[10] P. Szymański, M. Markowicz, E. Mikiciuk-Olasik, Adaptation of high-throughput screening in drug discovery—toxicological screening tests, Int. J. Mol. Sci. 13 (1) (2011) 427–452, https://doi.org/10.3390/ijms13010427.
[11] J.-H. Zhang, T.D.Y. Chung, K.R. Oldenburg, A simple statistical parameter for use in evaluation and validation of high throughput screening assays, SLAS Discov. 4 (2) (1999) 67–73, https://doi.org/10.1177/108705719900400206.
[12] X.D. Zhang, A new method with flexible and balanced control of false negatives and false positives for hit selection in RNA interference high-throughput screening assays, SLAS Discov. 12 (5) (2007) 645–655, https://doi.org/10.1177/1087057107300645.
[13] Y. Choi, Y. Kawazoe, K. Murakami, H. Misawa, M. Uesugi, Identification of bioactive molecules by adipogenesis profiling of organic compounds, J. Biol. Chem. 278 (9) (2003) 7320–7324, https://doi.org/10.1074/jbc.M210283200.
[14] T.H. Nguyen Vo, N. Tran, D. Nguyen, L. Le, An in silico study on antidiabetic activity of bioactive compounds in Euphorbia thymifolia Linn, Springerplus 5 (1) (2016), https://doi.org/10.1186/s40064-016-2631-5.
[15] M. Salman Khan, S. Akhtar, O.A. Al-Sagair, J.M. Arif, Protective effect of dietary tocotrienols against infection and inflammation-induced hyperlipidemia: an in vivo and in silico study, Phytother. Res. 25 (11) (2011) 1586–1595, https://doi.org/10.1002/ptr.3448.
[16] C. McInnes, Virtual screening strategies in drug discovery, Curr. Opin. Chem. Biol. 11 (5) (2007) 494–502, https://doi.org/10.1016/j.cbpa.2007.08.033.
[17] L. Scotti, F. Mendonca Junior, H. Ishiki, F. Ribeiro, R. Singla, J. Filho, et al., Docking studies for multi-target drugs, Curr. Drug Targets 18 (5) (2017) 592–604, https://doi.org/10.2174/1389450116666150825111818.
[18] P.D. Lyne, Structure-based virtual screening: an overview, Drug Discov. Today 7 (20) (2002) 1047–1055, https://doi.org/10.1016/s1359-6446(02)02483-2.

[19] T.K. Romano, Structure-based drug design: docking and scoring, Curr. Protein Pept. Sci. 8 (4) (2007) 312–328, https://doi.org/10.2174/138920307781369382.

[20] B.K. Shoichet, Virtual screening of chemical libraries, Nature 432 (7019) (2004) 862–865, https://doi.org/10.1038/nature03197.

[21] S. Kalyaanamoorthy, Y.-P.P. Chen, Structure-based drug design to augment hit discovery, Drug Discov. Today 16 (17-18) (2011) 831–839, https://doi.org/10.1016/j.drudis.2011.07.006.

[22] A.N. Jain, Surflex: fully automatic flexible molecular docking using a molecular similarity-based search engine, J. Med. Chem. 46 (4) (2003) 499–511, https://doi.org/10.1021/jm020406h.

[23] M. Rarey, B. Kramer, T. Lengauer, G. Klebe, A fast flexible docking method using an incremental construction algorithm, J. Mol. Biol. 261 (3) (1996) 470–489, https://doi.org/10.1006/jmbi.1996.0477.

[24] T.A. Halgren, R.B. Murphy, R.A. Friesner, H.S. Beard, L.L. Frye, W.T. Pollard, et al., Glide: a new approach for rapid, accurate docking and scoring. 2. Enrichment factors in database screening, J. Med. Chem. 47 (7) (2004) 1750–1759, https://doi.org/10.1021/jm030644s.

[25] T.J.A. Ewing, S. Makino, A.G. Skillman, I.D. Kuntz, DOCK 4.0: search strategies for automated molecular docking of flexible molecule databases, J. Comput. Aided Mol. Des. 15 (5) (2001) 411–428, https://doi.org/10.1023/a:1011115820450.

[26] M.R. McGann, H.R. Almond, A. Nicholls, J.A. Grant, F.K. Brown, Gaussian docking functions, Biopolymers 68 (1) (2003) 76–90, https://doi.org/10.1002/bip.10207.

[27] G. Jones, P. Willett, R.C. Glen, A.R. Leach, R. Taylor, Development and validation of a genetic algorithm for flexible docking 1 1Edited by F.E. Cohen, J. Mol. Biol. 267 (3) (1997) 727–748, https://doi.org/10.1006/jmbi.1996.0897.

[28] G.M. Morris, D.S. Goodsell, R.S. Halliday, R. Huey, W.E. Hart, R.K. Belew, et al., Automated docking using a Lamarckian genetic algorithm and an empirical binding free energy function, J. Comput. Chem. 19 (14) (1998) 1639–1662, https://doi.org/10.1002/(sici)1096-987x(19981115)19:14<1639::Aid-jcc10>3.0.Co;2-b.

[29] C.M. Venkatachalam, X. Jiang, T. Oldfield, M. Waldman, LigandFit: a novel method for the shape-directed rapid docking of ligands to protein active sites, J. Mol. Graph. Model. 21 (4) (2003) 289–307, https://doi.org/10.1016/s1093-3263(02)00164-x.

[30] J. Finn, Application of SBDD to the discovery of new antibacterial drugs, in: Structure-Based Drug Discovery, 2012, pp. 291–319.

[31] E. Jenwitheesuk, R. Samudrala, Virtual screening of HIV-1 protease inhibitors against human cytomegalovirus protease using docking and molecular dynamics, AIDS 19 (5) (2005) 529–531, https://doi.org/10.1097/01.aids.0000162343.96674.4c.

[32] D. Kuck, N. Singh, F. Lyko, J.L. Medina-Franco, Novel and selective DNA methyltransferase inhibitors: docking-based virtual screening and experimental evaluation, Bioorg. Med. Chem. 18 (2) (2010) 822–829, https://doi.org/10.1016/j.bmc.2009.11.050.

[33] C.L. Pierri, G. Parisi, V. Porcelli, Computational approaches for protein function prediction: a combined strategy from multiple sequence alignment to molecular docking-based virtual screening, Biochim. Biophys. Acta 1804 (9) (2010) 1695–1712, https://doi.org/10.1016/j.bbapap.2010.04.008.

[34] R.K. Singla, X. He, H. Chopra, C. Tsagkaris, L. Shen, M.A. Kamal, et al., Natural products for the prevention and control of the COVID-19 pandemic: sustainable bioresources, Front. Pharmacol. 12 (2021), https://doi.org/10.3389/fphar.2021.758159.

[35] R.D. Taylor, P.J. Jewsbury, J.W. Essex, A review of protein-small molecule docking methods, J. Comput. Aided Mol. Des. 16 (3) (2002) 151–166, https://doi.org/10.1023/a:1020155510718.

[36] D. Wang, F. Wang, Y. Tan, L. Dong, L. Chen, W. Zhu, et al., Discovery of potent small molecule inhibitors of DYRK1A by structure-based virtual screening and

bioassay, Bioorg. Med. Chem. Lett. 22 (1) (2012) 168–171, https://doi.org/10.1016/j.bmcl.2011.11.043.
[37] B. Waszkowycz, Structure-based approaches to drug design and virtual screening, Curr. Opin. Drug Discov. Devel. 5 (3) (2002) 407–413.
[38] S. Ghosh, A. Nie, J. An, Z. Huang, Structure-based virtual screening of chemical libraries for drug discovery, Curr. Opin. Chem. Biol. 10 (3) (2006) 194–202, https://doi.org/10.1016/j.cbpa.2006.04.002.
[39] G.L. Warren, C.W. Andrews, A.-M. Capelli, B. Clarke, J. LaLonde, M.H. Lambert, et al., A critical assessment of docking programs and scoring functions, J. Med. Chem. 49 (20) (2005) 5912–5931, https://doi.org/10.1021/jm050362n.
[40] R. Kumar Singla, R. Singh, A. Kumar Dubey, Important aspects of post-prandial antidiabetic drug, Acarbose, Curr. Top. Med. Chem. 16 (23) (2016) 2625–2633, https://doi.org/10.2174/1568026616666160414123500.
[41] R.K. Singla, L. Scotti, A.K. Dubey, In silico studies revealed multiple neurological targets for the antidepressant molecule ursolic acid, Curr. Neuropharmacol. 15 (8) (2017), https://doi.org/10.2174/1570159x14666161229115508.
[42] M.A. Murcko, in: K.B. Lipkowitz, D.B. Boyd (Eds.), Reviews in Computational Chemistry, John Wiley & Sons, Inc., Hoboken, NJ, USA, 2007, pp. 1–67.
[43] R.K. Singla, M. Ali, M.A. Kamal, A.K. Dubey, Isolation and characterization of nuciferoic acid, a novel keto fatty acid with hyaluronidase inhibitory activity from Cocos nucifera Linn. Endocarp, Curr. Top. Med. Chem. 18 (27) (2019) 2367–2378, https://doi.org/10.2174/1568026619666181224111319.
[44] P. Ehrlich, Über den jetzigen Stand der Chemotherapie, Ber. Dtsch. Chem. Ges. 42 (1) (1909) 17–47, https://doi.org/10.1002/cber.19090420105.
[45] P. Gund, Three-Dimensional Pharmacophoric Pattern Searching, in: Progress in Molecular and Subcellular Biology, 1977, pp. 117–143.
[46] F. Caporuscio, A. Tafi, Pharmacophore modelling: a forty year old approach and its modern synergies, Curr. Med. Chem. 18 (17) (2011) 2543–2553, https://doi.org/10.2174/092986711795933669.
[47] O. Guner, O. Clement, Y. Kurogi, Pharmacophore modeling and three dimensional database searching for drug design using catalyst: recent advances, Curr. Med. Chem. 11 (22) (2004) 2991–3005, https://doi.org/10.2174/0929867043364036.
[48] K.-H. Kim, N.D. Kim, B.-L. Seong, Pharmacophore-based virtual screening: a review of recent applications, Expert Opin. Drug Discovery 5 (3) (2010) 205–222, https://doi.org/10.1517/17460441003592072.
[49] G. Melagraki, A. Afantitis, Ligand and structure based virtual screening strategies for hit-finding and optimization of hepatitis C virus (HCV) inhibitors, Curr. Med. Chem. 18 (17) (2011) 2612–2619, https://doi.org/10.2174/092986711795933759.
[50] H. Sun, Pharmacophore-based virtual screening, Curr. Med. Chem. 15 (10) (2008) 1018–1024, https://doi.org/10.2174/092986708784049630.
[51] G. Jones, P. Willett, R.C. Glen, in: O.F. Güner (Ed.), Pharmacophore Perception, Development and Use in Drug Design, International University Line, La Jolla, CA, 2000, pp. 85–86.
[52] S.-K. Lin, Pharmacophore perception, development and use in drug design, Molecules 5 (12) (2000) 987–989, https://doi.org/10.3390/50700987.
[53] E.A. Hecker, C. Duraiswami, T.A. Andrea, D.J. Diller, Use of catalyst pharmacophore models for screening of large combinatorial libraries, J. Chem. Inf. Comput. Sci. 42 (5) (2002) 1204–1211, https://doi.org/10.1021/ci020368a.
[54] S.L. Dixon, A.M. Smondyrev, S.N. Rao, PHASE: a novel approach to pharmacophore modeling and 3D database searching, Chem. Biol. Drug Design 67 (5) (2006) 370–372, https://doi.org/10.1111/j.1747-0285.2006.00384.x.
[55] S.L. Cheong, S. Federico, G. Venkatesan, P. Paira, Y.-M. Shao, G. Spalluto, et al., Pharmacophore elucidation for a new series of 2-aryl-pyrazolo-triazolo-pyrimidines

as potent human A3 adenosine receptor antagonists, Bioorg. Med. Chem. Lett. 21 (10) (2011) 2898–2905, https://doi.org/10.1016/j.bmcl.2011.03.073.
[56] T.A. Halgren, Merck molecular force field. I. Basis, form, scope, parameterization, and performance of MMFF94, J. Comput. Chem. 17 (5-6) (1996) 490–519, https://doi.org/10.1002/(sici)1096-987x(199604)17:5/6<490::Aid-jcc1>3.0.Co;2-p.
[57] T. Seidel, G. Ibis, F. Bendix, G. Wolber, Strategies for 3D pharmacophore-based virtual screening, Drug Discov. Today Technol. 7 (4) (2010) e221–e228, https://doi.org/10.1016/j.ddtec.2010.11.004.
[58] G. Wolber, A.A. Dornhofer, T. Langer, Efficient overlay of small organic molecules using 3D pharmacophores, J. Comput. Aided Mol. Des. 20 (12) (2006) 773–788, https://doi.org/10.1007/s10822-006-9078-7.
[59] G. Wolber, T. Langer, LigandScout: 3-D pharmacophores derived from protein-bound ligands and their use as virtual screening filters, J. Chem. Inf. Model. 45 (1) (2004) 160–169, https://doi.org/10.1021/ci049885e.
[60] S. Distinto, F. Esposito, J. Kirchmair, M.C. Cardia, M. Gaspari, E. Maccioni, et al., Identification of HIV-1 reverse transcriptase dual inhibitors by a combined shape-, 2D-fingerprint- and pharmacophore-based virtual screening approach, Eur. J. Med. Chem. 50 (2012) 216–229, https://doi.org/10.1016/j.ejmech.2012.01.056.
[61] S.M. Noha, A.G. Atanasov, D. Schuster, P. Markt, N. Fakhrudin, E.H. Heiss, et al., Discovery of a novel IKK-β inhibitor by ligand-based virtual screening techniques, Bioorg. Med. Chem. Lett. 21 (1) (2011) 577–583, https://doi.org/10.1016/j.bmcl.2010.10.051.
[62] S.M. Noha, B. Jazzar, S. Kuehnl, J.M. Rollinger, H. Stuppner, A.M. Schaible, et al., Pharmacophore-based discovery of a novel cytosolic phospholipase A2α inhibitor, Bioorg. Med. Chem. Lett. 22 (2) (2012) 1202–1207, https://doi.org/10.1016/j.bmcl.2011.11.093.
[63] D. Schuster, D. Kowalik, J. Kirchmair, C. Laggner, P. Markt, C. Aebischer-Gumy, et al., Identification of chemically diverse, novel inhibitors of 17β-hydroxysteroid dehydrogenase type 3 and 5 by pharmacophore-based virtual screening, J. Steroid Biochem. Mol. Biol. 125 (1-2) (2011) 148–161, https://doi.org/10.1016/j.jsbmb.2011.01.016.
[64] D. Schuster, P. Markt, U. Grienke, J. Mihaly-Bison, M. Binder, S.M. Noha, et al., Pharmacophore-based discovery of FXR agonists. Part I: model development and experimental validation, Bioorg. Med. Chem. 19 (23) (2011) 7168–7180, https://doi.org/10.1016/j.bmc.2011.09.056.
[65] B. Waltenberger, K. Wiechmann, J. Bauer, P. Markt, S.M. Noha, G. Wolber, et al., Pharmacophore modeling and virtual screening for novel acidic inhibitors of microsomal prostaglandin E2 synthase-1 (mPGES-1), J. Med. Chem. 54 (9) (2011) 3163–3174, https://doi.org/10.1021/jm101309g.
[66] R.A. Jose, A. Voet, K. Broos, A.J. Jakobi, G. Bruylants, B. Egle, et al., An integrated fragment based screening approach for the discovery of small molecule modulators of the VWF-GPIbα interaction, Chem. Commun. 48 (92) (2012), https://doi.org/10.1039/c2cc35269a.
[67] M.J. McGregor, S.M. Muskal, Pharmacophore fingerprinting. 1. Application to QSAR and focused library design, J. Chem. Inf. Comput. Sci. 39 (3) (1999) 569–574, https://doi.org/10.1021/ci980159j.
[68] M.J. McGregor, S.M. Muskal, Pharmacophore fingerprinting. 2. Application to primary library design, J. Chem. Inf. Comput. Sci. 40 (1) (1999) 117–125, https://doi.org/10.1021/ci990313h.
[69] T.T. Luu, N. Malcolm, K. Nadassy, Pharmacophore modeling methods in focused library selection—applications in the context of a new classification scheme, Comb.

Chem. High Throughput Screen. 14 (6) (2011) 488–499, https://doi.org/10.2174/138620711795767820.
[70] V. Hähnke, G. Schneider, Pharmacophore alignment search tool: influence of scoring systems on text-based similarity searching, J. Comput. Chem. 32 (8) (2011) 1635–1647, https://doi.org/10.1002/jcc.21741.
[71] G. Jones, P. Willett, R.C. Glen, A genetic algorithm for flexible molecular overlay and pharmacophore elucidation, J. Comput. Aided Mol. Des. 9 (6) (1995) 532–549, https://doi.org/10.1007/bf00124324.
[72] A.R.D. Voet, A. Kumar, F. Berenger, K.Y.J. Zhang, Combining in silico and in cerebro approaches for virtual screening and pose prediction in SAMPL4, J. Comput. Aided Mol. Des. 28 (4) (2014) 363–373, https://doi.org/10.1007/s10822-013-9702-2.
[73] J. Desaphy, K. Azdimousa, E. Kellenberger, D. Rognan, Comparison and druggability prediction of protein-ligand binding sites from pharmacophore-annotated cavity shapes, J. Chem. Inf. Model. 52 (8) (2012) 2287–2299, https://doi.org/10.1021/ci300184x.
[74] M.P.A. Sanders, R. McGuire, L. Roumen, I.J.P. de Esch, J. de Vlieg, J.P.G. Klomp, et al., From the protein's perspective: the benefits and challenges of protein structure-based pharmacophore modeling, Med. Chem. Commun. 3 (1) (2012) 28–38, https://doi.org/10.1039/c1md00210d.
[75] C. Barillari, G. Marcou, D. Rognan, Hot-spots-guided receptor-based pharmacophores (HS-Pharm): a knowledge-based approach to identify ligand-anchoring atoms in protein cavities and prioritize structure-based pharmacophores, J. Chem. Inf. Model. 48 (7) (2008) 1396–1410, https://doi.org/10.1021/ci800064z.
[76] H.-J. Bohm, The computer program LUDI: a new method for the de novo design of enzyme inhibitors, J. Comput. Aided Mol. Des. 6 (1) (1992) 61–78, https://doi.org/10.1007/bf00124387.
[77] P.J. Goodford, A computational procedure for determining energetically favorable binding sites on biologically important macromolecules, J. Med. Chem. 28 (7) (2002) 849–857, https://doi.org/10.1021/jm00145a002.
[78] C. Helsen, T. Van den Broeck, A. Voet, S. Prekovic, H. Van Poppel, S. Joniau, et al., Androgen receptor antagonists for prostate cancer therapy, Endocr. Relat. Cancer 21 (4) (2014) T105–T118, https://doi.org/10.1530/erc-13-0545.
[79] C. Tintori, V. Corradi, M. Magnani, F. Manetti, M. Botta, Targets looking for drugs: a multistep computational protocol for the development of structure-based pharmacophores and their applications for hit discovery, J. Chem. Inf. Model. 48 (11) (2008) 2166–2179, https://doi.org/10.1021/ci800105p.
[80] A. Voet, C. Helsen, K.Y.J. Zhang, F. Claessens, The discovery of novel human androgen receptor antagonist chemotypes using a combined pharmacophore screening procedure, ChemMedChem 8 (4) (2013) 644–651, https://doi.org/10.1002/cmdc.201200549.
[81] X. Liu, F. Zhu, H. Ma, Z. Shi, S.Y. Yang, Y.Q. Wei, et al., Predicting targeted polypharmacology for drug repositioning and multi-target drug discovery, Curr. Med. Chem. 20 (13) (2013) 1646–1661, https://doi.org/10.2174/0929867311320130005.
[82] K.-M. Thai, T.-D. Ngo, T.-D. Tran, M.-T. Le, Pharmacophore modeling for antitargets, Curr. Top. Med. Chem. 13 (9) (2013) 1002–1014, https://doi.org/10.2174/1568026611313090004.
[83] A. Kumar, K.Y.J. Zhang, Hierarchical virtual screening approaches in small molecule drug discovery, Methods 71 (2015) 26–37, https://doi.org/10.1016/j.ymeth.2014.07.007.
[84] S.A. Hindle, M. Rarey, C. Buning, T. Lengauer, Flexible docking under pharmacophore type constraints, J. Comput. Aided Mol. Des. 16 (2) (2002) 129–149, https://doi.org/10.1023/a:1016399411208.

[85] B. Hu, M.A. Lill, Protein pharmacophore selection using hydration-site analysis, J. Chem. Inf. Model. 52 (4) (2012) 1046–1060, https://doi.org/10.1021/ci200620h.
[86] B. Hu, M.A. Lill, PharmDock: a pharmacophore-based docking program, J. Cheminform. 6 (1) (2014), https://doi.org/10.1186/1758-2946-6-14.
[87] J. Goto, R. Kataoka, N. Hirayama, Ph4Dock: pharmacophore-based protein−ligand docking, J. Med. Chem. 47 (27) (2004) 6804–6811, https://doi.org/10.1021/jm0493818.
[88] D.L. Mobley, S. Liu, N.M. Lim, K.L. Wymer, A.L. Perryman, S. Forli, et al., Blind prediction of HIV integrase binding from the SAMPL4 challenge, J. Comput. Aided Mol. Des. 28 (4) (2014) 327–345, https://doi.org/10.1007/s10822-014-9723-5.
[89] M.S. Alavijeh, A.M. Palmer, The pivotal role of drug metabolism and pharmacokinetics in the discovery and development of new medicines, IDrugs 7 (8) (2004) 755–763.
[90] J.H. Lin, A.Y. Lu, Role of pharmacokinetics and metabolism in drug discovery and development, Pharmacol. Rev. 49 (4) (1997) 403–449.
[91] R.K. Singla, R. Gupta, S. Joon, A.K. Gupta, B. Shen, Isolation, docking and in silico ADME-T studies of acacianol: novel antibacterial isoflavone analogue isolated from Acacia leucophloea Bark, Curr. Drug Metab. 22 (11) (2021) 893–904, https://doi.org/10.2174/1389200222666211005091417.
[92] R.K. Singla, B. Shen, In silico ADMET evaluation of natural DPP-IV inhibitors for rational drug design against diabetes, Curr. Drug Metab. 21 (10) (2020) 768–777, https://doi.org/10.2174/1389200221999200901202945.
[93] O. Guner, J. Bowen, Pharmacophore modeling for ADME, Curr. Top. Med. Chem. 13 (11) (2013) 1327–1342, https://doi.org/10.2174/15680266113139990037.
[94] F. Yamashita, M. Hashida, In silico approaches for predicting ADME properties of drugs, Drug Metabol. Pharm. 19 (5) (2004) 327–338, https://doi.org/10.2133/dmpk.19.327.
[95] E. Tanaka, Clinically important pharmacokinetic drug-drug interactions: role of cytochrome P450 enzymes, J. Clin. Pharm. Ther. 23 (6) (1998) 403–416, https://doi.org/10.1046/j.1365-2710.1998.00086.x.
[96] M.J. de Groot, S. Ekins, Pharmacophore modeling of cytochromes P450, Adv. Drug Deliv. Rev. 54 (3) (2002) 367–383, https://doi.org/10.1016/s0169-409x(02)00009-1.
[97] S. Ekins, M.J. de Groot, J.P. Jones, Pharmacophore and three-dimensional quantitative structure activity relationship methods for modeling cytochrome p450 active sites, Drug Metab. Dispos. 29 (7) (2001) 936–944.
[98] C.M. Masimirembwa, M. Ridderström, I. Zamora, T.B. Andersson, Combining pharmacophore and protein modeling to predict CYP450 inhibitors and substrates, Methods Enzymol. (2002) 133–144.
[99] D. Schuster, C. Laggner, T. Steindl, T. Langer, Development and validation of an in silico P450 profiler based on pharmacophore models, Curr. Drug Discov. Technol. 3 (1) (2006) 1–48, https://doi.org/10.2174/157016306776637609.
[100] M.J. Keiser, B.L. Roth, B.N. Armbruster, P. Ernsberger, J.J. Irwin, B.K. Shoichet, Relating protein pharmacology by ligand chemistry, Nat. Biotechnol. 25 (2) (2007) 197–206, https://doi.org/10.1038/nbt1284.
[101] M.J. Sorich, J.O. Miners, R.A. McKinnon, P.A. Smith, Multiple pharmacophores for the investigation of human UDP-glucuronosyltransferase isoform substrate selectivity, Mol. Pharmacol. 65 (2) (2004) 301–308, https://doi.org/10.1124/mol.65.2.301.
[102] M.J. Sorich, P.A. Smith, R.A. McKinnon, J.O. Miners, Pharmacophore and quantitative structure activity relationship modelling of UDP-glucuronosyltransferase 1A1 (UGT1A1) substrates, Pharmacogenetics 12 (8) (2002) 635–645, https://doi.org/10.1097/00008571-200211000-00008.

[103] A. Koutsoukas, B. Simms, J. Kirchmair, P.J. Bond, A.V. Whitmore, S. Zimmer, et al., From in silico target prediction to multi-target drug design: current databases, methods and applications, J. Proteome 74 (12) (2011) 2554–2574, https://doi.org/10.1016/j.jprot.2011.05.011.
[104] J. Rollinger, D. Schuster, B. Danzl, S. Schwaiger, P. Markt, M. Schmidtke, et al., In silico target fishing for rationalized ligand discovery exemplified on constituents of Ruta graveolens, Planta Med. 75 (03) (2008) 195–204, https://doi.org/10.1055/s-0028-1088397.
[105] Y. Hu, J. Bajorath, Polypharmacology directed compound data mining: identification of promiscuous chemotypes with different activity profiles and comparison to approved drugs, J. Chem. Inf. Model. 50 (12) (2010) 2112–2118, https://doi.org/10.1021/ci1003637.
[106] J. Kirchmair, C. Laggner, G. Wolber, T. Langer, Comparative analysis of protein-bound ligand conformations with respect to catalyst's conformational space subsampling algorithms, J. Chem. Inf. Model. 45 (2) (2005) 422–430, https://doi.org/10.1021/ci049753l.
[107] J. Kirchmair, G. Wolber, C. Laggner, T. Langer, Comparative performance assessment of the conformational model generators omega and catalyst: a large-scale survey on the retrieval of protein-bound ligand conformations, J. Chem. Inf. Model. 46 (4) (2006) 1848–1861, https://doi.org/10.1021/ci060084g.
[108] F. Christ, A. Voet, A. Marchand, S. Nicolet, B.A. Desimmie, D. Marchand, et al., Rational design of small-molecule inhibitors of the LEDGF/p75-integrase interaction and HIV replication, Nat. Chem. Biol. 6 (6) (2010) 442–448, https://doi.org/10.1038/nchembio.370.
[109] L. De Luca, M.L. Barreca, S. Ferro, F. Christ, N. Iraci, R. Gitto, et al., Pharmacophore-based discovery of small-molecule inhibitors of protein-protein interactions between HIV-1 integrase and cellular cofactor LEDGF/p75, ChemMedChem 4 (8) (2009) 1311–1316, https://doi.org/10.1002/cmdc.200900070.
[110] R.E. Vancraenenbroeck, J. De Raeymaecker, E. Lobbestael, F. Gao, M. De Maeyer, A. Voet, et al., In silico, in vitro and cellular analysis with a kinome-wide inhibitor panel correlates cellular LRRK2 dephosphorylation to inhibitor activity on LRRK2, Front. Mol. Neurosci. 7 (2014), https://doi.org/10.3389/fnmol.2014.00051.
[111] K.T. Schomburg, S. Bietz, H. Briem, A.M. Henzler, S. Urbaczek, M. Rarey, Facing the challenges of structure-based target prediction by inverse virtual screening, J. Chem. Inf. Model. 54 (6) (2014) 1676–1686, https://doi.org/10.1021/ci500130e.
[112] M. Bredel, E. Jacoby, Chemogenomics: an emerging strategy for rapid target and drug discovery, Nat. Rev. Genet. 5 (4) (2004) 262–275, https://doi.org/10.1038/nrg1317.
[113] A. Wuster, M. Madan Babu, Chemogenomics and biotechnology, Trends Biotechnol. 26 (5) (2008) 252–258, https://doi.org/10.1016/j.tibtech.2008.01.004.
[114] A. Engelberg, Iconix Pharmaceuticals, Inc.—removing barriers to efficient drug discovery through chemogenomics, Pharmacogenomics 5 (6) (2004) 741–744, https://doi.org/10.1517/14622416.5.6.741.
[115] B. Bhattacharjee, Chemogenomics profiling of drug targets of peptidoglycan biosynthesis pathway in leptospira interrogans by virtual screening approaches, J. Microbiol. Biotechnol. 23 (6) (2013) 779–784, https://doi.org/10.4014/jmb.1206.06050.
[116] K. Cheung-Ong, K.T. Song, Z. Ma, D. Shabtai, A.Y. Lee, D. Gallo, et al., Comparative chemogenomics to examine the mechanism of action of DNA-targeted platinum-acridine anticancer agents, ACS Chem. Biol. 7 (11) (2012) 1892–1901, https://doi.org/10.1021/cb300320d.
[117] F. Mohd Fauzi, A. Koutsoukas, R. Lowe, K. Joshi, T.-P. Fan, R.C. Glen, et al., Chemogenomics approaches to rationalizing the mode-of-action of traditional chinese and

ayurvedic medicines, J. Chem. Inf. Model. 53 (3) (2013) 661–673, https://doi.org/10.1021/ci3005513.
[118] Y. Yamanishi, M. Araki, A. Gutteridge, W. Honda, M. Kanehisa, Prediction of drug-target interaction networks from the integration of chemical and genomic spaces, Bioinformatics 24 (13) (2008) i232–i240, https://doi.org/10.1093/bioinformatics/btn162.
[119] V.C. Wasinger, S.J. Cordwell, A. Cerpa-Poljak, J.X. Yan, A.A. Gooley, M.R. Wilkins, et al., Progress with gene-product mapping of the Mollicutes:Mycoplasma genitalium, Electrophoresis 16 (1) (1995) 1090–1094, https://doi.org/10.1002/elps.11501601185.
[120] M.R. Wilkins, J.-C. Sanchez, A.A. Gooley, R.D. Appel, I. Humphery-Smith, D.F. Hochstrasser, et al., Progress with proteome projects: why all proteins expressed by a genome should be identified and how to do it, Biotechnol. Genet. Eng. Rev. 13 (1) (1996) 19–50, https://doi.org/10.1080/02648725.1996.10647923.
[121] J. Cox, M. Mann, Is proteomics the new genomics? Cell 130 (3) (2007) 395–398, https://doi.org/10.1016/j.cell.2007.07.032.
[122] E.S. Lander, L.M. Linton, B. Birren, C. Nusbaum, M.C. Zody, J. Baldwin, et al., Initial sequencing and analysis of the human genome, Nature 409 (6822) (2001) 860–921, https://doi.org/10.1038/35057062.
[123] A. Pandey, M. Mann, Proteomics to study genes and genomes, Nature 405 (6788) (2000) 837–846, https://doi.org/10.1038/35015709.
[124] E.T. Maggio, K. Ramnarayan, Recent developments in computational proteomics, Drug Discov. Today 6 (19) (2001) 996–1004, https://doi.org/10.1016/s1359-6446(01)02003-7.
[125] D.A. Jeffery, M. Bogyo, Chemical proteomics and its application to drug discovery, Curr. Opin. Biotechnol. 14 (1) (2003) 87–95, https://doi.org/10.1016/s0958-1669(02)00010-1.
[126] S. Goldsmith-Fischman, B. Honig, Structural genomics: computational methods for structure analysis, Protein Sci. 12 (9) (2003) 1813–1821, https://doi.org/10.1110/ps.0242903.
[127] R. Linding, L.J. Jensen, F. Diella, P. Bork, T.J. Gibson, R.B. Russell, Protein disorder prediction, Structure 11 (11) (2003) 1453–1459, https://doi.org/10.1016/j.str.2003.10.002.
[128] S. Renfrey, J. Featherstone, Structural proteomics, Nat. Rev. Drug Discov. 1 (3) (2002) 175–176, https://doi.org/10.1038/nrd766.
[129] A. Sali, R. Glaeser, T. Earnest, W. Baumeister, From words to literature in structural proteomics, Nature 422 (6928) (2003) 216–225, https://doi.org/10.1038/nature01513.
[130] W. Schubert, Topological proteomics, toponomics, MELK-technology, in: Proteomics of Microorganisms, 2003, pp. 189–209.
[131] D.J. Duggan, M. Bittner, Y. Chen, P. Meltzer, J.M. Trent, Expression profiling using cDNA microarrays, Nat. Genet. 21 (S1) (1999) 10–14, https://doi.org/10.1038/4434.
[132] M. Schena, D. Shalon, R.W. Davis, P.O. Brown, Quantitative monitoring of gene expression patterns with a complementary DNA microarray, Science 270 (5235) (1995) 467–470, https://doi.org/10.1126/science.270.5235.467.
[133] E. Kopf, D. Shnitzer, D. Zharhary, Panorama™ ab microarray cell signaling kit: a unique tool for protein expression analysis, Proteomics 5 (9) (2005) 2412–2416, https://doi.org/10.1002/pmic.200401305.
[134] I. Sielaff, A. Arnold, G. Godin, S. Tugulu, H.-A. Klok, K. Johnsson, Protein function microarrays based on self-immobilizing and self-labeling fusion proteins, ChemBioChem 7 (1) (2006) 194–202, https://doi.org/10.1002/cbic.200500278.

[135] P. Kralik, M. Ricchi, A basic guide to real time PCR in microbial diagnostics: definitions, parameters, and everything, Front. Microbiol. 8 (2017), https://doi.org/10.3389/fmicb.2017.00108.

[136] N.L. Anderson, J. Taylor, A.E. Scandora, B.P. Coulter, N.G. Anderson, The TYCHO system for computer analysis of two-dimensional gel electrophoresis patterns, Clin. Chem. 27 (11) (1981) 1807–1820.

[137] P.H. O'Farrell, High resolution two-dimensional electrophoresis of proteins, J. Biol. Chem. 250 (10) (1975) 4007–4021.

[138] P.G. Righetti, A. Castagna, P. Antonioli, E. Boschetti, Prefractionation techniques in proteome analysis: the mining tools of the third millennium, Electrophoresis 26 (2) (2005) 297–319, https://doi.org/10.1002/elps.200406189.

[139] T. Stasyk, L.A. Huber, Zooming in: fractionation strategies in proteomics, Proteomics 4 (12) (2004) 3704–3716, https://doi.org/10.1002/pmic.200401048.

[140] X. Sun, J.-F. Chiu, Q.-Y. He, Application of immobilized metal affinity chromatography in proteomics, Expert Rev. Proteom. 2 (5) (2014) 649–657, https://doi.org/10.1586/14789450.2.5.649.

[141] J.N. Adkins, S.M. Varnum, K.J. Auberry, R.J. Moore, N.H. Angell, R.D. Smith, et al., Toward a human blood serum proteome, Mol. Cell. Proteomics 1 (12) (2002) 947–955, https://doi.org/10.1074/mcp.M200066-MCP200.

[142] S. Gu, Y. Du, J. Chen, Z. Liu, E.M. Bradbury, C.-A.A. Hu, et al., Large-scale quantitative proteomic study of PUMA-induced apoptosis using two-dimensional liquid chromatography–mass spectrometry coupled with amino acid-coded mass tagging, J. Proteome Res. 3 (6) (2004) 1191–1200, https://doi.org/10.1021/pr049893a.

[143] G. Heine, M. Raida, W.-G. Forssmann, Mapping of peptides and protein fragments in human urine using liquid chromatography-mass spectrometry, J. Chromatogr. A 776 (1) (1997) 117–124, https://doi.org/10.1016/s0021-9673(97)00440-8.

[144] H. Skalnikova, P. Halada, P. Dzubak, M. Hajduch, H. Kovarova, Protein fingerprints of anti-cancer effects of cyclin-dependent kinase inhibition: identification of candidate biomarkers using 2-D liquid phase separation coupled to mass spectrometry, Technol. Cancer Res. Treat. 4 (4) (2016) 447–454, https://doi.org/10.1177/153303460500400412.

[145] K.-H. Song, H.-M. An, H.-J. Kim, S.-H. Ahn, S.-J. Chung, C.-K. Shim, Simple liquid chromatography-electrospray ionization mass spectrometry method for the routine determination of salmon calcitonin in serum, J. Chromatogr. B 775 (2) (2002) 247–255, https://doi.org/10.1016/s1570-0232(02)00316-1.

[146] M. Karas, F. Hillenkamp, Laser desorption ionization of proteins with molecular masses exceeding 10,000 daltons, Anal. Chem. 60 (20) (2002) 2299–2301, https://doi.org/10.1021/ac00171a028.

[147] J.B. Fenn, M. Mann, C.K. Meng, S.F. Wong, C.M. Whitehouse, Electrospray ionization for mass spectrometry of large biomolecules, Science 246 (4926) (1989) 64–71, https://doi.org/10.1126/science.2675315.

[148] P. Kebarle, A brief overview of the present status of the mechanisms involved in electrospray mass spectrometry, J. Mass Spectrom. 35 (7) (2000) 804–817, https://doi.org/10.1002/1096-9888(200007)35:7<804::Aid-jms22>3.0.Co;2-q.

[149] F. Valianpour, R.J. Wanders, P.G. Barth, H. Overmars, A.H. van Gennip, Quantitative and compositional study of cardiolipin in platelets by electrospray ionization mass spectrometry: application for the identification of Barth syndrome patients, Clin. Chem. 48 (9) (2002) 1390–1397.

[150] C.M. Whitehouse, R.N. Dreyer, M. Yamashita, J.B. Fenn, Electrospray interface for liquid chromatographs and mass spectrometers, Anal. Chem. 57 (3) (2002) 675–679, https://doi.org/10.1021/ac00280a023.

[151] H.J. Issaq, T.D. Veenstra, T.P. Conrads, D. Felschow, The SELDI-TOF MS approach to proteomics: protein profiling and biomarker identification, Biochem. Biophys. Res. Commun. 292 (3) (2002) 587–592, https://doi.org/10.1006/bbrc.2002.6678.

[152] S. Vorderwülbecke, S. Cleverley, S.R. Weinberger, A. Wiesner, Protein quantification by the SELDI-TOF-MS-based ProteinChip system, Nat. Methods 2 (5) (2005) 393–395, https://doi.org/10.1038/nmeth0505-393.

[153] C. Liu, The application of SELDI-TOF-MS in clinical diagnosis of cancers, J. Biomed. Biotechnol. 2011 (2011) 1–6, https://doi.org/10.1155/2011/245821.

[154] F. Simpkins, J.A. Czechowicz, L. Liotta, E.C. Kohn, SELDI-TOF mass spectrometry for cancer biomarker discovery and serum proteomic diagnostics, Pharmacogenomics 6 (6) (2005) 647–653, https://doi.org/10.2217/14622416.6.6.647.

[155] A.I. Archakov, V.M. Govorun, A.V. Dubanov, Y.D. Ivanov, A.V. Veselovsky, P. Lewi, et al., Protein-protein interactions as a target for drugs in proteomics, Proteomics 3 (4) (2003) 380–391, https://doi.org/10.1002/pmic.200390053.

[156] P.R. Graves, J.J. Kwiek, P. Fadden, R. Ray, K. Hardeman, A.M. Coley, et al., Discovery of novel targets of quinoline drugs in the human purine binding proteome, Mol. Pharmacol. 62 (6) (2002) 1364–1372, https://doi.org/10.1124/mol.62.6.1364.

[157] K.K. Kopec, D. Bozyczko-Coyne, M. Williams, Target identification and validation in drug discovery: the role of proteomics, Biochem. Pharmacol. 69 (8) (2005) 1133–1139, https://doi.org/10.1016/j.bcp.2005.01.004.

[158] T. Imamura, F. Kanai, T. Kawakami, J. Amarsanaa, H. Ijichi, Y. Hoshida, et al., Proteomic analysis of the TGF-β signaling pathway in pancreatic carcinoma cells using stable RNA interference to silence Smad4 expression, Biochem. Biophys. Res. Commun. 318 (1) (2004) 289–296, https://doi.org/10.1016/j.bbrc.2004.04.029.

[159] R.S. Boyd, P.J. Adam, S. Patel, J.A. Loader, J. Berry, N.T. Redpath, et al., Proteomic analysis of the cell-surface membrane in chronic lymphocytic leukemia: identification of two novel proteins, BCNP1 and MIG2B, Leukemia 17 (8) (2003) 1605–1612, https://doi.org/10.1038/sj.leu.2402993.

[160] W. Hu, W. Wu, C.F. Verschraegen, L. Chen, L. Mao, S.-C.J. Yeung, et al., Proteomic identification of heat shock protein 70 as a candidate target for enhancing apoptosis induced by farnesyl transferase inhibitor, Proteomics 3 (10) (2003) 1904–1911, https://doi.org/10.1002/pmic.200300547.

[161] M. Takashima, Y. Kuramitsu, Y. Yokoyama, N. Iizuka, T. Toda, I. Sakaida, et al., Proteomic profiling of heat shock protein 70 family members as biomarkers for hepatitis C virus-related hepatocellular carcinoma, Proteomics 3 (12) (2003) 2487–2493, https://doi.org/10.1002/pmic.200300621.

[162] P.J. Adam, R. Boyd, K.L. Tyson, G.C. Fletcher, A. Stamps, L. Hudson, et al., Comprehensive proteomic analysis of breast cancer cell membranes reveals unique proteins with potential roles in clinical cancer, J. Biol. Chem. 278 (8) (2003) 6482–6489, https://doi.org/10.1074/jbc.M210184200.

[163] H. Towbin, K.W. Bair, J.A. DeCaprio, M.J. Eck, S. Kim, F.R. Kinder, et al., Proteomics-based target identification, J. Biol. Chem. 278 (52) (2003) 52964–52971, https://doi.org/10.1074/jbc.M309039200.

[164] J.K. Kumar, S. Tabor, C.C. Richardson, Proteomic analysis of thioredoxin-targeted proteins in Escherichia coli, Proc. Natl. Acad. Sci. 101 (11) (2004) 3759–3764, https://doi.org/10.1073/pnas.0308701101.

[165] K. Godl, J. Wissing, A. Kurtenbach, P. Habenberger, S. Blencke, H. Gutbrod, et al., An efficient proteomics method to identify the cellular targets of protein kinase inhibitors, Proc. Natl. Acad. Sci. 100 (26) (2003) 15434–15439, https://doi.org/10.1073/pnas.2535024100.

[166] M. Okada, H. Itoh, T. Hatakeyama, H. Tokumitsu, R. Kobayashi, Hsp90 is a direct target of the anti-allergic drugs disodium cromoglycate and amlexanox, Biochem. J. 374 (2) (2003) 433–441, https://doi.org/10.1042/bj20030351.

[167] K.E. Luker, M.C.P. Smith, G.D. Luker, S.T. Gammon, H. Piwnica-Worms, D. Piwnica-Worms, Kinetics of regulated protein-protein interactions revealed with firefly luciferase complementation imaging in cells and living animals, Proc. Natl. Acad. Sci. 101 (33) (2004) 12288–12293, https://doi.org/10.1073/pnas.0404041101.
[168] I.G. Serebriiskii, O. Mitina, E.N. Pugacheva, E. Benevolenskaya, E. Kotova, G.G. Toby, et al., Detection of peptides, proteins, and drugs that selectively interact with protein targets, Genome Res. 12 (11) (2002) 1785–1791, https://doi.org/10.1101/gr.450702.
[169] M. Rodriguez, S.S.C. Li, J.W. Harper, Z. Songyang, An oriented peptide array library (OPAL) strategy to study protein-protein interactions, J. Biol. Chem. 279 (10) (2004) 8802–8807, https://doi.org/10.1074/jbc.M311886200.
[170] D.B. Longley, P.G. Johnston, Molecular mechanisms of drug resistance, J. Pathol. 205 (2) (2005) 275–292, https://doi.org/10.1002/path.1706.
[171] Y. Wang, Q.-Y. He, C.-M. Che, J.-F. Chiu, Proteomic characterization of the cytotoxic mechanism of gold (III) porphyrin 1a, a potential anticancer drug, Proteomics 6 (1) (2006) 131–142, https://doi.org/10.1002/pmic.200402027.
[172] J.P. MacKeigan, C.M. Clements, J.D. Lich, R.M. Pope, Y. Hod, J.P. Ting, Proteomic profiling drug-induced apoptosis in non-small cell lung carcinoma: identification of RS/DJ-1 and RhoGDIalpha, Cancer Res. 63 (20) (2003) 6928–6934.
[173] E. O'Neill, L. Rushworth, M. Baccarini, W. Kolch, Role of the kinase MST2 in suppression of apoptosis by the proto-oncogene product Raf-1, Science 306 (5705) (2004) 2267–2270, https://doi.org/10.1126/science.1103233.
[174] D. Brehmer, Z. Greff, K. Godl, S. Blencke, A. Kurtenbach, M. Weber, et al., Cellular targets of gefitinib, Cancer Res. 65 (2) (2005) 379–382.
[175] B. Sitek, O. Apostolov, K. Stühler, K. Pfeiffer, H.E. Meyer, A. Eggert, et al., Identification of dynamic proteome changes upon ligand activation of Trk-receptors using two-dimensional fluorescence difference gel electrophoresis and mass spectrometry, Mol. Cell. Proteomics 4 (3) (2005) 291–299, https://doi.org/10.1074/mcp.M400188-MCP200.
[176] Y. Shiio, K.S. Suh, H. Lee, S.H. Yuspa, R.N. Eisenman, R. Aebersold, Quantitative proteomic analysis of Myc-induced apoptosis, J. Biol. Chem. 281 (5) (2006) 2750–2756, https://doi.org/10.1074/jbc.M509349200.
[177] M.L. Reyzer, R.L. Caldwell, T.C. Dugger, J.T. Forbes, C.A. Ritter, M. Guix, et al., Early changes in protein expression detected by mass spectrometry predict tumor response to molecular therapeutics, Cancer Res. 64 (24) (2004) 9093–9100, https://doi.org/10.1158/0008-5472.Can-04-2231.
[178] N. Li, R. Guo, W. Li, J. Shao, S. Li, K. Zhao, et al., A proteomic investigation into a human gastric cancer cell line BGC823 treated with diallyl trisulfide, Carcinogenesis 27 (6) (2006) 1222–1231, https://doi.org/10.1093/carcin/bgi306.
[179] E.-K. Yim, K.-H. Lee, J.S. Bae, S.-E. Namkoong, S.-J. Um, J.-S. Park, Proteomic analysis of antiproliferative effects by treatment of 5-fluorouracil in cervical cancer cells, DNA Cell Biol. 23 (11) (2004) 769–776, https://doi.org/10.1089/dna.2004.23.769.
[180] J. Chen, Q.-Y. He, A.P.-W. Yuen, J.-F. Chiu, Proteomics of buccal squamous cell carcinoma: the involvement of multiple pathways in tumorigenesis, Proteomics 4 (8) (2004) 2465–2475, https://doi.org/10.1002/pmic.200300762.
[181] A.T.Y. Lau, Q.-Y. He, J.-F. Chiu, A proteome analysis of the arsenite response in cultured lung cells: evidence for in vitro oxidative stress-induced apoptosis, Biochem. J. 382 (2) (2004) 641–650, https://doi.org/10.1042/bj20040224.
[182] S.T. Nawrocki, J.S. Carew, M.S. Pino, R.A. Highshaw, K. Dunner, P. Huang, et al., Bortezomib sensitizes pancreatic cancer cells to endoplasmic reticulum stress-mediated apoptosis, Cancer Res. 65 (24) (2005) 11658–11666, https://doi.org/10.1158/0008-5472.Can-05-2370.

[183] A. Venkatraman, A. Landar, A.J. Davis, L. Chamlee, T. Sanderson, H. Kim, et al., Modification of the mitochondrial proteome in response to the stress of ethanol-dependent hepatotoxicity, J. Biol. Chem. 279 (21) (2004) 22092–22101, https://doi.org/10.1074/jbc.M402245200.

[184] Y. Yamazaki, M. Tsuruga, D. Zhou, Y. Fujita, X. Shang, Y. Dang, et al., Cytoskeletal disruption accelerates caspase-3 activation and alters the intracellular membrane reorganization in DNA damage-induced apoptosis, Exp. Cell Res. 259 (1) (2000) 64–78, https://doi.org/10.1006/excr.2000.4970.

[185] Y. Yan, V.M. Weaver, I.A. Blair, Analysis of protein expression during oxidative stress in breast epithelial cells using a stable isotope labeled proteome internal standard, J. Proteome Res. 4 (6) (2005) 2007–2014, https://doi.org/10.1021/pr050175d.

[186] S.K. Niture, C.E. Doneanu, C.S. Velu, N.I. Bailey, K.S. Srivenugopal, Proteomic analysis of human O6-methylguanine-DNA methyltransferase by affinity chromatography and tandem mass spectrometry, Biochem. Biophys. Res. Commun. 337 (4) (2005) 1176–1184, https://doi.org/10.1016/j.bbrc.2005.09.177.

[187] M.A. Jordan, L. Wilson, Microtubules and actin filaments: dynamic targets for cancer chemotherapy, Curr. Opin. Cell Biol. 10 (1) (1998) 123–130, https://doi.org/10.1016/s0955-0674(98)80095-1.

[188] N.M. Verrills, B.J. Walsh, G.S. Cobon, P.G. Hains, M. Kavallaris, Proteome analysis of vinca alkaloid response and resistance in acute lymphoblastic leukemia reveals novel cytoskeletal alterations, J. Biol. Chem. 278 (46) (2003) 45082–45093, https://doi.org/10.1074/jbc.M303378200.

[189] H. Bernstein, C.M. Payne, K. Kunke, C.L. Crowley-Weber, C.N. Waltmire, K. Dvorakova, et al., A proteomic study of resistance to deoxycholate-induced apoptosis, Carcinogenesis 25 (5) (2004) 681–692, https://doi.org/10.1093/carcin/bgh072.

[190] A. Castagna, P. Antonioli, H. Astner, M. Hamdan, S.C. Righetti, P. Perego, et al., A proteomic approach to cisplatin resistance in the cervix squamous cell carcinoma cell line A431, Proteomics 4 (10) (2004) 3246–3267, https://doi.org/10.1002/pmic.200400835.

[191] J.E. Celis, H. Wolf, M. Østergaard, Bladder squamous cell carcinoma biomarkers derived from proteomics, Electrophoresis 21 (11) (2000) 2115–2121, https://doi.org/10.1002/1522-2683(20000601)21:11<2115::Aid-elps2115>3.0.Co;2-k.

[192] Q.-Y. He, G.K.K. Lau, Y. Zhou, S.-T. Yuen, M.C. Lin, H.-F. Kung, et al., Serum biomarkers of hepatitis B virus infected liver inflammation: a proteomic study, Proteomics 3 (5) (2003) 666–674, https://doi.org/10.1002/pmic.200300394.

[193] M. Mayr, J. Zhang, A.S. Greene, D. Gutterman, J. Perloff, P. Ping, Proteomics-based development of biomarkers in cardiovascular disease, Mol. Cell. Proteomics 5 (10) (2006) 1853–1864, https://doi.org/10.1074/mcp.R600007-MCP200.

[194] Q.-Y. He, J. Chen, H.-F. Kung, A.P.-W. Yuen, J.-F. Chiu, Identification of tumor-associated proteins in oral tongue squamous cell carcinoma by proteomics, Proteomics 4 (1) (2004) 271–278, https://doi.org/10.1002/pmic.200300550.

[195] V. Paradis, F. Degos, D. Dargère, N. Pham, J. Belghiti, C. Degott, et al., Identification of a new marker of hepatocellular carcinoma by serum protein profiling of patients with chronic liver diseases, Hepatology 41 (1) (2005) 40–47, https://doi.org/10.1002/hep.20505.

[196] K.-S. Park, H. Kim, N.-G. Kim, S.Y. Cho, K.-H. Choi, J.K. Seong, et al., Proteomic analysis and molecular characterization of tissue ferritin light chain in hepatocellular carcinoma, Hepatology 35 (6) (2002) 1459–1466, https://doi.org/10.1053/jhep.2002.33204.

[197] S.-J. Ding, Y. Li, Y.-X. Tan, M.-R. Jiang, B. Tian, Y.-K. Liu, et al., From proteomic analysis to clinical significance, Mol. Cell. Proteomics 3 (1) (2004) 73–81, https://doi.org/10.1074/mcp.M300094-MCP200.

[198] M.A. Comunale, M. Lowman, R.E. Long, J. Krakover, R. Philip, S. Seeholzer, et al., Proteomic analysis of serum associated fucosylated glycoproteins in the development of primary hepatocellular carcinoma, J. Proteome Res. 5 (2) (2006) 308–315, https://doi.org/10.1021/pr050328x.
[199] H.J. An, D.S. Kim, Y.K. Park, S.K. Kim, Y.P. Choi, S. Kang, et al., Comparative proteomics of ovarian epithelial tumors, J. Proteome Res. 5 (5) (2006) 1082–1090, https://doi.org/10.1021/pr050461p.
[200] E.F. Petricoin, A.M. Ardekani, B.A. Hitt, P.J. Levine, V.A. Fusaro, S.M. Steinberg, et al., Use of proteomic patterns in serum to identify ovarian cancer, Lancet 359 (9306) (2002) 572–577, https://doi.org/10.1016/s0140-6736(02)07746-2.
[201] B.-L. Adam, A. Vlahou, O.J. Semmes, J.G.L. Wright, Proteomic approaches to biomarker discovery in prostate and bladder cancers, Proteomics 1 (10) (2001) 1264–1270, https://doi.org/10.1002/1615-9861(200110)1:10<1264::Aid-prot1264>3.0.Co;2-r.
[202] H.B. Grossman, Surveillance for recurrent bladder cancer using a point-of-care proteomic assay, JAMA 295 (3) (2006), https://doi.org/10.1001/jama.295.3.299.
[203] T. Yoshiki, Y. Arai, A. Terai, K. Yoshimura, K. Kontani, Y. Okada, et al., Identification by proteomic analysis of calreticulin as a marker for bladder cancer and evaluation of the diagnostic accuracy of its detection in urine, Clin. Chem. 50 (5) (2004) 857–866, https://doi.org/10.1373/clinchem.2003.027425.
[204] E.F. Petricoin, D.K. Ornstein, L.A. Liotta, Clinical proteomics: applications for prostate cancer biomarker discovery and detection, Urol. Oncol. 22 (4) (2004) 322–328, https://doi.org/10.1016/j.urolonc.2004.04.011.

CHAPTER 4

Artificial intelligence (AI) and machine learning in the treatment of various diseases

Pooja Mittal[a], Rajat Goyal[b], Ramit Kapoor[c], and Rupesh Kumar Gautam[d]
[a]Chitkara College of Pharmacy, Chitkara University, Rajpura, Punjab, India
[b]MM College of Pharmacy, Maharishi Markandeshwar (Deemed to be University), Mullana, Ambala, Haryana, India
[c]Clarivate India Pvt. Ltd, Noida, Uttar Pradesh, India
[d]Department of Pharmacology, Indore Institute of Pharmacy, IIST Campus, Indore, Madhya Pradesh, India

1. Introduction

Artificial Intelligence (AI) and Machine Learning (ML) have significant ability in improving the health care research. The adoption of AI-driven technologies can aid in the elimination of health disparities and reduce the load on healthcare systems [1]. AI and ML and even could be utilized to treat a wide range of disorders such as

- **Infectious diseases**: Despite advancements in healthcare sectors, infectious illnesses such as Spanish flu, tuberculosis, Ebola, SARS, and influenza have remained among the major reasons of mortality worldwide, particularly in low-income nations. Healthcare organizations and academics have devised novel approaches to enhance the health-care industry, particularly attempts to track the transmission of infectious illnesses. ML and AI are currently modifying the manner in which diseases are treated by predicting the virus's path and devising novel containment approaches. While national authorities across the world work with local authorities and health professionals to track, respond to, and halt the exposure of infectious diseases, health specialists use statistical models to enhance existing interventions and prevent additional infections. The advancement of mathematical techniques helps researchers to effectively anticipate the spread of infectious disease, take into account the unique characteristics of every pathogen, and determine vaccine distribution priorities. Advanced analytics could be extremely

Computational Approaches in Drug Discovery, Development and Systems Pharmacology
https://doi.org/10.1016/B978-0-323-99137-7.00010-1

useful in reacting to fatal epidemics because they can assess enormous amounts of data, such as health data, human behavior patterns, and environmental variables. [1,2]

- **Chronic airway diseases**: Severe respiratory disorders are marked by inflammation, blockage, and remodeling of the airways, and they are common, specifically in developing nations. Asthma and chronic obstructive pulmonary disease (COPD) have the largest global morbidity and economic impact [2]. Regardless of the fact that there are several protocols for the prevention, timely detection, and appropriate treatment of various chronic illnesses, their utility in precision medicine is limited. ML and AI strategies have developed as viable tools for mining and synthesizing significant, heterogeneous medical information for clinical practice, and various AI and ML technologies have recently been used to treat asthma and COPD. Yet, just a few approaches have had a substantial impact on clinical practice. [3]
- **Ophthalmic disorders**: AI, ML, and Deep Learning (DL) methods have already been demonstrated to be efficient diagnostic tools for recognizing and diagnosing several eye disorders in ophthalmic health care services in a number of recent research. Because of the widespread usage of ophthalmic pictures, which offer a vast amount of information to a computer algorithm, ophthalmology, in contrast to other medical specialities, adapts itself very well to AI-, ML-, and DL-assisted automated screening and diagnosing. [4]
- **Diabetic retinopathy**: Both the diabetic retinopathy and DME lead to impairment of the central vision because of the increasing retinal microvascular problems and leakage of fluid from aberrant blood vessels in retinas of the persons suffering from diabetes. As a result, large-scale DR screening is urgently needed to identify potential changes that could be life threatening at an initial stage, which would be helpful for better monitoring and treatment. Moreover, early intervention is well considered as being the most cost-effective approach. Timely screening of DR and DME by regular and careful monitoring by clinical assessment or evaluation of retinal images is thus critical in order to avoid vision loss due to sight-threatening retinopathy. Periodic retinal screening using fundus digital photography, fundus luorescein angiography, and optical coherence tomography (OCT) is encouraged; however, in many countries, this is a significant difficulty and an issue. According to data provided on worldwide incidence of diabetes and diabetes-related vision loss, as well as the lack of ophthalmologists, retina specialists, and

qualified human graders, providing adequate diabetic screening will be a difficult task for current global health-care administration. Analyzing the pictures takes time, money, and is exposed to human error. As a result, these problems may be handled exclusively through unmanned automated implementations of revolutionary ways of analysis that do not require the involvement of human experts. [1]

- **AMD**: AMD is an irreversible severe disorder that is marked by drusen, retinal pigment alterations, choroidal neovascularization, hemorrhage, exudation, and occasionally geographic atrophy. It affects the elderly, causing vision impairment, anxiety, a decrease in quality of life, and eventually death. Generally, drusen either in or out of retinal pigment epithelium trigger macular degeneration, which leads to visual impairment in AMD. Hard drusen and soft drusen are the two main forms of drusen. Soft drusen, on the other hand, is more common in the adult population and can cause choroidal neovascularization, which can lead to vision loss. As a result, monitoring drusen quantitatively is critical for preventing macular degeneration. Traditional manual drusen measures with current visual evaluation, on the other hand, consumes significant time, involves a lot of work, and yield a less reliable result. As a result, assumptions centered on drusen may be made using AI, ML, and DL algorithms to make customized AMD forecasts. In the case of AMD, these complex algorithms can anticipate drusen beneath the retina. By utilizing retinal pictures and spectral-domain OCT, AI, ML, and DL algorithms offer automatic identification of drusen, fluid, and geographical atrophy in AMD lesions, allowing for better AMD diagnosis and therapy. Automatic drusen identification using AI, ML, and DL is anticipated to aid ophthalmologists in improving fundus imaging diagnostic performance. [4]
- **Glaucoma**: Glaucoma is characterized by progressive neurodegeneration of retinal ganglion cells and permanent loss of axons from the optic nerve, making it the second most frequent reason of blindness in the world. The importance of early glaucoma identification and treatment in avoiding probable blindness cannot be overstated. For early glaucoma diagnosis, the optic nerve head (ONH) and retinal nerve fiber layer (RNFL) around the optic disk must be examined. OCT allows for a quantitative assessment of glaucomatous structural alterations. In both industrialized and developing nations, however, the scarcity of retinal imaging technologies, retina specialists, general ophthalmologists, ophthalmologic graders, eye clinics, and healthcare facilities is a major issue.

Furthermore, glaucoma sufferers, particularly in developing nations, have issues with the accessibility, availability, cost, and stability of ocular health care services. It is consequently critical for AI, ML, and DL to diagnose glaucoma automatically. VFs, fundus pictures, and OCT scans were utilized to build the AI-, ML-, and DL-based glaucomatous diagnosis systems. However, a set of standardized VF test is significant in the diagnosis and monitoring of glaucoma, and it takes a long time and requires a lot of resources. Furthermore, such a patient-performed manual method is subjective and has proven difficult to study in epidemiological research. AI, ML, and DL techniques, on the other hand, have demonstrated great performance in the categorization of glaucoma and healthy eyes in a short amount of time. Ophthalmologists can use these automated data to help them make improved therapeutic judgments. AI, ML, and deep learning are thought to have the potential to revolutionize glaucoma screening, diagnosis, and classification. [1] [4]

2. Types of artificial intelligence with respect to healthcare

AI is not only a single technology, rather than it is a network of various aspects that uses their principles and are relevant in the field of medicine and are helpful for the treatment and detection principles of the disease. Some of the important attributes of AI w.r.t healthcare are mentioned below:

- ML, Neural Networking (NN), and DL: ML, NN, and DL are the main techniques of AI. These concepts uses the data and put that data in statistical models to estimate the attributes. The most common application of ML is the precision medicine, which is derived from the traditional medicine. In precision medicine, it is depicted that which treatment protocol is going to work best in context to the various patient attributes. Majority of ML and precision medicine require the training database for which the outcome is known. That data set is called as supervised learning. The more complex part of ML is NN, which was developed in 1960s and now it is completely established in the healthcare field. NN is applied for the categorization applications like whether the patient will get this disease or not whose decisions are taken by the software based on the data inputs and outputs. It works similarly like the neurons work in human brain and take the decisions of the human body, so the name is NN. The higher level of difficulty arises with deep learning where NN exists with many levels or variables that predict the outcome. The most common application of DL in healthcare and medicine is the identification of cancerous tissue in the scanning images. Also, the DL is being applied in the radiology where it is being applied to perceive the data which is out of sight of the human eye. Hence, the DL, NN, and ML are found in the detection and diagnosis of cancer [1,2,4,5]. This application of AI founds to be more promising tool for the detection of cancers rather than any available tool. It is also being utilized for the speech identification by using other tool known as Natural Language Processing (NLP).

- Natural Language Processing: NLP involves the applications such as recognition of human speech, speech analysis, and translation. In pharmaceutical field or in healthcare department, NLP involves the formation of clinical documents, their understanding, classification, and to publish the research work. NLP systems can analyze the unstructured data, they can prepare reports, and can conduct the conversational AI [6,7].
- Robotic systems: Now a days, we all are familiar with the physical robots, according to study, each year about 200,000 robots are being installed throughout the world. Robots can perform the task that are predefined like they can be used to deliver the supplies in the hospital, welding, or assembling objects. Now a days, robots are becoming more intelligent with the collaboration of AI capabilities in their brains and are even getting more collaborative with the humans, getting trained easily while moving them through the desired task. Even, surgical robots were approved in U.S. in 2000 who enhanced the power of the surgeons because of their ability to create more precise incision, improved the ability to see inside the body so that the surgery can be more successful, stitching of the cuts precisely, etc.; however, the important decisions are still taken by the human doctors not by the robots. The various surgical procedures involving surgical robots are prostrate surgery, gynecological surgery, many cancer radiological surgeries, and head and neck surgery as well [2,6,8].

3. Role of AI in drug research and development

AI is caughting up the roots of each and every sector particularly in healthcare and pharmaceutical industry. It is being implemented in various sectors such as pharmaceutical drug discovery, development, drug repurposing, improved drug therapy, clinical trials, and drug designing, the use of AI in these field can enhance the precision and accuracy and can reduce the human errors and make the work easier and more convenient. By using AI in drug designing and development, we can easily identify the targets and can develop the target susceptible drugs only which will reduce the wastage of time and money. In earlier time, the vast chemical space leads to the problems in the drug development, but now a days, the use of AI can solve this problem. AI can easily identify the drug target, identify the drug lead, and can provide the quick drug target validation. Inspite of these applications, the AI faces some big challenges such as uncertainty and diversity in the database. Quantitative structure-activity relationship (QSAR) based data base can rapidly predict the vast number of molecules and can also predict the various physicochemical properties of the molecules like Log P, etc. from the available database and physicochemical properties of the compounds, these database can also predict various other properties such as biological activities and efficacy of the compounds; moreover, these systems are still associated with some drawbacks such as lack of data base for specificity and validation of the approaches. To overcome the existing problems of QSAR, AI has developed the other approaches such as ML, DL, and NN, which can be applied for safety and toxicity evaluation of drug molecules. The virtual space suggests the geographical map of the molecules by demonstration of their molecules and their corresponding properties. The chemical space collects the information about the molecules within the space for the active compounds, and therefore, the virtual screening identifies the molecules and helps in further screening. Several chemical spaces are PubChem, ChemBank, DrugBank, and ChemDB, etc. [9–12] (Fig. 1).

- **AI in drug screening**: The process of drug screening and development approximately takes about 15 years and billions of dollars on average. Then too, 9 out of 10 molecules did not pass the phase II clinical trials and some fails the regulatory approvals. Many algorithms such as Nearest-Neighbors classifiers, extreme learning machines, and deep neural networks have been explored in these cases for the virtual space-based screening. Many of the pharmaceutical companies like Roche, Pfizer, and Bayer's have tied up with IT companies for these virtual space-based work. AI in short can be used in each and every aspect of drug designing. Role of AI in the prediction of physicochemical properties cannot be ignored as the physicochemical properties like Log *P*, solubility, partition coefficient, and intrinsic permeability of the drug directly affect the pharmacokinetics of the drug, and pharmacokinetics is directly related to the bioavailability and efficacy of the drug, hence

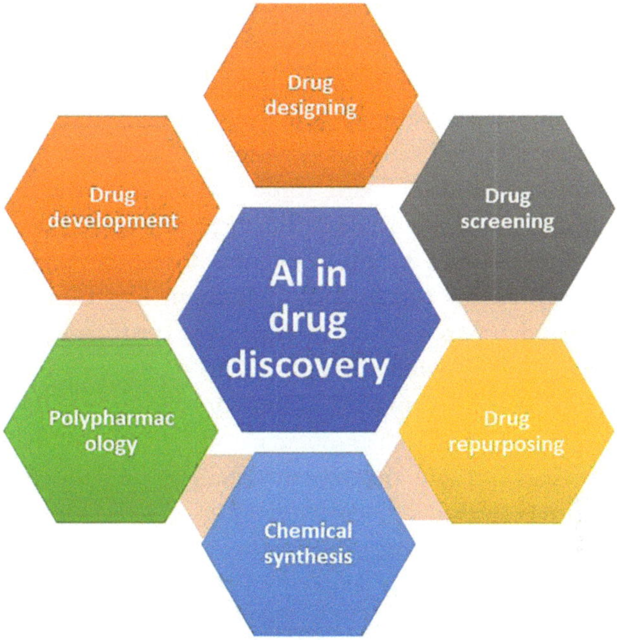

Fig. 1 AI in various fields of drug discovery.

it must be consider during the target identification. Different AI-based tools can predict the physicochemical properties of the target molecules [3–6,13].

- **Bioactivity prediction**: For the drugs to be biologically active, it is essential that the developed molecule should interact with the target protein or receptor. The more the drug target interaction, the higher is the bioactivity of the drug. Sometime, it also happens that the developed molecules do not have any interaction for the target protein and sometimes the interaction of the drug with the target can leads to the toxicity as well. Hence, it is essential to conduct the drug target-binding affinity (DTBA) studies so that the estimate of Drug-Target can be made. AI and its techniques can made these estimations by considering the features or the similarities in the structures of drug and its targets. In feature-based interactions, feature vectors are being determined by considering the chemical moieties of the drugs and the targets while in similarities based interactions, the similarities that exist between the drug and the targets are being considered. A number of web applications like ChemMapper and the similarity ensemble approach (SEA) are there for this work.

A number of tools are there to determine the DTBA like KronRLS, SimBoost, DeepDTA, and PADME [8–10,14].

- **Toxicity prediction**: Prediction of the drug receptor toxicity is a very important step in the development of a new drug molecule. Normally, it can be measured by cell assay, in vitro cell line analysis followed by animal based in vivo studies. These studies when performed on each and every individual molecule lead to the increased expense of the research. To cut the cost, AI-based tools can be used here, and many web-based tools are available for the toxicity estimation like LimTox, pkCSM, admetSAR, and Toxtree. These tools provide the toxicity-related information based on the input data about the compound. For example: DeepTox performs the toxicity evaluation studies by identification of the chemical properties such as molecular weight and vander walls forces of the molecules and gave the toxicity details on predefined toxicophore features [1,11,12,15,16]
- **AI in drug development**:

  Identification of drug target structure: It is necessary to find the right target for the drug or we can also say that is essential to assign the right drug to its compatible target. Then only the drug can be bioactive if it having the good binding capacity to its target. A number of proteins are involved when a disease occurs and some of the proteins are overexpressed, and our work is to find out the overexpressed receptors for that particular disease and target the drug to that receptors only. Hence, it is essential to find out the structure of the target protein so that the selective targeting can be made successfully. AI can play a vital role in this part as it can help in determination of the 3D structure of the target protein, and the design will be in accordance to the chemical environment of the drug, hence the safety and efficacy considerations can be predicted easily. The AI-based tool AlphaFold that works on the DNN basis determines the distance between the amino acids and the angles of the peptide bonds so that the 3D structure of the protein can be determined [1,6,10–12,16,17].
- **AI in determination of drug-protein interactions**: To know the interactions between the drugs and the proteins is very important aspect in the case of drug development. It is essential to determine the safety, efficacy, and effectiveness of the drug as well as it plays an important role in drug repurposing and polypharmacology. Various methods are being utilized to accurately predict the interactions between ligand and proteins among them one is approach SVM which is trained on 15,000

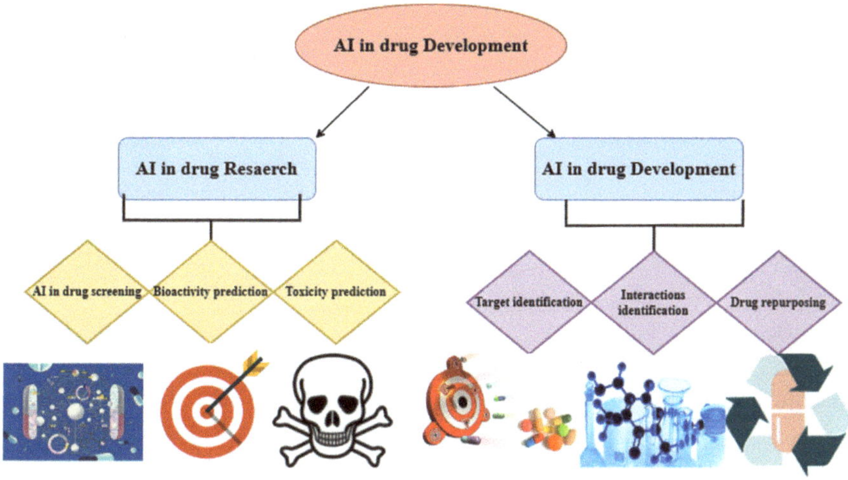

Fig. 2 Role of AI in drug development and drug designing.

protein and ligand interactions. The AI-based prediction of drug target interactions can also be utilized in the field of drug repurposing and avoiding of the polypharmacology. Repurposing of an approved existing drug makes it qualified for directly the clinical trial phase II and reduces the expenditure upto 4.8 million US dollars. For repurposing of a drug, various ML-based techniques can be implemented such as SVM, NN, DL, and logistic regression. Other logistic regression-based techniques such as PREDICT, DSPACE, and other approaches consider the similarity between drug-drug and receptor-receptor, target molecule similarity, etc. [1,8,9,17–20] (Fig. 2).

4. Role of AI in detection of diseases

Detection of disease is an important aspect in healthcare. Without the assessment of disease, no healthcare person can track the disease. However, detection of disease is a long process and involves the long practices and is very time consuming. Here, the demand exceeds far than the supply. This situation has put the doctors under strain which often delay the life saving and this situation leads to life threatening. ML- and AI-based tools can now be utilized in this aspect also which made the diagnosis cost effective and more accessible. MI-based tools also work on the way as doctors work, and they used to diagnose the disease based on the pattern similarity of various factors but they see the similarity of the pattern on number of examples such as

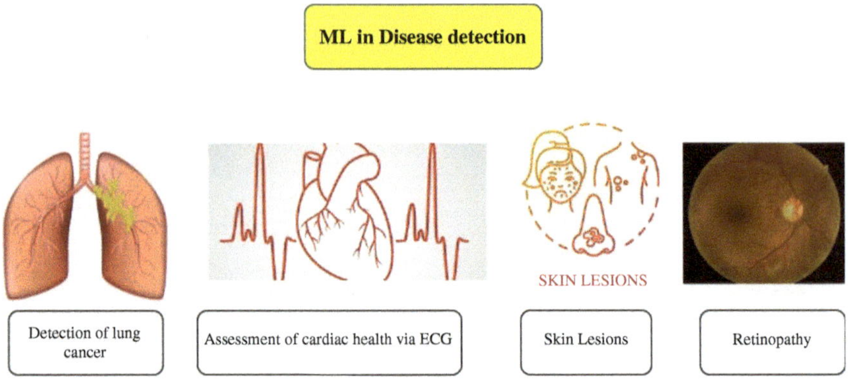

Fig. 3 Role of ML and AI in detection of the disease.

thousands and even more from the stored data. Hence, ML can help only where the diagnostic information is already digitalized for example in case of CT scanning, PET scan, ECG images, MRI data, skin images, and eye images, etc. [16,18,21–24] (Fig. 3).

5. AI and ML in clinical trial research

Clinical trials are no longer an exception; therefore, technology has been progressively used in recent years to help them operate more successfully, accurately, and dynamically. A variety of technical advances have made this feasible, but two in particular—AI and ML—are driving industry-wide revolution[5]. Clinical trials are an important part of the pharmaceutical medication development phase. Clinical trials are significant research that are conducted to evaluate if a medical therapy or equipment is safe and efficacious in individuals. Although the pharmaceutical medication sector has seen its ups and downs, it is still a lucrative field. Global prescription drug spending is anticipated to exceed $1.5 trillion by 2021, as per Quintiles IMS Holding.

Generally, most of the cases associated with the usage of AI and developing new technologies for clinical trials seem to be focused on three main applications: Patient Recruitment, Designing of the Clinical Trials and Optimization of the Clinical Trials [25–28] (Fig. 4).

(A) Patient recruitment

ML and AI really have started to improve the healthcare industry. ML algorithms are being used to fix out some of the major healthcare issues, and AI's uses in health care system now range from information management to establishing treatment programs to genetic analysis. Apart from the optimistic influence that AI seems to have had on

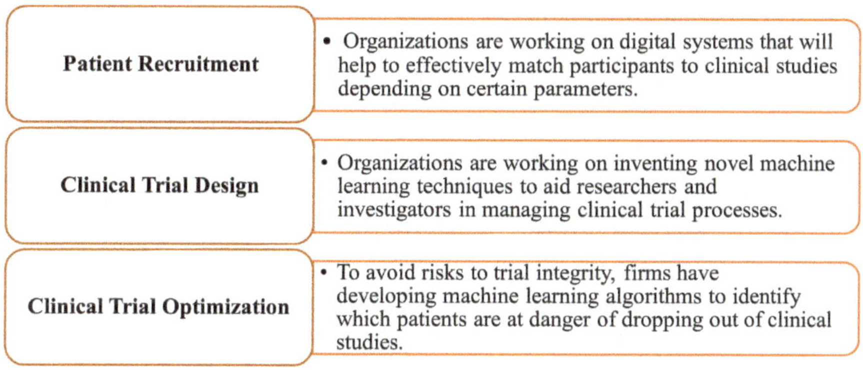

Fig. 4 Role of AI in clinical trials.

the healthcare society at vast, clinical studies have been slow in adopting these technological advances, even after its potential to improve patient outcomes. Patient recruitment, in general, appears to be a key stumbling barrier to success. In the modern era, traditional recruitment techniques have become largely ineffective, and prices have skyrocketed as a by-product.

Following are some number of ways that AI technology might help in the coming years with patient recruiting difficulties:

(1) Advanced digital advertising approaches

Clinical study enrolment is already being accelerated by modern advertising platforms like Google and Facebook. Sponsors and CROs can launch programs that focus study participants based on important inclusion/exclusion variables instead of putting advertisements physically or digitally where they assume their patients would be. Targets may now be identified by the applications they utilize, the digital groups which they attend, former ads in which they acted on, and their purchase history, in addition to their age, locality, and sexual identity. For instance, Facebook's website may compare advertising effectiveness statistics to individuals' geographical information and shown interests, which therefore could be used to find additional prospects that are similar. Additionally, it allows you to discover formerly unexplored groups of eligible participants by dynamically expanding your audience in the most precise possible way. Another advantage of Google AdWords is that it combines research data with user preferences. It enables you to target advertising to potential participants whose web searches suggest that they are close to finalizing a treatment choice. This improves the probability that they will be interested in a new clinical opportunity, which enhances the conversion rate of your ad campaign and, as a result, your ROI [29–33].

(2) Anticipating enrollment outcomes

- Experts at Cincinnati Children's Hospital Medical Centre are developing a novel machine-learning algorithm aimed at improving clinical trial participation by analyzing why the affected patients accept or refuse requests to related research studies.
- To put it another way, the algorithm "analyses, correlates, and interprets data from various sources in order to anticipate particular patient decision-making." The concept is that by using an automated system designed to examine patient's individual data to obtain a better knowledge of their particular prejudices and/or interests, accurate "patient-directed recruiting tactics to enhance participation" may be developed [30,32,34,35].
- This research technology is constantly being used at the hospital's Emergency Department as part of an in-person, per-patient recruitment campaign. Patients reached using standard recruiting techniques accept invites approximately 60% of the time, according to the creators, but the algorithms raise that figure to more than 70%, that will also probably rise as the technology continues to improve [32,33,36].

(3) Patient matching platforms

- Over the past few years, the broad use of EHRs has paved the way for healthcare technology firms to boost novel technology meant that could replace lengthy medical procedures—and the recruiting for the clinical research is no different.
- Leading firms such as Mendel.ai and Deep 6 AI have been developing AI-powered systems that link eligible patients with appropriate medical research possibilities. Patients are only matched with studies that they qualify for, saving time and energy for all concerned stakeholders. Sponsors and CROs acquire listings of participants that perfectly fit their requirements, and patients are only matched with studies that they compatible for.
- The disadvantage of this technique is that participants nowadays have the opportunity of self-selecting. Patients then must upload their own medical information to either of these platforms or grant their physician consent to do so — and individuals who are typically unaware that clinical trials are a legitimate therapeutic option are unlikely to feel obliged to do so. However, if these platforms can build solid collaborations with health care professionals in order to obtain that patient information, they may soon become an effective patient recruiting tool [37–39].

- One thing is obvious, at the end of the day that if clinical studies really require a noticeable change in the domain of recruitment of the participants, they have to begin looking at novel technology and out-of-the-box approaches. AI and ML technology has shown to be a big game-changer in basically all other sector on the globe, therefore I believe it is past time we took a closer look at innovation and advancement. [40]

(B) Clinical trial design

Because of the confluence of vast new digital data sets, computer capacity to find therapeutically significant patterns in the information utilizing effective AI and machine-learning methodologies, and regulatory encouraging this innovation through comprehensive intervention, the prospect of clinical research is on the approach of a transformation. From the academia, the biotechnology sector, nonprofit organizations, regulators, and technology firms, this viewpoint highlights ideas, current advances, and suggestions for integrating insightful algorithmic data into clinical development and health care. Machine-learning frameworks are used to analyze and improve from publicly accessible biomedical and healthcare trial sets of data, direct proof from devices, and medical histories. Through recently disclosed regulatory routes at the US Food and Drug Administration, approaches for upgrading the novel clinical process of development by integrating AI- and ML-based digital techniques and secure networking technologies are presented. Finally, we explore the uses and effect of digital algorithmic evidence in improving patient care [38,40,41].

Over the past 30 years, clinical drug research has stayed mostly constant. This is because of absence of appropriate useful medical and biological sources of data and advanced analytical insights to create theories that could encourage the research and advancement of new diagnostic methods and treatments, as well as regulatory uncertainties, risk reluctance, and skepticism about rapidly developing, yet primarily unsubstantiated innovations (including ML and wireless health monitoring devices and sensors). Because present medicines have been found to only effective for a small percentage of individuals, evaluating novel biomedical therapies for safety and efficacy will necessitate new techniques. However, the use of new technological advances like next-generation sequencing has enhanced both our knowledge of disease processes and the possibility for generating customized treatments in a broader group of patients. The majority of novel compounds authorized by the FDA in recent times, for instance, were developed to target particular abnormalities involved in disease onset and preservation characteristic of targeted therapy, which attempts to personalize treatments based on unique patient features.

Another significant issue in the biomedical research process is presenting the outcomes of most traditional clinical studies on average therapeutic outcomes, which may not effectively transfer into generating customized treatment decisions at the time of care. Further standardized procedures, exploitation of new digital clinical studies and therapeutic response biomarkers susceptible to similar and effective monitoring (such as circulating tumor DNA), enhance safety and effectiveness while also significantly lowering toxic effects and adverse reactions, and increased insights into the patient 's journey via detectors, and low-cost imaging are all appealing strategies to tackle this challenging task [41–43].

Safeguarding, standardizing, and improving routinely obtained information of EHR as a source of reliable clinical findings focused on RWD can help with clinical trial management at the point-of-care and should enhance the process of clinical development [44,45].

ML and computer vision have also improved several aspects of human visual perception in order to discover clinically relevant characteristics in, for example, imaging data, and neural networks have been utilized for a number of objectives specifically for medical picture segmentation to clinical data creation, categorization, and forecasting. Scientific research laboratories, biotech firms, and technology companies have all been experimenting with AI and ML in three main areas:

(1) Utilizing ML to anticipate pharmacological characteristics of chemical compounds and targets for drug development;

(2) Using sequence identification and segmentation methods to diagnostic images (from, for example, retinal scans, pathology slides, and body surfaces, bones, and internal organs) to enable quicker diagnosis and disease progression monitoring and generating algorithms for computer augmentation of current clinical and imaging statistical data.

(3) Detecting novel predictive models using deep-learning algorithms on diverse information sources, such as integrating genetic and clinical evidence [42–44,46].

Considering these predictions, there have been few effective applications of ML in scientific research. These modest results have been ascribed to a lack of time after the emergence of modern techniques, as well as the inability of modern computer science deep learning and related ML methods to generalize increasingly complicated and authentic medical data sources and tasks. The lack of huge amounts of high-quality labeled data, fledgling laws, and ethical and legal issues regarding data sharing are all major obstacles that limit the use of AI/ML approaches in medicinal research. Various learning approaches that take use of the human brain's neocortex and learn from fewer instances have been considered as substitutes to deep learning, but they have yet to gain traction. Insights and commentaries on DNN's approach to imaging data sets, pharmacological characteristics of substances, clinical diagnostics and genomics, computer vision uses for medical imaging, and Natural Language Processing approaches to EHR have recently been demonstrated. [45–48]

(C) Clinical trial optimization

AI and ML technologies, particularly natural language processing (NLP), show a lot of potential for assisting and optimizing clinical research. However, only businesses with the right tools, skills, and partners will be able to reap the full benefits of AI and ML. Clinical research may be improved using AI and ML technologies that analyze research data more effectively for hazards and allow for speedier trial design and study. Those that do not use AI and ML in clinical research may discover that their competitors do, and that as a consequence, they are bringing new medications and goods to market sooner and with larger revenues due to reduced research time and safer procedures. [44,47–49]

6. Epidemic outbreak predictions via AI

In the epidemiological discipline, AI is frequently utilized to avoid, manage, monitor, and forecast disease transmission. AI is having the greatest influence on emerging epidemics, like as the ongoing coronavirus pandemic. We know that BlueDot, a Canadian AI start-up, had previously triggered an early alert about the mysterious virus even before announcement of the Corona virus epidemic became public. It focuses on the surveillance of infectious diseases. In terms of predicting epidemics and comprehending their dynamics, AI has gone a considerable way. Furthermore, the firm anticipated that the epidemic will spread to locations like Tokyo, Bangkok, Seoul, and Taipei after studying worldwide airline booking statistics. AI assisted in tracking the exact bat species that were transmitters in the 2018 Nipah virus epidemic in Kerala [43].

6.1 Artificial intelligence for virus detection and epidemic prediction

To begin with, AI and ML algorithms can detect any disease epidemic even before it occurs. BlueDot, for instance, employed an AI-driven system to avoid risk zones by scanning through foreign language news stories, flora and fauna disease databases, and other official resources. Healthcare providers can use preventive measures for cardiac arrest, strokes, infections, and other severe disorders in times of emergency. [37]

To monitor anthrax epidemic in Mongolia, ML was utilized to build a model using NLP. Researchers take over when the automatic data filtering is completed. The finalized analysis is provided to the authorities or clients once it has been checked from a scientific standpoint.

6.2 Research using artificial intelligence to develop treatments and vaccines

AI was involved not just in Corona virus epidemic but also in the Zika virus outbreak. ML models can assist in identifying viral carriers. Only two monkey species have been confirmed to be viral carriers worldwide. The investigators attempted to expand on a small corpus. One is based on multiple assertions made, while the other is based on MICE. Missing data may be replaced in two different ways using multiple imputations. Alternatively, Bayesian multilabel ML or replaced variables that represent ambiguity around the real values. The MICE, or multiply imputed chained equations, is a second algorithmic system.

This MICE system can filter through data sources looking for environmental and physical characteristic connections between organisms and infer missing data from those associations.

In recent years, AI has aided researchers in the discovery of cures, particular patterns of disease, and therapies. Because these viruses can evolve, it is critical to recognize these alterations and eliminate them as soon as possible.

It is an accomplishment in and of itself that experts were able to develop a novel gene sequencing technology. This demonstrates that, even with limited data, AI can detect trends and provide alarms before a major event occurs. As a result, AI can successfully assist in epidemic outbreak predictions [36,50].

7. Challenges in adopting the AI in healthcare

The whole success of the AI system depends upon the availability of the data as this data is only used by the AI based software's to conduct the substantial research and provide the results. The data access poses extra cost on the company also, and the data should be of high quality and reliable for the accurate data prediction. Another challenge that leads to the difficulty in adoption of AI in healthcare is the lack of skilled persons who can easily understand and operate AI platforms, and run the softwares with accuracy with the limited budget. Automation of various steps of drug development like manufacturing, clinical trials, sale will takes place but with a slower pace as these all falls under the category of narrow AI. Here, the AI has to be trained on a larger amount of data so that it can be suitable for the particular task. Therefore, human involvement is mandatory for the lucrative implementation of the AI platform in all the stages. Moreover, the fear of getting jobless is just a myth in adaption of AI, the only change that will come in adoption of AI will be the changed job profile while leaving scope for human intelligence to be used for developing more complicated insights and creativity [34,35,51].

8. Conclusion

AI is a branch of research in which computers are programmed to perform tasks that people accomplish. Computer systems are clearly speedier when it comes to calculations and analytic skills, yet they could not indeed make judgments on their own, since they lack the capacity to do so. Artificial intellect is the process of allowing computers to make decisions based on their own intelligence. Today, AI has a broad range of usage in nearly every sector, which appears to be beneficial and is displacing human professions that may be deemed unfavorable.

AI is already a part of our daily life; Alexa and Google Home, both of which are quite easy to utilize and deliver practically precise outcomes. The suggestion to finish sentences may be seen in email writing. AI systems are aiding in military action, warfare tactics, and weapon technology, in addition to our everyday lives. AI has improved cybersecurity to the point that protection systems can now detect a sequence of hacking attempts and build a tactical counterattack security program to manage them.

In the fields of healthcare and pharmaceuticals, AI is playing a pivotal role. Currently, in breast cancer diagnosis studies, Google's Deep Mind outperformed physicians. In the pharmaceutical industry, new combinations and results may be achieved in a fraction of the time and with more precision than ever before. [32,36]

References

[1] A. Bohr, K. Memarzadeh, Artificial Intelligence in Healthcare, Academic Press, 2020.

[2] J. Amann, A. Blasimme, E. Vayena, D. Frey, V.I. Madai, Explainability for artificial intelligence in healthcare: a multidisciplinary perspective, BMC Med. Inform. Decis. Mak. 20 (1) (2020) 1–9.

[3] K. Bera, K.A. Schalper, D.L. Rimm, V. Velcheti, A. Madabhushi, Artificial intelligence in digital pathology—new tools for diagnosis and precision oncology, Nat. Rev. Clin. Oncol. 16 (11) (2019) 703–715.

[4] A.R.M. Al-shamasneh, U.H.B. Obaidellah, Artificial intelligence techniques for cancer detection and classification: review study, Eur. Sci. J. 13 (3) (2017) 342–370.

[5] O.I. Abiodun, A. Jantan, A.E. Omolara, K.V. Dada, N.A. Mohamed, H. Arshad, State-of-the-art in artificial neural network applications: a survey, Heliyon 4 (11) (2018), e00938.

[6] R. Bhardwaj, A.R. Nambiar, D. Dutta (Eds.), A study of machine learning in healthcare, 2017 IEEE 41st Annual Computer Software and Applications Conference (COMPSAC), IEEE, 2017.

[7] J.S. Almeida, Predictive non-linear modeling of complex data by artificial neural networks, Curr. Opin. Biotechnol. 13 (1) (2002) 72–76.

[8] R. Burbidge, M. Trotter, B. Buxton, S. Holden, Drug design by machine learning: support vector machines for pharmaceutical data analysis, Comput. Chem. 26 (1) (2001) 5–14.

[9] A. Callahan, N.H. Shah, Machine learning in healthcare, in: Key Advances in Clinical Informatics, Elsevier, 2017, pp. 279–291.

[10] H. Chen, O. Engkvist, Y. Wang, M. Olivecrona, T. Blaschke, The rise of deep learning in drug discovery, Drug Discov. Today 23 (6) (2018) 1241–1250.

[11] I.Y. Chen, E. Pierson, S. Rose, S. Joshi, K. Ferryman, M. Ghassemi, Ethical machine learning in healthcare, Annu. Rev. Biomed. Data Sci. 4 (2021) 123–144.

[12] M. Chen, M. Decary (Eds.), Artificial Intelligence in Healthcare: An Essential Guide for Health Leaders, SAGE Publications Sage CA, Los Angeles, CA, 2020. Healthcare management forum.

[13] M.A. Ahmad, C. Eckert, A. Teredesai (Eds.), Interpretable machine learning in healthcare, Proceedings of the 2018 ACM international conference on bioinformatics, computational biology, and health informatics, 2018.

[14] E. Byvatov, U. Fechner, J. Sadowski, G. Schneider, Comparison of support vector machine and artificial neural network systems for drug/nondrug classification, J. Chem. Inf. Comput. Sci. 43 (6) (2003) 1882–1889.

[15] A. Dhillon, A. Singh, Machine learning in healthcare data analysis: a survey, J. Biol. Today's World 8 (6) (2019) 1–10.

[16] T. Davenport, R. Kalakota, The potential for artificial intelligence in healthcare, Future Healthc. J. 6 (2) (2019) 94.

[17] C.W. Coley, W. Jin, L. Rogers, T.F. Jamison, T.S. Jaakkola, W.H. Green, et al., A graph-convolutional neural network model for the prediction of chemical reactivity, Chem. Sci. 10 (2) (2019) 370–377.

[18] R. Gupta, D. Srivastava, M. Sahu, S. Tiwari, R.K. Ambasta, P. Kumar, Artificial intelligence to deep learning: machine intelligence approach for drug discovery, Mol. Divers. 25 (3) (2021) 1315–1360.
[19] J. Guan, Artificial intelligence in healthcare and medicine: promises, ethical challenges and governance, Chin. Med. Sci. J. 34 (2) (2019) 76–83.
[20] E. Gawehn, J.A. Hiss, G. Schneider, Deep learning in drug discovery, Mol. Inf. 35 (1) (2016) 3–14.
[21] S. Dua, U.R. Acharya, P. Dua, Machine Learning in Healthcare Informatics, Springer, 2014.
[22] Y. Horie, T. Yoshio, K. Aoyama, S. Yoshimizu, Y. Horiuchi, A. Ishiyama, et al., Diagnostic outcomes of esophageal cancer by artificial intelligence using convolutional neural networks, Gastrointest. Endosc. 89 (1) (2019) 25–32.
[23] G. Hessler, K.-H. Baringhaus, Artificial intelligence in drug design, Molecules 23 (10) (2018) 2520.
[24] O. Iliashenko, Z. Bikkulova, A. Dubgorn (Eds.), Opportunities and challenges of artificial intelligence in healthcare, E3S Web of Conferences, EDP Sciences, 2019.
[25] F. Jiang, Y. Jiang, H. Zhi, Y. Dong, H. Li, S. Ma, et al., Artificial intelligence in healthcare: past, present and future, Stroke Vasc. Neurol. 2 (4) (2017).
[26] J. Jiménez, S. Doerr, G. Martínez-Rosell, A.S. Rose, G. De Fabritiis, DeepSite: protein-binding site predictor using 3D-convolutional neural networks, Bioinformatics 33 (19) (2017) 3036–3042.
[27] M.-C. Laï, M. Brian, M.-F. Mamzer, Perceptions of artificial intelligence in healthcare: findings from a qualitative survey study among actors in France, J. Transl. Med. 18 (1) (2020) 1–13.
[28] G. Klambauer, T. Unterthiner, A. Mayr, S. Hochreiter, Self-normalizing neural networks, Adv. Neural Inf. Proces. Syst. 30 (2017).
[29] A. Lavecchia, Machine-learning approaches in drug discovery: methods and applications, Drug Discov. Today 20 (3) (2015) 318–331.
[30] Y.-C. Lo, S.E. Rensi, W. Torng, R.B. Altman, Machine learning in chemoinformatics and drug discovery, Drug Discov. Today 23 (8) (2018) 1538–1546.
[31] X. Li, B. Hu, H. Li, B. You, Application of artificial intelligence in the diagnosis of multiple primary lung cancer, Thorac. Cancer 10 (11) (2019) 2168–2174.
[32] K.-K. Mak, M.R. Pichika, Artificial intelligence in drug development: present status and future prospects, Drug Discov. Today 24 (3) (2019) 773–780.
[33] M. Mozaffari-Kermani, S. Sur-Kolay, A. Raghunathan, N.K. Jha, Systematic poisoning attacks on and defenses for machine learning in healthcare, IEEE J. Biomed. Health Inform. 19 (6) (2014) 1893–1905.
[34] A. Qayyum, J. Qadir, M. Bilal, A. Al-Fuqaha, Secure and robust machine learning for healthcare: a survey, IEEE Rev. Biomed. Eng. 14 (2020) 156–180.
[35] M. Ragoza, J. Hochuli, E. Idrobo, J. Sunseri, D.R. Koes, Protein-ligand scoring with convolutional neural networks, J. Chem. Inf. Model. 57 (4) (2017) 942–957.
[36] S. Reddy, J. Fox, M.P. Purohit, Artificial intelligence-enabled healthcare delivery, J. R. Soc. Med. 112 (1) (2019) 22–28.
[37] S. Ruder, An overview of multi-task learning in deep neural networks, arXiv (2017). preprint arXiv:170605098.
[38] S. Secinaro, D. Calandra, A. Secinaro, V. Muthurangu, P. Biancone, The role of artificial intelligence in healthcare: a structured literature review, BMC Med. Inform. Decis. Mak. 21 (1) (2021) 1–23.
[39] M.H. Segler, T. Kogej, C. Tyrchan, M.P. Waller, Generating focused molecule libraries for drug discovery with recurrent neural networks, ACS Cent. Sci. 4 (1) (2018) 120–131.

[40] K. Shailaja, B. Seetharamulu, M. Jabbar (Eds.), Machine learning in healthcare: a review, 2018 Second international conference on electronics, communication and aerospace technology (ICECA), IEEE, 2018.
[41] S. Shanmuganathan, Artificial Neural Network Modelling: An Introduction. Artificial Neural Network Modelling, Springer, 2016, pp. 1–14.
[42] S. Siddique, J.C. Chow, Machine learning in healthcare communication, Encyclopedia 1 (1) (2021) 220–239.
[43] S. Sunarti, F.F. Rahman, M. Naufal, M. Risky, K. Febriyanto, R. Masnina, Artificial intelligence in healthcare: opportunities and risk for future, Gac. Sanit. 35 (2021) S67–S70.
[44] K.-H. Yu, A.L. Beam, I.S. Kohane, Artificial intelligence in healthcare, Nat. Biomed. Eng. 2 (10) (2018) 719–731.
[45] V.V. Zernov, K.V. Balakin, A.A. Ivaschenko, N.P. Savchuk, I.V. Pletnev, Drug discovery using support vector machines. The case studies of drug-likeness, agrochemical-likeness, and enzyme inhibition predictions, J. Chem. Inf. Comput. Sci. 43 (6) (2003) 2048–2056.
[46] L. Zhang, J. Tan, D. Han, H. Zhu, From machine learning to deep learning: progress in machine intelligence for rational drug discovery, Drug Discov. Today 22 (11) (2017) 1680–1685.
[47] J. Zou, Y. Han, S.-S. So, Overview of artificial neural networks, Artif. Neural Netw. (2008) 14–22.
[48] A. Zhavoronkov, Artificial Intelligence for Drug Discovery, Biomarker Development, and Generation of Novel Chemistry, ACS Publications, 2018, pp. 4311–4313.
[49] J. Vamathevan, D. Clark, P. Czodrowski, I. Dunham, E. Ferran, G. Lee, et al., Applications of machine learning in drug discovery and development, Nat. Rev. Drug Discov. 18 (6) (2019) 463–477.
[50] G. Rong, A. Mendez, E.B. Assi, B. Zhao, M. Sawan, Artificial intelligence in healthcare: review and prediction case studies, Engineering 6 (3) (2020) 291–301.
[51] S. Reddy, Use of artificial intelligence in healthcare delivery, in: eHealth-Making Health Care Smarter, IntechOpen, 2018.

CHAPTER 5

Pharmacophore modeling

Maheshkumar Borkar[a], Arati Prabhu[a], Abhishek Kanugo[b], and Rupesh Kumar Gautam[c]

[a]SVKM's Dr. Bhanuben Nanavati College of Pharmacy, Mumbai, Maharashtra, India
[b]SVKM's NMIMS School of Pharmacy and Technology Management, Shirpur, Dhule, Maharashtra, India
[c]Department of Pharmacology, Indore Institute of Pharmacy, IIST Campus, Indore, Madhya Pradesh, India

1. Introduction to pharmacophore modeling

The concept of pharmacophore was first coined by Paul Ehrlich in 1909 [1], who defined the pharmacophore as "a molecular framework that carries the essential features responsible (phoros) for a drug's (pharmacon) therapeutic activity." However, the physico-chemical concept of pharmacophore was introduced by Lemont Kier [2,3]. Peter Günd has broadly reviewed the evolution and history of the pharmacophore concept [4]. Since 1997, the International Union of Pure and Applied Chemistry defined pharmacophore as "an ensemble of steric and electronic features that is necessary to ensure the optimal supramolecular interactions with a specific biological target and to trigger (or block) its biological response." [5] A pharmacophore is a part of the three-dimensional structure of a chemical or a drug, which is responsible for the biological activity. Pharmacophore is the illustration of specific groups and stearic arrangement of the molecules, which are needed for the better interaction with the specific target.

Pharmacophore is the ligand-based or structure-based model, which is based on the 3D shape of the target protein. In ligand-based model, all the biologically active molecules are superimposed and the common features of all the molecules, which are essential for biological activity are extracted [6,7]. However, in structural approach, the interactions between the target and the ligands are examined that are further used to construct the pharmacophore [8–10]. Both of these approaches are discussed in detail in Section 2. Pharmacophores are broadly used in the rational drug design, making them an important tool in CADD. Some well-known applications of this concept are virtual screening, de novo design, lead optimization, target identification, side effect, ADME-tox modeling, and off-target prediction. Detailed descriptions are given in Section 5.

Computational Approaches in Drug Discovery, Development and Systems Pharmacology
https://doi.org/10.1016/B978-0-323-99137-7.00004-6

In pharmacophore modeling, chemical groups in a molecule that are responsible for molecular recognition are replaced with abstract "features," which represent functionalities important for binding with the macromolecular target. These molecular patterns that are labeled as hydrogen bond donors, hydrogen-bond acceptors, positively or negatively charged groups, and aromatic or hydrophobic moieties represent different types of nonbonded protein-ligand interactions, which contribute to the binding affinity of the ligand [4,11].

Earlier, simple interactive molecular graphics visualization tools were utilized for the manual development of pharmacophore models. In the past few decades, with the advances in CADD development, pharmacophore modeling automated tools and applications have emerged [12]. A list of structure/ligand-based pharmacophore modeling software/tools is given in Table 1.

2. Types of pharmacophores

In ligand-based model, all the biologically active molecules are superimposed and the common features of all the molecules that are essential for biological activity are extracted [6,7]. However, in structural approach, the interactions between the target and the ligands are examined that are further used to construct the pharmacophore [8–10]. The schematic presentation of types of pharmacophores modeling and its uses are depicted in Fig. 1.

2.1 Ligand-based pharmacophore modeling

Ligand-based pharmacophore modeling is an essential step for drug discovery, especially when the 3D macromolecular target structure in not available. This method involves the extraction of common features from the known ligands with similar or different scaffolds after molecular alignment [6,7,13,14]. The elucidation of the superimposed molecules will happen in two stages. First, as the bioactive conformations of flexible molecules are unknown, the conformational space of the molecules must be thoroughly studied. Second, common pharmacophore features that can be preserved in a 3D model must be used to align the conformers to each other. Structural information of the inactive analogs must also be taken into consideration during the training of the pharmacophore model [14]. A perusal of the literature reveals that ligand-based pharmacophore models do not gave the detailed information, which is required for the lead optimization. Thus,

Table 1 List of the structure/ligand-based pharmacophore modeling software.

Software name	Details	Format	Availability	URL
Align-it (Pharao)	Pharmacophore alignment	Standalone	Free	http://silicos-it.be
Catalyst	Pharmacophore modeling	Standalone	Commercial	http://accelrys.com/products/discovery-studio/pharmacophore.html
CATSlight2	Topological pharmacophore descriptor for scaffold hopping and target identification	Web service	Free	http://modlab-cadd.ethz.ch/software/catslight2/
e-Pharmacophore	Pharmacophore modeling	Standalone	Commercial	https://www.schrodinger.com/products/e-pharmacophores
FLAP	Fingerprints using pharmacophoric features	Standalone	Commercial	http://www.moldiscovery.com/software/flap/
LigandScout	Pharmacophore modeling	Standalone	Commercial	http://www.inteligand.com/ligandscout/
MOE	Pharmacophore modeling	Standalone	Commercial	http://www.chemcomp.com/MOE-Pharmacophore_Discovery.htm
MolSign	Pharmacophore modeling	Standalone	Commercial	http://www.vlifesciences.com/products/Functional_products/Molsign.php
PharmaGist	Pharmacophore detection	Standalone/Web service	Free	http://bioinfo3d.cs.tau.ac.il/pharma/
Pharmer	Pharmacophore search	Standalone	Free	http://smoothdock.ccbb.pitt.edu/pharmer/
PharmMapper	Drug target identification	Web service	Free	http://59.78.96.61/pharmmapper
Phase	Pharmacophore modeling	Standalone	Commercial	http://www.schrodinger.com/Phase/

Continued

Table 1 List of the structure/ligand-based pharmacophore modeling software—cont'd

Software name	Details	Format	Availability	URL
Pocket v.2	Pharmacophore modeling	Standalone/ Web service	Free	http://www.pkumdl.cn:8080/pocketv2.html
Quasi	Pharmacophore modeling	Standalone	Commercial	http://www.denovopharma.com/page2.asp?PageID=485
UNITY	Pharmacophore modeling	Standalone	Commercial	http://www.certara.com/products/molmod/sybyl-x/simpharm/
ZincPharmer	Pharmacophore search for purchasable compounds from ZINC database	Web service	Free	http://zincpharmer.csb.pitt.edu

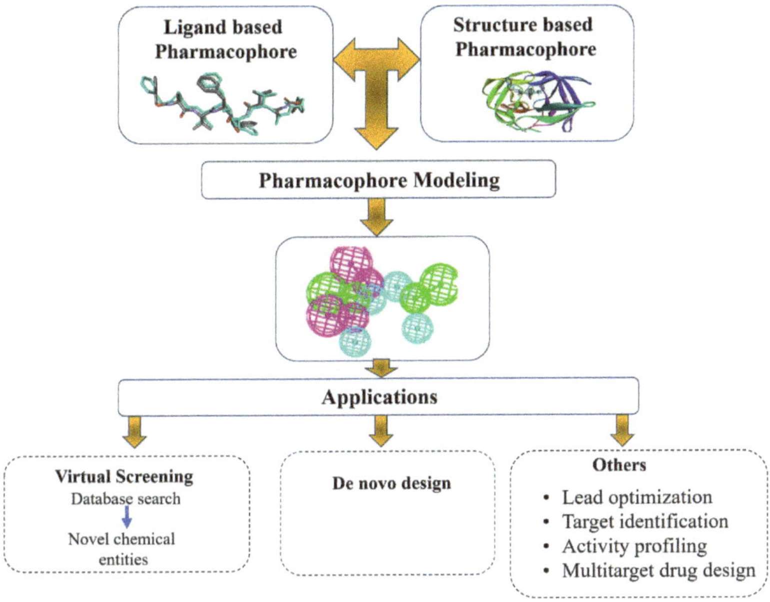

Fig. 1 Types of pharmacophores modeling.

conventional ligand-based pharmacophores screening has the inherent limitation of yielding a higher proportion of false positives [15].

2.2 Structure-based pharmacophore modeling

In structure-based modeling, the 3D structure of the macromolecular ligand is studied, and the chemical features as well as stearic artefacts are produced. This technique investigates the interactions between the target and the ligand, which we can get by two approaches [8–10]. The first one includes the 3D crystal structures of targets along with the co-crystalized ligands that describe the principal interactions between the protein and ligand. In this approach, information about hydrogen bond interactions and the charges are plotted on the bioactive conformation of the ligand to generate feature-based pharmacophores [10,14]. X-ray crystallographic structures, nuclear magnetic resonance data of protein, and validated homology models are generally used for the determination of 3D structures of the molecular targets [14]. Various free as well as commercial software/tools are available for pharmacophore modeling via structures and virtual screening [14–16]. Some of these software's are depicted in Table 1.

Second approach in which apo structures of the biological target without complexed ligands have been used for generation of structure-based pharmacophores. This method includes the calculation of all the possible interactions at the active site. The binding site feature information is subjected to clustering algorithms in order to intelligently reduce the search space and the pharmacophore models are generated then. Such models are based on target structure information such as potential interaction residues and the shape of binding cavities and hence overcome the limitations of conventional ligand-based pharmacophores.

3. Selection of pharmacophores

Pharmacophore modeling takes place in various stages. The stages in the development of pharmacophore models involve the library designing of the active ligands, conformational analysis, molecular superimposition, abstraction/generation of 3D pharmacophore, selection of pharmacophore hypothesis, and validation of the pharmacophore model. The schematic representation of the stages in the development of pharmacophore model is depicted in Fig. 2.

(1) **Design of the library of active ligands**: The first step in any pharmacophore development is the design of a set of structurally diverse active ligands. The set of molecules should cover a broad range of biological activities and should include highly active and moderately active ligands as well as inactive compounds. This increases the applicability domain of the pharmacophore model and enables it to distinguish between active and inactive molecules. The selection of ligand type, data set size, and its chemical diversity should be done carefully as it affects the quality of the final pharmacophore model. Inclusion of a structurally diverse data set, which will bind to the similar binding pocket in the molecular target protein, will improves the robustness of the pharmacophore model [15].

(2) **Conformational analysis**: The most important aspect in the pharmacophore model building is conformational search of the ligand. In this step, low-energy conformations are generated for each of the selected molecules that are likely to contain the bioactive conformation. Several algorithms have been developed for performing an exhaustive conformational search: clustering; the torsional space systematic search; stochastic methods, like Monte Carlo (MC), molecular

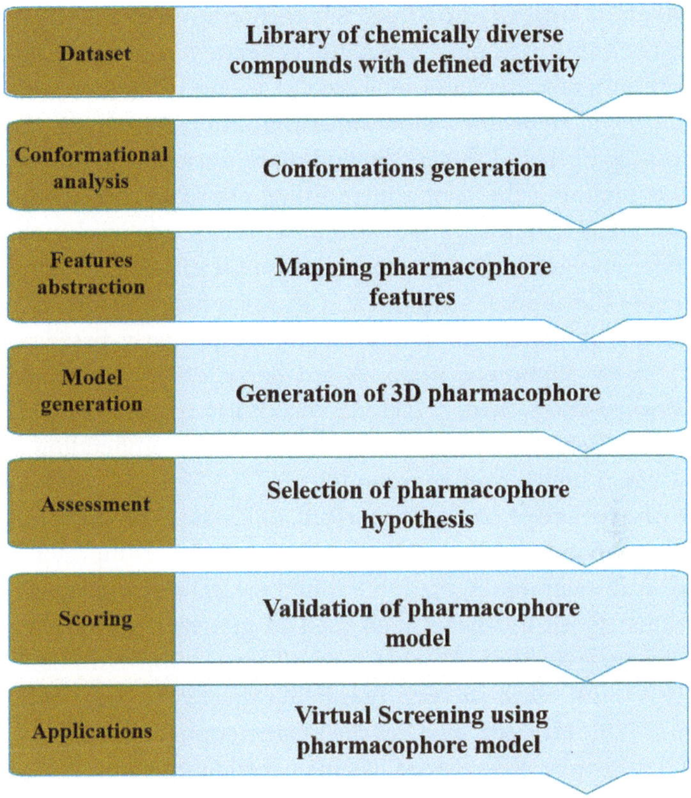

Fig. 2 Steps involved in the pharmacophore model development.

dynamics; and sampling and Poling [17,18]. Commonly used conformational search programs are FAST, Catalyst's BEST, and conformer algorithms, which are based on the recursive build up and energy screening CAESAR (Conformer Algorithm based on Energy Screening and Recursive Build-up) [19]. They all produce conformations that gave wide coverage of the conformational space. The BEST method uses Poling algorithm, which will perform a meticulous minimization of the energy and will find out the conformations through Cartesian space. In comparison, the FAST method utilizes lesser time and optimizes the conformations in torsion space only. CAESAR approach is the combination of local and rotational summary which to reject the duplicate conformation, which arises due to topological symmetry [20].

(3) Molecular superimposition: Superimposition or alignment of low-energy conformations of molecules generated in the previous step are commonly done using point-based or property-based strategies [21]. Point-based algorithms allow superimposition of pairs of atoms, fragments, or chemical feature (including bioisosteric functional groups) points retaining the least-square fitting approach [22]. This method is associated with a drawback that it requires predefined anchor points as different ligands might contain different feature points. However, to generate the alignments, the set of gaussian function-based molecular field descriptors are being utilized by the property-based algorithms [18]. New alignment methods are being developed for improved superimposition, which includes fuzzy pattern recognition, atomic property field [23] [24], stochastic proximity embedding [25], and grid-based interaction energies [8].

(4) 3D pharmacophore abstraction: Following superimposition, the subsequent stage is the transformation of the superimposed molecules into an abstract representation to build the 3D pharmacophore model. Various algorithms have been used to generate the pharmacophore model such as HipHop [13], HypoGen [20,26], MPHIL [27], and RAPID [28]. with the first two being the two most preferred algorithms [29]. HipHop develop the pharmacophore models by utilizing the data from a different set of active compounds to drive a common feature hypothesis. HipHop algorithm recognized different configurations of chemical features by treating each molecule as template and common configurations are identified. Lastly, the resulting pharmacophores are ranked using various scoring metrics [18]. Finding the maximum common substructure (MCS) is the most common method for defining a pattern. This strategy has been implemented in DISCO [30], RAPID [28], GAMMA [31], and GASP [13]. In the HypoGen [20,26] algorithm, the known activity of the training set ligands used to create hypotheses and build 3D pharmacophore models. In the constructive step, it recognizes and examines all permitted pharmacophores, which are consisting of approximately five features among the two most active compounds. The next is the subtractive stage, in which redundant pharmacophore candidates identified and removed those that are present in more than half of the least active ligands. The optimization stage is the final step, in which attempts are made to increase the score of a pharmacophore candidate that has passed the subtractive stage. A set of ten pharmacophore models are generated for each run which are then optimized by utilizing simulated annealing algorithm. Pharmacophore develop by HypoGen consists of various pharmacophoric features (i) hydrogen bond donor (HBD), e.g., hydroxyl or amine groups; (ii) hydrogen bond acceptor (HBA) (e.g., hydroxyl or carbonyl groups); (iii) hydrophobic (aliphatic), e.g., cyclohexyl or long alkyl chain and hydrophobic (aromatic), e.g., phenyl or heterocyclic ring system; (iv) negative charge, e.g., carboxylates; (v) negative ionizable; (vi) positive charge, e.g., guanidines, ammonium; and (vii) positive ionizable [15,18]. The model is classified as three-point (three features) or four-point (four features) pharmacophore based on the number of features present in the final pharmacophore. A hypothetical example defining the common pharmacophore features is depicted in Fig. 3.

Pharmacophore fingerprints: These are pharmacophore features that allow a molecule to be annotated as a unique data string [11,32]. A binary bitstring (0 or 1) identifies the pharmacophore features, where one indicates the presence of a potential feature and zero indicates the absence. Fingerprints are built for each molecule by collecting all the feature bitstrings. Pharmacophore fingerprints are used to measure molecular similarity, diversity assessments, and designing libraries [15]. Chem-X is a well-known programme for defining pharmacophore fingerprints [33].

(5) Assessment and selection of pharmacophore hypothesis: Catalyst/Hypogen algorithm is used to assess the quality of the generated

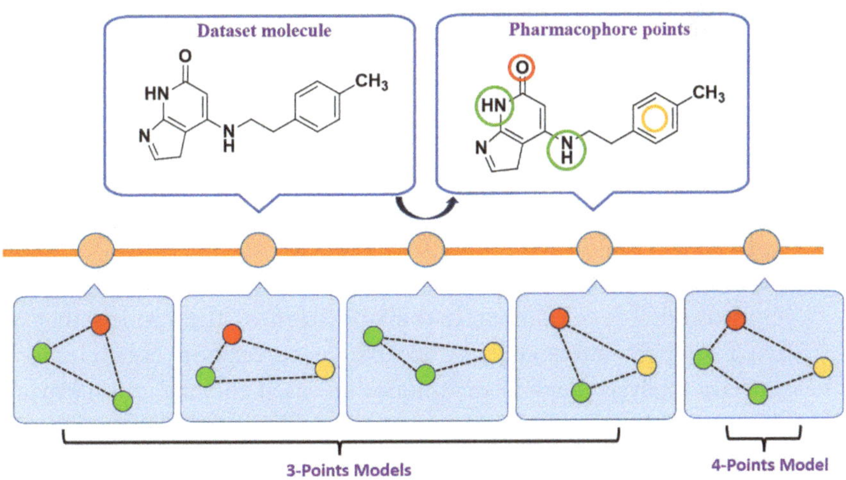

Fig. 3 A hypothetical example defining the common pharmacophore features.

pharmacophore hypothesis. Eq. (1) is used to calculate the cost (total cost) of a hypothesis.

$$\text{cost} = eE + wW + cC \tag{1}$$

where e=coefficient of error (E), w=coefficient of weight (W), c=coefficient of configuration (C) component [34].

Another two important cost calculations are "Fixed cost" and "null cost." Eq. (2) represents the fixed cost, while the Eq. (3) represents the null cost. The Eq. (2) shows the simple model that fits all the data, while the Eq. (3) concludes that data sets are not related, and all the experimental activities are distributed normally to their average value. As the null pharmacophore exhibits none of the features, zero contribution from the weight or configuration component was levied [34].

$$\text{Fixed cost} = eE(x = 0) + wW(x = 0) + cC \tag{2}$$

where x denotes the variation from the usual values of weight and error.

$$\text{Null cost} = eE\left(\chi_{est} = \overline{\chi}\right) \tag{3}$$

where χ_{est} denotes the average scaled activity of all the molecules present in training set.

For a credible pharmacophore model, the cost difference in the test hypothesis and the null hypothesis should be significant (higher difference is required). For example, if the difference is 40–60, it implies that there are 75%–90% of chances that the true correlation data is being used. The value of the total cost should be nearer to the fixed cost in order for the model to be meaningful. Additionally, two more output parameters are also assessed, viz., the error cost and the configuration cost. A configuration cost more than 17 implies that the generated pharmacophore is most likely due to chance. The value of the root mean square (RMS) is directly proportional to error the cost, which helps to assess the quality of the correlation between the actual and the estimated activity data [18,34].

(6) Validation of pharmacophore model: The last step in pharmacophore model development is the validation of the models that are based on parameters such as acceptable correlation coefficient (R) and cost analysis. Several techniques are used to validate pharmacophore models.

(a) Fischer's randomization test: The CatScramble technique in Catalyst [26] has been developed to assess the quality of the pharmacophore. In this method, the activity has been randomized among the training set molecules and assigning them new values. A new pharmacophore hypothesis has been developed employing the identical parameters to the initial hypothesis. If the randomized sets produce pharmacophores with similar or better cost values, rms, and correlation, the original pharmacophore can be assumed to have been created by chance [35].

(b) Test set prediction: In this method, the external test set molecules are used to check the correctness of activity predictions and ability of the model to discriminate between active and inactive molecules. The predictive R^2 values are used to assess the models' prediction ability. (R^2_{pred} with a threshold value of 0.5).

(c) Guner Henry (GH) scoring method: The method is used to quantify the goodness of hit and it gives the quantitative measurement of model selectivity, activity space coverage while mining of database, similarity search in the database, which contains both quantitatively measures structural and biological data. It helps to assess the quality of the pharmacophore models using the known actives and inactive as test set molecules. The parameters mentioned below can be measured using the GH scoring method where the database based percent yield of actives (%Y) mentioned in Eq. (4), the hit list based percent ratio of actives (%A, precision) mentioned in Eq. (5), the enrichment factor E mentioned in Eq. (6), and the GH score mentioned in Eq. (7), are used and the value of 1 signifies the ideal model [18,36–38].

$$\text{Percent yield of the actives} : \%Y = \frac{H_a}{H_t} \times 100 \tag{4}$$

$$\text{Percent ratio of the actives in the hit list} : \%A = \frac{H_a}{A} \times 100 \tag{5}$$

$$\text{Enrichment (enhancement)} : E = \frac{H_a/H_t}{A/D} = \frac{H_a \times D}{H_t \times A} \tag{6}$$

$$\text{GH Score} : \text{GH} = \left[\frac{H_a(3A + H_t)}{4HtA}\right]\left(1 - \frac{H_t - H_a}{D - A}\right) \tag{7}$$

$$\text{False negatives} = A - H_a \tag{8}$$

$$\text{False positives} = H_t - H_a \tag{9}$$

where "D" represents the database no. of compounds, "A" represents the number of active present in the database, "H_t" is the number of hits recovered, and "H_a" represents the active compounds present in the hit list. "E" denotes the active concentrations of model's enrichment across random screening without the involvement of any pharmacophoric methodology [18,36–38].

4. Pharmacophore-based ligand profiling

Ligand profiling is the process of extrapolating information about all probable molecular targets of a compound based on its structural attributes. In silico chemogenomic approaches such as compound similarity screenings and reverse docking are widely used for predicting bimolecular targets of small-molecule compounds [39–41]. Thierry Langer was the first to concretize the concept of pharmacophore-based ligand profiling with the explicit purpose of identifying new molecular targets for bioactive compounds, based on their pharmacophore complementarity [42].

This technique, which attempts to match ligand and target pharmacophoric space, has a great potential in drug repurposing [43], design of selective modulators [44,45], polypharmacology, and predictive toxicology. Ligand profiling methods [46] help in predicting novel targets of existing drugs [41,47,48] and aid in deducing their mechanism of action. This can open up new avenues for orphan bioactive ligands [49]. Metabolic pathways, antitargets, and secondary off-target effects that may results undesired side effects and adverse reactions have also been identified from these screening methods [50–56].

Pharmacophore-based ligand profiling starts with the construction of a database of the macromolecular target-binding pharmacophores from a wide array of protein-ligand complex structures. The significance of the targets in the disease context must be validated and the active site/allosteric site must be thoroughly mapped. Target-based pharmacophores are created via careful representation of ligand-receptor interactions. The pharmacophore hypotheses are validated on the basis of their abilities to map the original crystal structure ligand and discriminate other actives from inactive molecules. After that, the external test set is validated. These molecules are subjected to structure optimization and conformer generation and screened against the target-based pharmacophore models in accordance with various search algorithms. The results are analyzed and compiled in visual color-coded hit maps.

The validated protocol is used for rapid, automated, parallel screening of compound molecules against all target-based models. The hit set of matching pharmacophores acts as a guide to link small molecules to their biological targets. The pharmacophore profile of the molecule thus acts as an excellent guide to predict the pharmacological profile of the compound.

Langer et al. [42] conducted initial proof of principle studies for this virtual activity profiling technique using 100 antiviral compounds database. Parallel screening of these compounds against a library of 50 pharmacophore models generated from multiple antiviral targets gave excellent enrichment, pointing to successful virtual activity profiling for 90% of tested molecules. Pharmacophore databases derived from HIV proteases [42] and peroxisome proliferator activator receptors [57] have been successfully used for automatic large-scale profiling of compounds. Despite utilizing a parallel screening methodology, the technique demonstrated excellent differentiating ability between different levels of activity of compounds. The steps involved in pharmacophore-based ligand profiling are depicted in Fig. 4.

This technique has shown promise in other domains such as target-based profiling of plant extracts and compounds in natural product research. For evaluating prospective therapeutic targets for secondary plant metabolites, a

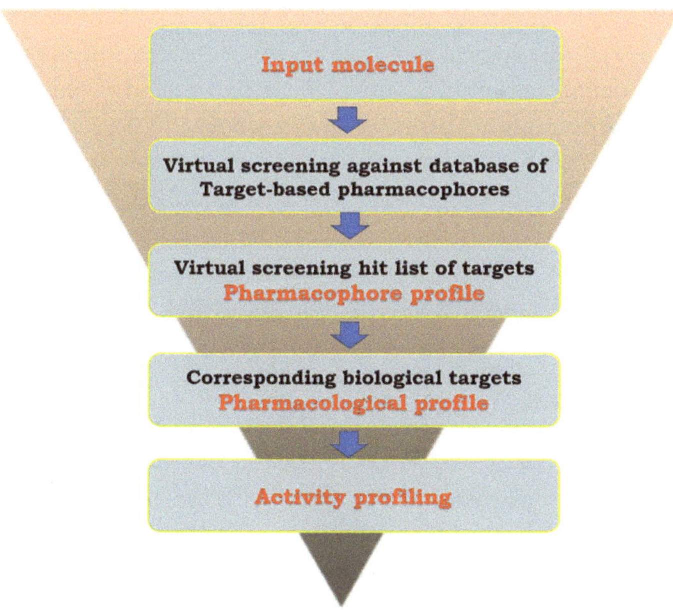

Fig. 4 Pharmacophore-based ligand profiling.

parallel screening methodology was used [58]. The metabolite compounds' conformer libraries were created, and their possible targets were predicted using a large database of varied target-based pharmacophore models. Based on the ligand profile output and subsequent experimental testing, many compounds were identified with potent activity against three biological targets, *viz.* CB2 receptor, HRV coat protein, and acetylcholinesterase.

5. Applications of pharmacophore modeling

Pharmacophore modeling has evolved as a cornerstone computational strategy in rational drug discovery. This technique has wide applications and has been successfully employed in virtual screening for lead identification, de novo drug design, scaffold hopping, selectivity profiling, multitarget drug design, fragment-based drug design, diversity assessment, ADME profiling, as well as identification of toxicophores and olfactophores.

5.1 Pharmacophore-based virtual screening

Lead identification has been touted as the best application of pharmacophore-based design strategies. This approach has revolutionized the early phases of drug discovery by expediting the initial selection of hit compound classes in drug discovery projects. Pharmacophore models mapped to specific biological activities have been used for mining structural libraries to identify promising, novel bioactive ligands. This method is known as pharmacophore-based virtual screening. The virtual hits fulfil the requirements of the pharmacophore model and have a higher likelihood of testing positive in biological assays. Virtual screening has successfully identified novel lead molecules for many therapeutic diseases [59–66]. Virtual screening protocols using a pharmacophore-based approach are superior to structure-based algorithms in their ability to rapidly screen multiconformational mega compound databases in comparatively shorter timespans and pave the way for structurally diverse leads [18].

5.2 De novo design based on pharmacophore

The de novo design platform can be fitted with the concept of pharmacophore. This method uses a collection of disjointed molecular groupings that are in alignment with the input pharmacophore model. Excluded volumes are integrated in the pharmacophore model to simulate the binding surface residues. To create the novel compounds, various linkers are connected to the hit fragments who possess the structural compliance with the added pharmacophore. Huang et al. [67] have developed a program called PhDD (a pharmacophore-based de novo design method of drug like molecules), which has helped in the identification of druglike molecules that comply with the constraints of an input pharmacophore hypothesis.

5.3 Hopping of the Scaffold

Scaffold hopping refers to the process of replacing the chemical core of the molecule with a novel structural scaffold, while retaining its biological activity. This strategy is extremely useful in generating novel intellectual property and may be indispensable while dealing with chemotypes with metabolic or toxicological liabilities. Pharmacophores derived from pharmacologically active compounds or from the bound ligand poses in co-crystallized protein complexes define the geometric set of chemical features necessary for pharmacological effect without incorporating the actual functional groups and chemical units of the molecule. Thus, pharmacophore-based virtual screening is the perfect strategy for scaffold hopping and has been used to identify novel molecules with promising biological activity [68,69]. Scaffold hopping hits present structurally diverse starting points for further lead optimization [69].

5.4 Selectivity profiling and multitarget drug design

Pharmacophores can be used to develop molecules that exhibit isoform-specific activity. Different pharmacophore models can be built for binding to the various enzyme isoforms and used in a filter-based virtual screening paradigm to identify molecules with a specific selectivity profile [70]. A conceptually opposite strategy can be used to combine pharmacophores from different macromolecular targets to develop molecules that can simultaneously interact with many macromolecular targets with resultant multifunctional biological profile. Sequential combination protocols developed from different pharmacophore models integrated into virtual screening lead to molecules with polypharmacological potential [71].

5.5 Fragment-based drug design

Fragment-based drug design is an approach that is based on identification of small weakly binding chemical fragments that are then combined to design a lead with a higher affinity for the target protein. Pharmacophore models developed from ligand-receptor complexes can be broken down to produce smaller receptor segment grids, each focused on a subset of binding site amino acid residues. These smaller pharmacophore subsets are then used for mining fragment libraries in order to identify novel fragments. The construction of a novel library of tailored molecules with the ability to bind to the selected target is achieved by combining several hit fragments across the whole binding site via diverse linker groups [72–74].

5.6 Diversity assessment

Jon Mason and co-workers generated 3D pharmacophoric keys to determine structural diversity [75]. 3-Center and 4-center pharmacophore feature subsets within molecules are treated as descriptors and used for assessment for molecular similarity and diversity [32]. Total pharmacophore diversity can be computed using distance-based approaches, which have been demonstrated to be more effective than 2D binary fingerprints for molecular recognition [76].

5.7 Drug designing based on natural products

Phyto products are conformationally more compliant and have high complexity in structure and highly polar than small organic molecules, which are usually developed in drug discovery projects.

This domain represents novel chemical space and has the capacity to drive innovative drug design. When the pharmacophore modeling, which was developed for synthetic drug like molecules, applied to the natural products, it come up with many important leads that can be applied for the treatment of various diseases [77–82]. Pharmacophore- based virtual screening of natural product libraries is done, and the hit molecules are then subjected to extensive biological testing.

5.8 ADME profiling

One of the major contributors to high drug attrition rates during clinical phases is poor ADME-tox properties [20,83]. Early identification of these liabilities is crucial to smooth drug development. Pharmacophore modeling approaches are widely used for in silico ADME-tox profiling [84]. Ligand-based pharmacophores for various physicochemical and pharmacokinetic attributes have been developed that help in building the ADME profile of compounds under development [85]. Target-based pharmacophores with drug-metabolizing proteins such as CYP enzymes have also been developed and form the basis of various algorithms which predict the metabolic liabilities and drug-drug interaction potential of compounds [86–88]. Sean Ekins developed a combinatorial pharmacophore grid-based algorithm for identifying potential drug-drug interactions of molecules [89]. Based on the hit list that is obtained after screening of libraries against pharmacophore models of various CYP enzymes, an affinity matrix can be established that helps in identification of compounds with pharmacokinetic liabilities. The versatility of the pharmacophore approach enables the development of predictive models for both CYP substrates as well as inhibitors [90–94].

5.9 Toxicity profiling

Pharmacophore models can be developed for various adverse events. Such toxicophores can be used for antitarget screening and are invaluable in identifying preclinical compounds with the predisposition toward serious adverse events. Antitarget screening facilitates the identification of molecules with predisposition toward binding with macromolecules that mediate potentially harmful effects. Such protocols help in early identification of the toxicity potential of molecules. This strategy has been successfully applied to identify hERG inhibition potential of promising compounds, which led to the prediction of their cardiotoxic potential [95].

5.10 Olfactophores: Pharmacophores in perfume industry

Three-dimensional pharmacophore models can be used to capture the crucial structural hypotheses of various fragrances. Distinct olfactophores have been developed for numerous fragrances such as sandalwood, amber, fruity pear odorants, lily flowers, pineapple-like, and musk odorants [96–99]. A three-dimensional electron topological approach has been explored for odor prediction of garlic aroma [100] and meat odor [101]. This concept of an olfactophore has been utilized in developing the chemistry of odorants with applications in the fragrances and flavors industry.

6. Conclusion and future perspectives

Pharmacophore modeling has evolved as a burgeoning, versatile technique for the identification of active compounds. Crystallizing the complexity of functional groups linked via molecular graphs into a set of abstract features culminates in the pharmacophore approach that is simple to use, easy to interpret, and practically feasible for rapid lead identification. A logical extension of the development of a 3D pharmacophore is virtual screening of molecule databases, with the ultimate purpose of identifying a diverse set of novel molecules that possess key pharmacophore features crucial for biological activity. The simplicity of ligand-based algorithm enables rapid, exhaustive searches of mega-sized databases. This versatile method has wide applications in various medicinal approaches to drug design, macromolecular target identification, selectivity profiling, ADMET profiling, and diversity estimation.

Advances in molecular alignment algorithms, efficient manipulation of ligand flexibility, and exhaustive model optimization have overcome some of the limitations of the early model building approaches. More recently, deep learning techniques such as convoluted neural networks (CNN) and graph-based deep generative models have been used to integrate and expand the applicability of pharmacophoric motifs for enhanced exploration of activity-focused chemical space. In another development, Weider et al. have used molecular dynamics (MD) simulations of ligand-bound biomolecules to generate a family of dynamic pharmacophores [102]. The original PDB pharmacophore was supplemented with the consensus MD trajectory pharmacophore and used for virtual screening exercises. Such merged pharmacophores are thought to overcome the lower applicability of static pharmacophores obtained from rigid protein ligand complexes.

Starting from a simple concept, the pharmacophore has now become indispensable to modern day drug design. In the field of drug discovery and development, pharmacophore modeling is widely employed and continues to expand in allied domains such as the fragrance industry and biologically active natural products.

References

[1] P. Ehrlich, Über den jetzigen Stand der Chemotherapie, Ber. Dtsch. Chem. Ges. 42 (1909) 17–47.
[2] L.B. Kier, Molecular orbital calculation of preferred conformations of acetylcholine, muscarine, and muscarone, Mol. Pharmacol. 3 (1967) 487–494.
[3] L.B. Kier, MO Theory in Drug Research, Academic Press, New York, NY, 1971.
[4] P. Gund, Evolution of the pharmacophore concept in pharmaceutical research, in: O.F. Güner (Ed.), Pharmacophore Perception, Development, and Use in Drug Design, Internat'l University Line, La Jolla, 2000.
[5] C.-G. Wermuth, C.R. Ganellin, P. Lindberg, L.A. Mitscher, Glossary of terms used in medicinal chemistry (IUPAC Recommendations 1997), Annu. Rep. Med. Chem. 33 (1998) 385–395.
[6] T. Langer, E.M. Krovat, Chemical feature-based pharmacophores and virtual library screening for discovery of new leads, Curr. Opin. Drug Discov. Devel. 6 (2003) 370–376.

[7] Y. Kurogi, O.F. Guner, Pharmacophore modeling and three-dimensional database searching for drug design using catalyst, Curr. Med. Chem. 8 (2001) 1035–1055.
[8] M. Baroni, G. Cruciani, S. Sciabola, F. Perruccio, J.S. Mason, A common reference framework for analyzing/comparing proteins and ligands. Fingerprints for Ligands and Proteins (FLAP): theory and application, J. Chem. Inf. Model. 47 (2007) 279–294.
[9] H.J. Böhm, The computer program LUDI: a new method for the de novo design of enzyme inhibitors, J. Comput. Aided Mol. Des. 6 (1992) 61–78.
[10] J. Chen, L. Lai, Pocket v., Pocket v.2: further developments on receptor-based pharmacophore modeling, J. Chem. Inf. Model. 46 (2006) 2684–2691.
[11] X. Qing, X.Y. Lee, J. De Raeymaecker, J.R. Tame, K.Y. Zhang, M. De Maeyer, A. Voet, Pharmacophore modeling: advances, limitations, and current utility in drug discovery, J. Rec. Ligand Channel Res. 7 (2014) 81–92.
[12] A.R. Leach, V.J. Gillet, R.A. Lewis, R. Taylor, Three-dimensional pharmacophore methods in drug discovery, J. Med. Chem. 53 (2010) 539–558.
[13] G. Jones, P. Willett, R.C. Glen, A genetic algorithm for flexible molecular overlay and pharmacophore elucidation, J. Comput. Aided Mol. Des. 9 (1995) 532–549.
[14] A. Gaurav, V. Gautam, Structure-based three-dimensional pharmacophores as an alternative to traditional methodologies, J. Rec. Ligand Channel Res. 7 (2014) 27–38.
[15] S.A. Khedkar, A.K. Malde, E.C. Coutinho, S. Srivastava, Pharmacophore modeling in drug discovery and development: an overview, Med. Chem. 3 (2007) 187–197.
[16] J. Desaphy, K. Azdimousa, E. Kellenberger, D. Rognan, Comparison and Druggability Prediction of Protein-Ligand Binding Sites From Pharmacophore-Annotated Cavity Shapes, ACS Publications, 2012.
[17] A. Smellie, S.L. Teig, P. Towbin, Poling: promoting conformational variation, J. Comput. Chem. 16 (1995) 171–187.
[18] K. Roy, Understanding the Basics of QSAR for Applications in Pharmaceutical Sciences and Risk Assessment, Academic Press, 2015.
[19] R. Kristam, V.J. Gillet, R.A. Lewis, D. Thorner, Comparison of conformational analysis techniques to generate pharmacophore hypotheses using catalyst, J. Chem. Inf. Model. 45 (2005) 461–476.
[20] J. Li, T. Ehlers, J. Sutter, S. Varma-O'Brien, J. Kirchmair, CAESAR: a new conformer generation algorithm based on recursive buildup and local rotational symmetry consideration, J. Chem. Inf. Model. 47 (2007) 1923–1932.
[21] G. Wolber, T. Seidel, F. Bendix, T. Langer, Molecule-pharmacophore superpositioning and pattern matching in computational drug design, Drug Discov. Today 13 (2008) 23–29.
[22] O. Dror, A. Shulman-Peleg, R. Nussinov, H.J. Wolfson, Predicting molecular interactions in silico: I. an updated guide to pharmacophore identification and its applications to drug design, Front. Med. Chem. 551 (2006) 551–584.
[23] M. Totrov, Atomic property fields: generalized 3D pharmacophoric potential for automated ligand superposition, pharmacophore elucidation and 3D QSAR, Chem. Biol. Drug Des. 71 (2008) 15–27.
[24] J.H. Nettles, J.L. Jenkins, C. Williams, A.M. Clark, A. Bender, Z. Deng, J.W. Davies, M. Glick, Flexible 3D pharmacophores as descriptors of dynamic biological space, J. Mol. Graph. Model. 26 (2007) 622–633.
[25] D. Bandyopadhyay, D.K. Agrafiotis, A self-organizing algorithm for molecular alignment and pharmacophore development, J. Comput. Chem. 29 (2008) 965–982.
[26] Accelrys Inc, Discovery Studio 2.1, 2009. San Diego, CA.
[27] J.D. Holliday, P. Willett, Using a genetic algorithm to identify common structural features in sets of ligands, J. Mol. Graph. Model. 15 (1997) 221–232.
[28] P.W. Finn, L.E. Kavraki, J.-C. Latombe, R. Motwani, C. Shelton, S. Venkatasubramanian, A. Yao, Rapid: randomized pharmacophore identification for

drug design, in: Proceedings of the Thirteenth Annual Symposium on Computational Geometry, 1997, pp. 324–333.
[29] O.F. Güner, Pharmacophore Perception, Development, and Use in Drug Design, vol. 2, Internat'l University Line, 2000.
[30] Y. Martin, in: C. Hansch, T. Fujita (Eds.), Classical and 3D QSAR in Agrochemistry, American Chemical Society, Washington, DC, 1995.
[31] S. Handschuh, M. Wagener, J. Gasteiger, Superposition of three-dimensional chemical structures allowing for conformational flexibility by a hybrid method, J. Chem. Inf. Comput. Sci. 38 (1998) 220–232.
[32] J.S. Mason, I. Morize, P.R. Menard, D.L. Cheney, C. Hulme, R.F. Labaudiniere, New 4-point pharmacophore method for molecular similarity and diversity applications: overview of the method and applications, including a novel approach to the design of combinatorial libraries containing privileged substructures, J. Med. Chem. 42 (1999) 3251–3264.
[33] J.H. Van Drie, D. Weininger, Y.C. Martin, ALADDIN: an integrated tool for computer-assisted molecular design and pharmacophore recognition from geometric, steric, and substructure searching of three-dimensional molecular structures, J. Comput. Aided Mol. Des. 3 (1989) 225–251.
[34] J.G. Sutter, Güner, R. Hoffman, H. Li, M. Waldman, Effect of variable weight and tolerances on predictive model generation, in: O.F. Guner (Ed.), Pharmacophore Perception, Development, and Use in Drug Design, International University Line, La Jolla, CA, 1999, pp. 501–511.
[35] A.K. Debnath, Generation of predictive pharmacophore models for CCR5 antagonists: study with piperidine- and piperazine-based compounds as a new class of HIV-1 entry inhibitors, J. Med. Chem. 46 (2003) 4501–4515.
[36] O. Güner, D.R. Henry, Metric for analyzing hit lists and pharmacophores, in: Pharmacophore Perception, Development, and Use in Drug Design, 2000, pp. 195–213.
[37] O. Güner, M. Waldman, R. Hoffmann, J. Kim, Strategies for database mining and pharmacophore development, in: Pharmacophore Perception, Development, and Use in Drug Design, first ed., IUL Biotechnology Series, 2000, pp. 213–236.
[38] O.O. Clement, C.M. Freeman, R.W. Hartmann, V.D. Handratta, T.S. Vasaitis, A.M. Brodie, V.C. Njar, Three dimensional pharmacophore modeling of human CYP17 inhibitors. Potential agents for prostate cancer therapy, J. Med. Chem. 46 (2003) 2345–2351.
[39] G. Schneider, Virtual screening: an endless staircase? Nat. Rev. Drug Discov. 9 (2010) 273–276.
[40] A. Koutsoukas, B. Simms, J. Kirchmair, P.J. Bond, A.V. Whitmore, S. Zimmer, M.P. Young, J.L. Jenkins, M. Glick, R.C. Glen, From in silico target prediction to multi-target drug design: current databases, methods and applications, J. Proteome 74 (2011) 2554–2574.
[41] M.J. Keiser, V. Setola, J.J. Irwin, C. Laggner, A.I. Abbas, S.J. Hufeisen, N.H. Jensen, M.B. Kuijer, R.C. Matos, T.B. Tran, R. Whaley, R.A. Glennon, J. Hert, K.L. Thomas, D.D. Edwards, B.K. Shoichet, B.L. Roth, Predicting new molecular targets for known drugs, Nature 462 (2009) 175–181.
[42] T.M. Steindl, D. Schuster, C. Laggner, T. Langer, Parallel screening: a novel concept in pharmacophore modeling and virtual screening, J. Chem. Inf. Model. 46 (2006) 2146–2157.
[43] S. Ekins, A.J. Williams, M.D. Krasowski, J.S. Freundlich, In silico repositioning of approved drugs for rare and neglected diseases, Drug Discov. Today 16 (2011) 298–310.
[44] A.L. Hopkins, J.S. Mason, J.P. Overington, Can we rationally design promiscuous drugs? Curr. Opin. Struct. Biol. 16 (2006) 127–136.

[45] R. Morphy, Selectively nonselective kinase inhibition: striking the right balance, J. Med. Chem. 53 (2010) 1413–1437.
[46] D. Rognan, Structure-based approaches to target fishing and ligand profiling, Mol. Inform. 29 (2010) 176–187.
[47] H. Kubinyi, In search for new leads, in: EFMC–Yearbook 2003, 2004, pp. 14–28.
[48] H.J. Bohm, G. Klebe, H. Kubinyi, Wirkstoffdesign, Spektrum Akademischer Verlag GmbH, Heidelberg, Germany, 1996, pp. 451–466.
[49] P. Muller, G. Lena, E. Boilard, S. Bezzine, G. Lambeau, G. Guichard, D. Rognan, In silico-guided target identification of a scaffold-focused library: 1,3,5-Triazepan-2,6-diones as novel phospholipase A2 inhibitors, J. Med. Chem. 49 (2006) 6768–6778.
[50] L. Yang, K. Wang, J. Chen, A.G. Jegga, H. Luo, L. Shi, C. Wan, X. Guo, S. Qin, G. He, Exploring off-targets and off-systems for adverse drug reactions via chemical-protein interactome—clozapine-induced agranulocytosis as a case study, PLoS Comput. Biol. 7 (2011), e1002016.
[51] D. Schuster, T. Langer, The identification of ligand features essential for PXR activation by pharmacophore modeling, J. Chem. Inf. Model. 45 (2005) 431–439.
[52] M.C. Sanguinetti, J.S. Mitcheson, Predicting drug-hERG channel interactions that cause acquired long QT syndrome, Trends Pharmacol. Sci. 26 (2005) 119–124.
[53] O.O. Clement, O.F. Güner, Use of Pharmacophores in Predictive ADME, Wiley Online Library, 2006, pp. 381–393.
[54] T. Klabunde, A. Evers, GPCR antitarget modeling: pharmacophore models for biogenic amine binding GPCRs to avoid GPCR-mediated side effects, ChemBioChem 6 (2005) 876–889.
[55] U. Norinder, In silico modelling of ADMET—a minireview of work from 2000 to 2004, SAR QSAR Environ. Res. 16 (2005) 1–11.
[56] S. Oloff, S. Zhang, N. Sukumar, C. Breneman, A. Tropsha, Chemometric analysis of ligand receptor complementarity: identifying Complementary Ligands Based on Receptor Information (CoLiBRI), J. Chem. Inf. Model. 46 (2006) 844–851.
[57] P. Markt, D. Schuster, J. Kirchmair, C. Laggner, T. Langer, Pharmacophore modeling and parallel screening for PPAR ligands, J. Comput. Aided Mol. Des. 21 (2007) 575–590.
[58] J.M. Rollinger, D. Schuster, B. Danzl, S. Schwaiger, P. Markt, M. Schmidtke, J. Gertsch, S. Raduner, G. Wolber, T. Langer, In silico target fishing for rationalized ligand discovery exemplified on constituents of Ruta graveolens, Planta Med. 75 (2009) 195–204.
[59] M.S. Murgueitio, P. Henneke, H. Glossmann, S. Santos-Sierra, G. Wolber, Prospective virtual screening in a sparse data scenario: design of small-molecule TLR2 antagonists, ChemMedChem 9 (2014) 813–822.
[60] Y. Krautscheid, C.J.Å. Senning, S.B. Sartori, N. Singewald, D. Schuster, H. Stuppner, Pharmacophore modeling, virtual screening, and in vitro testing reveal haloperidol, eprazinone, and fenbutrazate as neurokinin receptors ligands, J. Chem. Inf. Model. 54 (2014) 1747–1757.
[61] J.Y. Joung, H.Y. Lee, J. Park, J.-Y. Lee, B.H. Chang, K.T. No, K.-Y. Nam, J.S. Hwang, Identification of novel rab27a/melanophilin blockers by pharmacophore-based virtual screening, Appl. Biochem. Biotechnol. 172 (2014) 1882–1897.
[62] P. Lu, Y. Wang, P. Kai Ouyang, J. She, M. He, 3d-qsar based pharmacophore modeling and virtual screening for identification of novel G protein-coupled receptor40 agonists, Curr. Comput. Aided Drug Des. 11 (2015) 51–56.
[63] N. Singh, S. Tiwari, K.K. Srivastava, M.I. Siddiqi, Identification of novel inhibitors of Mycobacterium tuberculosis PknG using pharmacophore based virtual screening,

docking, molecular dynamics simulation, and their biological evaluation, J. Chem. Inf. Model. 55 (2015) 1120–1129.
[64] V. Temml, C.V. Voss, V.M. Dirsch, D. Schuster, Discovery of new liver X receptor agonists by pharmacophore modeling and shape-based virtual screening, J. Chem. Inf. Model. 54 (2014) 367–371.
[65] H. Ha, B. Debnath, S. Odde, T. Bensman, H. Ho, P.M. Beringer, N. Neamati, Discovery of novel CXCR2 inhibitors using ligand-based pharmacophore models, J. Chem. Inf. Model. 55 (2015) 1720–1738.
[66] A. Lepailleur, T. Freret, S. Lemaître, M. Boulouard, F. Dauphin, A. Hinschberger, F. Dulin, A. Lesnard, R. Bureau, S. Rault, Dual histamine H3R/serotonin 5-HT4R ligands with antiamnesic properties: pharmacophore-based virtual screening and polypharmacology, J. Chem. Inf. Model. 54 (2014) 1773–1784.
[67] Q. Huang, L.-L. Li, S.-Y. Yang, PhDD: a new pharmacophore-based de novo design method of drug-like molecules combined with assessment of synthetic accessibility, J. Mol. Graph. Model. 28 (2010) 775–787.
[68] G. Hessler, K.-H. Baringhaus, The scaffold hopping potential of pharmacophores, Drug Discov. Today Technol. 7 (2010) e263–e269.
[69] D. Goldmann, P. Pakfeifer, S. Hering, G.F. Ecker, Novel scaffolds for modulation of TRPV1 identified with pharmacophore modeling and virtual screening, Future Med. Chem. 7 (2015) 243–256.
[70] L. Guasch, E. Sala, A. Castell-Auví, L. Cedó, K.R. Liedl, G. Wolber, M. Muehlbacher, M. Mulero, M. Pinent, A. Ardévol, Identification of PPARgamma partial agonists of natural origin (I): development of a virtual screening procedure and in vitro validation, PLoS One 7 (2012), e50816.
[71] D. Wei, X. Jiang, L. Zhou, J. Chen, Z. Chen, C. He, K. Yang, Y. Liu, J. Pei, L. Lai, Discovery of multitarget inhibitors by combining molecular docking with common pharmacophore matching, J. Med. Chem. 51 (2008) 7882–7888.
[72] A. Kumar, S. Rai, E. Rathi, P. Agarwal, S.G. Kini, Pharmacophore-guided fragment-based design of novel mammalian target of rapamycin inhibitors: extra precision docking, fingerprint-based 2D and atom-based 3D-QSAR modelling, J. Biomol. Struct. Dyn. 39 (2021) 1155–1173.
[73] C.P. Anju, S. Subhramanian, N. Sizochenko, A.R. Melge, J. Leszczynski, C.G. Mohan, Multiple e-Pharmacophore modeling to identify a single molecule that could target both streptomycin and paromomycin binding sites for 30S ribosomal subunit inhibition, J. Biomol. Struct. Dyn. 37 (2019) 1582–1596.
[74] A. Kumar, E. Rathi, S.G. Kini, E-pharmacophore modelling, virtual screening, molecular dynamics simulations and in-silico ADME analysis for identification of potential E6 inhibitors against cervical cancer, J. Mol. Struct. 1189 (2019) 299–306.
[75] S.D. Pickett, J.S. Mason, I.M. McLay, Diversity profiling and design using 3D pharmacophores: pharmacophore-derived queries (PDQ), J. Chem. Inf. Comput. Sci. 36 (1996) 1214–1223.
[76] G.M. Makara, Measuring molecular similarity and diversity: total pharmacophore diversity, J. Med. Chem. 44 (2001) 3563–3571.
[77] J. Gerstmeier, J. Seegers, F. Witt, B. Waltenberger, V. Temml, J.M. Rollinger, H. Stuppner, A. Koeberle, D. Schuster, O. Werz, Ginkgolic acid is a multi-target inhibitor of key enzymes in pro-inflammatory lipid mediator biosynthesis, Front. Pharmacol. 10 (2019) 797.
[78] U. Grienke, T. Kaserer, B. Kirchweger, G. Lambrinidis, R.T. Kandel, P.A. Foster, D. Schuster, E. Mikros, J.M. Rollinger, Steroid sulfatase inhibiting lanostane triterpenes—structure activity relationship and in silico insights, Bioorg. Chem. 95 (2020), 103495.

[79] P. Mutai, E. Pavadai, I. Wiid, A. Ngwane, B. Baker, K. Chibale, Synthesis, antimycobacterial evaluation and pharmacophore modeling of analogues of the natural product formononetin, Bioorg. Med. Chem. Lett. 25 (2015) 2510–2513.
[80] F. Ntie-Kang, C.V. Simoben, B. Karaman, V.F. Ngwa, P.N. Judson, W. Sippl, L.M. Mbaze, Pharmacophore modeling and in silico toxicity assessment of potential anticancer agents from African medicinal plants, Drug Des. Devel. Ther. 10 (2016) 2137–2154.
[81] J.M. Kratz, C.E. Mair, S.K. Oettl, P. Saxena, O. Scheel, D. Schuster, S. Hering, J.M. Rollinger, hERG channel blocking ipecac alkaloids identified by combined in silico-in vitro screening, Planta Med. 82 (2016) 1009–1015.
[82] F. La Porta, C.A. Taft, Emerging Research in Science and Engineering Based on Advanced Experimental and Computational Strategies, Springer Nature, 2020.
[83] M.S. Alavijeh, A.M. Palmer, The pivotal role of drug metabolism and pharmacokinetics in the discovery and development of new medicines, Curr. Opin. Investig. Drugs 5 (2004) 755–763.
[84] O.F. Guner, J.P. Bowen, Pharmacophore modeling for ADME, Curr. Top. Med. Chem. 13 (2013) 1327–1342.
[85] F. Yamashita, M. Hashida, In silico approaches for predicting ADME properties of drugs, Drug Metabol. Pharm. 19 (2004) 327–338.
[86] M.J. de Groot, S. Ekins, Pharmacophore modeling of cytochromes P450, Adv. Drug Deliv. Rev. 54 (2002) 367–383.
[87] C.M. Masimirembwa, M. Ridderström, I. Zamora, T.B. Andersson, Combining pharmacophore and protein modeling to predict CYP450 inhibitors and substrates, Methods Enzymol. 357 (2002).
[88] D. Schuster, C. Laggner, T.M. Steindl, T. Langer, Development and validation of an in silico P450 profiler based on pharmacophore models, Curr. Drug Discov. Technol. 3 (2006) 1–48.
[89] S. Ekins, B.J. Ring, G. Bravi, J.H. Wikel, S.A. Wrighton, Predicting drug-drug, in: Pharmacophore Perception, Development, and Use in Drug Design, vol. 2, 2000, p. 269.
[90] S. Ekins, G. Bravi, S. Binkley, J.S. Gillespie, B.J. Ring, J.H. Wikel, S.A. Wrighton, Three and four dimensional-quantitative structure activity relationship (3D/4D-QSAR) analyses of CYP2D6 inhibitors, Pharmacogenetics 9 (1999) 477–489.
[91] S. Ekins, G. Bravi, S. Binkley, J.S. Gillespie, B.J. Ring, J.H. Wikel, S.A. Wrighton, Three- and four-dimensional quantitative structure activity relationship analyses of cytochrome P-450 3A4 inhibitors, J. Pharmacol. Exp. Ther. 290 (1999) 429–438.
[92] S. Ekins, G. Bravi, B.J. Ring, T.A. Gillespie, J.S. Gillespie, M. Vandenbranden, S.A. Wrighton, J.H. Wikel, Three-dimensional quantitative structure activity relationship analyses of substrates for CYP2B6, J. Pharmacol. Exp. Ther. 288 (1999) 21–29.
[93] S. Ekins, G. Bravi, J.H. Wikel, S.A. Wrighton, Three-dimensional-quantitative structure activity relationship analysis of cytochrome P-450 3A4 substrates, J. Pharmacol. Exp. Ther. 291 (1999) 424–433.
[94] S. Ekins, G. Bravi, S. Binkley, J.S. Gillespie, B.J. Ring, J.H. Wikel, S.A. Wrighton, Three-and four-dimensional-quantitative structure activity relationship (3D/4D-QSAR) analyses of CYP2C9 inhibitors, Drug Metab. Dispos. 28 (2000) 994–1002.
[95] J.M. Kratz, D. Schuster, M. Edtbauer, P. Saxena, C.E. Mair, J. Kirchebner, B. Matuszczak, I. Baburin, S. Hering, J.M. Rollinger, Experimentally validated hERG pharmacophore models as cardiotoxicity prediction tools, J. Chem. Inf. Model. 54 (2014) 2887–2901.
[96] P. Kraft, J.A. Bajgrowicz, C. Denis, G. Frater, Odds and trends: recent developments in the chemistry of odorants, Angew. Chem. Int. Ed. 39 (2000) 2980–3010.

[97] M. Kansy, M. Ulmschneider, H. van de Waterbeemd, 3D structural databases in the olfactophore generation of musk odor, in: QSAR and Molecular Modelling: Concepts, Computational Tools, and Biological Applications, 1995, pp. 633–638.
[98] I. Bersuker, A. Dimoglo, M.Y. Gorbachov, P. Vlad, M. Pesaro, Origin of musk fragrance activity: the electron-topologic approach, New J. Chem. 1991 (15) (1987) 307–320.
[99] J. Bajgrowicz, G. Frater, Chiral recognition of sandalwood odorants, Enantiomer 5 (2000) 225–234.
[100] I. Bersuker, A. Dimoglo, M.Y. Gorbachov, A. Greni, L. Vysotskaya, T. Mikhailova, Study of the electronic and structural properties of the chemical compounds in garlic aroma, Food/Nahrung 33 (1989) 405–411.
[101] A. Dimoglo, M. Yu Gorbachov, I. Bersuker, A. Greni, L. Vysotskaya, O. Stepanova, E. Yu Lukash, Structural and electronic origin of meat odour of organic hetero-atomic compounds, Food/Nahrung 32 (1988) 461–473.
[102] M. Wieder, U. Perricone, T. Seidel, T. Langer, Pharmacophore models derived from molecular dynamics simulations of protein-ligand complexes: a case study, Nat. Prod. Commun. 11 (2016) 1499–1504.

CHAPTER 6

Target identification for potential drug discovery

Saurabh Sharma, J. Kumaravel, Gurjeet Kaur, Ajay Prakash, and Bikash Medhi
Department of Pharmacology, Postgraduate Institute of Medical Education and Research, Chandigarh, India

1. Introduction

Among more than 20,000 protein coding genes in the human genome, only 700 are known targets for FDA approved drugs [1]. Limited understanding of the causal genes and potential drug targets is a significant impediment to the process of drug discovery. It is common for drugs to fail because the drug target turns out to be unrelated to the phenotype [2]. The target selection strategy should be rational and consider the molecular mechanism of the disease so that the resources are allocated to the most promising drug targets [3].

Drug candidates may be discovered by two main methods: a target-based discovery and a phenotype-based discovery. In a target-based approach, the search starts with the selection of a target molecule that is validated in later stages. A phenotype approach relies on the development of an assay, whereby several phenotypes of the cell, such as receptor translocation, gene expression, and proliferation, are monitored. Recent advances in genomics, molecular biology as well as computer-aided drug design (CADD) has brought a lot of focus on target-based drug discovery. These are further facilitated by the establishment of large chemical libraries. While a target-based approach offers a cheaper and robust alternative to phenotype-based assays it cannot cover all the proteins that are potentially targeted by a drug molecule, thus failing to predict clinical phenotypes. Target deconvolution identifies molecular targets, helping with the prediction of possible adverse effects of the drugs. It also helps with the optimization of the drug molecule and elucidation of additional indications of the drug [4]. Target deconvolution may be implemented through a direct or indirect approach. Direct approaches seek to identify proteins which physically bind the target compound and may be done by: (1) cloning-based expression system, (2) protein microarray, or (3) chemical biology approaches.

Computational Approaches in Drug Discovery, Development and Systems Pharmacology
https://doi.org/10.1016/B978-0-323-99137-7.00008-3

Indirect approaches measure the differential gene expression profiles between test and known compounds. These include connectivity maps, Library of Integrated Network-Based Cellular Signatures (LINCS) and comprehensive screening methods like genome-wide RNAi and clustered regularly interspaced palindromic repeats (CRISPR)/Cas9. Indirect approach may also include the comparison of phenotype profiles between the test and known compounds, such as in BioMap database [5]. Connectivity maps include a database of gene expression profile changes in response to small molecules, which may be applied in a variety of ways. For example, connectivity maps revealed that gene expression signatures of gedunin were similar to geldanamycin, leading to its recognition as an HSP90 inhibitor [6].

Knowing the functions of various proteins and their possible role in the disease pathology plays an important role in drug target identification. Biological assays for identifying protein targets rely on the affinity of small molecules to their biological targets. Affinity chromatography-based approaches have been used extensively to find protein targets physically interacting with small ligand molecules. Similarly, expression-cloning-based methods like three-hybrid system, phage display, and mRNA display are used widely. Owing to complexity of function elucidation through experimental studies, the functions of many proteins are still unknown [7]. Large swathes of protein-protein interaction (PPI) data generated from high throughput experiments may also be used to elucidate possible targets by the application of mathematical modeling [8]. By quantifying the host interactome and integrating the expression data, drug targets can be identified in the human PPI network [9]. Identifying a target requires the integration of mechanistic understanding with a systems pharmacology approach. While modern high-throughput methods quickly produce gene and protein expression data, the gene regulatory network (GRN) elucidation remains a challenge [10]. Machine learning approaches leverage the power of predictive modeling to formulate accurate hypotheses of interaction networks. Machine learning enables the prediction of detailed downstream effects on a system [11]. Clustering algorithms like k-nearest neighbors (KNN), hierarchical clustering, dendrogram plus heat map visualization (tree view), k-medoid, and spectral clustering of protein sequences (SCPS) cluster similar proteins into groups offering wider choice of targets for further study [12].

2. Strategies for identification of targets

Ideal pharmacological targets are relevant to the disease phenotype, therapeutically targetable, and have minimal side effects. Good therapeutic targets tend to not affect the physiological functioning of the healthy tissues. The functional elucidation of potential therapeutic targets is an important first step in identification of the molecular targets of a drug molecule.

Rational drug discovery can be classified into:

Structure-based drug designing
Ligand-based drug designing
In silico drug designing
Homology modeling

Target identification may be classified as follows [13]

Target-based approach	Phenotype-based approach
Protein validation	Phenotype model
Assay development	Assay development
Target-based screening	Phenotype-based screening
Hit optimization	Hit optimization
Phenotype validation	Target validation

3. Advancements in identification of targets

Biological assays, drug target database, and machine learning-based methods offer an effective and time-saving method for identifying protein targets of small ligands. Biological assays include technologies like gene transfection, RNAi, DNA microarray, RT-PCR analysis, MARCM technique, and RNA sequencing. Drug target databases provide information on several aspects of small molecules, including the 3D structure, functional targets, and sequence of the ligand binding domains. Among the most promising technological developments in the field of target identification has been the application of machine learning and artificial intelligence for prediction of ligand targets as well as identification of druggable targets. Support vector machines (SVM) and random forest algorithms are commonly used for this application, even though several algorithms are available. Overall, these technologies can be used in combination to provide an effective way of target identification [14].

4. Application of machine learning for target-drug interaction

The function of a potential therapeutic target (gene/protein) and its role in the disease are the first steps in target identification and characterization. Following the identification of the target, the molecular mechanisms addressed by the target are characterized. A good target should be effective, safe, and druggable while also meeting clinical and commercial needs. Predicting drug-target interactions can aid in the screening of inappropriate compounds and is a crucial step in the creation of novel medications.

Biomedical trials that investigate drug-target interactions necessitate a significant amount of human, financial, and material resources. Machine learning technologies have been applied to drug-target interaction prediction to save resources. Availability of drug interaction data in large databases has enabled the utilization of machine learning techniques for predicting drug-target interaction. With evolving and innovative computer technologies, large data sets offer a fast and accurate workflow for drug-target prediction with machine learning [15].

Steps involved in current drug-target prediction procedures:

(1) Data set acquisition
(2) Feature extraction and processing
(3) Selection of task algorithms

For drug-target interaction prediction, a variety of task algorithms have been utilized, including classification algorithms, learning to rank algorithms, and deep learning algorithms [16–18].

The support vector machines (SVM) algorithm has been successfully applied to the drug development process. The SVM algorithm might classify a compound from a different database and forecast whether or not the item in question is active [19].

5. Steps for the in silico target identification

The exploration of protein-ligand, ligand-ligand interactions, biochemical mechanisms and drug repurposing can be studied by computational identification of biological targets. Biologically annotated chemical databases may be mapped into chemogenomical space, allowing the prediction of drug targets. Further, program failure at later stages of development such as clinical phases during drug discovery were extremely costly [20]. In most of the cases, the primary cause of failure was the lack of efficacy [21]. Efficacy failures can be due to a nonspecific linkage between the disease of interest and therapeutic drug target or the lack of a valid specific animal model of the disease [2]. Hence, identifying the optimal target for a disease in the early phases of drug discovery is critical to maximize the chances of success in the clinic phase and secure a long-term return on investment. Computational methods now complement (or replace) the laborious and expensive wet lab experiments, which are necessary for elucidation of drug targets. Such methods allow for a wider, and a more thorough search for molecular targets, which may then be validated in the laboratory [22–24]. Computational methods may be broadly classified into comparative network-based methods or genomics [10,25]. Infectious and noninfectious diseases are both amenable to network analysis. Comparative genomics is suitable only for the investigation of infectious diseases. Finding therapeutic targets is critical in case of pathogens where antimicrobial resistance has spread rapidly, and targeting novel targets may provide a viable solution. Comparative genomics can reveal targets in pathogens that are critical for their growth and reproduction in the host. Using comparative genomics, the genome of pathogens may be compared to the host, thus eliminating the targets that can affect the host and cause toxicity and side effects. Eliminating problematic drugs in the initial phase of the drug development increases the chances of success in subsequent phases of drug development [26].

Contemporary approaches integrate data from pathway information with biological networks to identify promising pathogen targets. The network-based strategies leverage several approaches like systems biology, network pharmacology, medicine, or biology, often integrating multiomics data. This strategy applies the network graph theory to biological molecular interaction networks, helping identify the components of functional importance in the network on the basis of the network topology or mechanistic importance. Network-based methods may reveal biomarkers and disease diagnosis targets apart from the components of biological networks that are functionally important. In network-based methods, all relevant data are mapped visually to a network. The highly connected nodes play an important role in the network and may be acting as essential proteins or genes for the pathogens. Nodes that are essential for the pathogens, but less so for the host, are considered to be ideal therapeutic targets and may be targeted without compromising the integrity of the physiological interaction network in the host.

Open targets collates and provides information of potential drug targets in several diseases [27]. DisGeNET platform aims to focus on gene-disease association. It contains "380,000 associations between >16,000 genes and

13,000 diseases" [28]. Many other similar web-based tools help identify potential drug targets. Drug targets may be computationally identified by two main strategies: Either based on the ligand or the receptor. Ligand-based methods are independent of the availability of the target protein structure and is a more approachable technique for relatively unskilled users. These methods can predict drug activity sufficiently accurately [29]. Receptor-based approaches rely on the target protein's structure to predict the drug-target interactions. Receptor-based techniques offer a more elaborate investigation into a target protein, enabling the examination of several binding modes, prediction of "off-targets," or a general understanding of the receptor. For the application of receptor-based techniques, it is critical to have access to an accurate three-dimensional (3D) model of the protein. This approach enables reverse docking, which looks for receptors for small ligands rather than small ligands that interact with receptors as in docking. Pharmacophore-based target identification is also accomplished in receptor-based approaches. Algorithms that can predict the placement of binding pockets on a protein can be used for receptor-based drug target identification [30].

Reverse docking predicts that all macromolecules will be interacting with a ligand, thus playing an important role in the process of drug optimization. However, due to being a computationally intensive task, it is not viable to have flexible receptors during reverse docking. Poor prediction performance is another issue that limits its wider application.

Apart from reverse docking, pharmacophore approaches have also been used widely for target and ligand identification. Certain structural moieties have high affinity for some targets and pharmacophore-based approaches virtually screens molecules to identify such structures [31]. An important web-based tool is TargetHunter (http://www.cbligand.org/TargetHunter). It utilizes a "MOst SImilar Counterparts" algorithm to predict the most probable targets of small molecules. The TargetHunter algorithm is trained on ChEMBL, the largest chemogenomical database. Considering the top three predictions on a predefined subset of high-potency compounds from the ChEMBL database, TargetHunter displayed an accuracy of 91.1%, outperforming other published algorithms. TargetHunter's BioassayGeoMap function can be used to find possible collaborator(s) who can test the projected target experimentally. As a result, in-silico drug design and discovery technologies have matured to the point that they can bridge a significant knowledge gap between biology and chemistry [32].

6. Target deconvolution for target discovery

A drug or small molecule initiates its biological effect by binding to protein targets and affecting pathways. The process of identifying the proteins binding with the drug and the pathways affected by the same is termed as "Drug Target Deconvolution." Identifying the targets for a drug helps infer the potential for toxicity and also the mechanism of action of the drug [33]. With the development of molecular biology and biochemistry, the elucidation of the molecular mechanism has historically been accomplished by a reductionist approach. However, target-based discovery has proven insufficient, leading to the resurgence of a holistic based approach, which seeks to unravel the effect of small ligands on the whole system, rather than individual genes. Target deconvolution approaches identify the molecular targets that lead to the phenotyping changes induced by the drug. Molecular targets that are linked with toxicity and side effects may be identified earlier and reduce later-stage "attrition." Most of the methods for target deconvolution depend upon the affinity of small organic molecules to the putative targets. Candidate genes are overexpressed by cloning, and resultant proteins are used in affinity chromatography, expression-based cloning methods, and the three hybrid systems. Other approaches utilize pooled libraries that increase the screening throughput [4].

7. Affinity chromatography methods

Affinity chromatography can identify the cellular target proteins of small ligand molecules by immobilization on solid support matrix through a linker. Linkage to the solid support is possible through introduction of an appropriate functional group to the ligand, which also helps with separation in the later phases. When incubated together, proteins with high affinity to the immobilized ligands attach to the same, while the unbound protein is washed off. The immobilized protein is subsequently identified by immunodetection or mass spectrometry. This method may be applied to any molecule that is amenable to synthesizing derivatives without affecting its biological activity, although each case has to be evaluated individually. With some molecules, there may be a problem with steric hindrance, while others may show non-specific binding. The nonspecific binding may be addressed by adding linkers that have polar functional groups. This has been commonly done by using biotin and polyethylene glycol as linkers [34].

However, the affinity chromatography methodology has some inherent drawbacks, mostly related to the attachment of a linker to the drug molecule. The attachment of a linker may lead to the modulation of the structure-activity relationship (SAR) of the drug molecule. The attachment is also not always straightforward and might require synthesis of a new molecule. Moreover, the linker has to be attached to alternate positions so as to not disrupt the SAR, but given that drugs may interact with the protein pocket with varying orientations, having the linker attached to a specific site (which also doesn't interfere with the SAR) leads to limitations on the application of this method [33].

8. Expression-cloning methods

Expression-cloning-based methods do utilize an affinity step, but address the problem associated with low protein concentrations inherent with regular affinity chromatography. This is done by expression of cDNA library constructs in methods like "Yeast three-hybrid and mammalian three-hybrid systems," "phage display," and "mRNA display."

8.1 Three-hybrid-system

Before the development of the three-hybrid system, receptors of small molecules were identified by in vitro biochemical methods like photocrosslinking, radiolabeled-ligand binding, and affinity chromatography. The difficulty in detecting low concentration proteins limits the application of affinity chromatography to target detection. Such shortcomings are addressed by the two-hybrid and the three-hybrid systems. The yeast three-hybrid system is a modification of the earlier two-hybrid systems whereby the synthetic heterodimer of two different small organic ligands acts as a third hybrid molecule. The yeast two-hybrid system combines the yeast genetics with synthetically generated heterodimeric hybrid ligands. While it proved to be an excellent method for detection of the protein-protein interaction, the three-hybrid modification enabled the screening for the protein targets of know ligands or the ligands of known receptors.

This system consists of three hybrids:

(1) A "DNA-binding domain" is bound to a "ligand-binding domain" in a hybrid protein,

(2) A cDNA library with potential protein targets linked to a transcriptional activation domain, and

(3) A molecule that connects the first and second hybrids by being covalently linked to a ligand.

The reported gene is activated on a successful trimeric complex formation and captured as an assay signal. DNA is extracted and sequenced from cells expressing the reported genes, and the target proteins are identified based on the sequence [35] (Fig. 1).

8.2 Phage display

Phage display overcomes some of the shortcomings of affinity chromatography. Due to the small size of the screened compounds, binding sites of some proteins may be sterically inaccessible to the drug molecule in case of affinity chromatography. Also, some protein molecules like cytokines and autocoids are underrepresented in the protein extract as they may form dime and tetramer complexes, or are expressed less, or simply degrade too

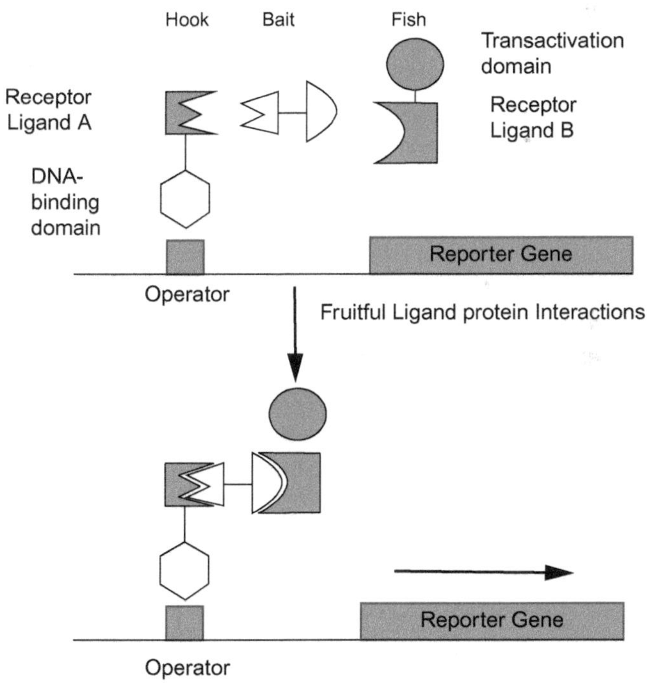

Fig. 1 Yeast three-hybrid system. "Bait": The Ligands connected with a linker. "Hook": Transcription factor fused with ligand A receptor through "DNA-binding domain." Fish: The transcription factor fused to ligand B receptor through a transactivation domain. On interaction between ligand and receptor, a trimeric complex is formed which leads to the activation of the reporter gene.

quickly. Membrane-associated receptors like GPCR are also problematic for affinity chromatography. Phage display offers an improvement over the range and types of protein and drug interactions. Phage display allows the analysis of GPCR, cytokines, and autocoids for interactions with drug molecules [36].

Initially developed for generation of antibodies, phage display is also used for identifying proteins binding to a specific drug. This is accomplished by cloning a library of DNA sequence into the phage genome so as to display the intended protein on the phage coat. The phage library is then co-incubated with immobilized small molecules of interest, leading to the capture of phages with affinity to the drug molecule. The bound phages are transfected into bacteria for amplification while the unbound ones are washed off.

A range of peptides may be displayed on the bacteriophage capsid protein. This array of the foreign protein displayed on the phage is referred to as the phage library. A target (peptide, antibodies, drug molecules, etc.) against which the phage library's affinity has to be tested is referred to as the bait. Phage display is commonly applied for identifying protein-protein interactions and also for target identification. This technique makes it possible to identify the whole array of proteins interacting with a drug molecule, thus revealing the entire interactome of the drug molecule of interest. Further, the drug's interactome helps decipher its "absorption, distribution, metabolism, excretion, and toxicity (ADMET)" parameters [36] (Fig. 2).

8.3 mRNA display

In mRNA display technique, translated proteins are individually attached to the protein-encoding mRNA sequence. The polypeptide chain is connected to the 3′-end of the mRNA through a terminal puromycin-containing DNA linker.

The puromycin molecule bonds with the growing polypeptide chain by entering the "ribosome-A" site during translation. By implementing this on a natural cDNA library, an entire proteome can be conjugated to its corresponding mRNAs. This practically connects the genotype and phenotype and allows the amplification of proteins with the required functions from a diverse library.

mRNA display technology may be applied for a variety of purposes, namely: elucidating several kinds of interactions like protein-protein, DNA-protein, enzyme-substrate, and peptide ligand-receptor. "Synthetic

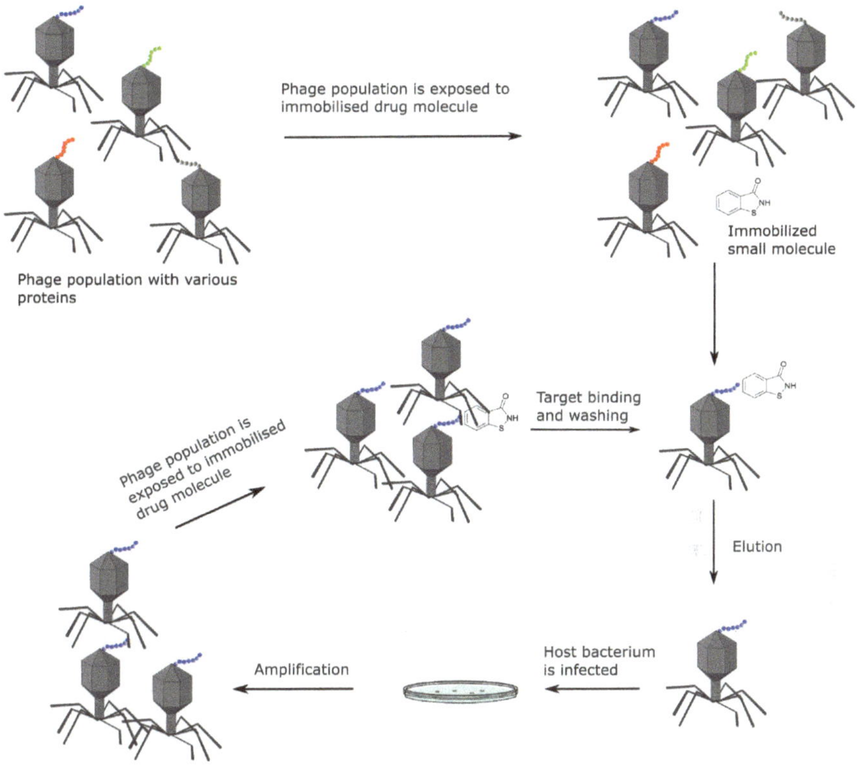

Fig. 2 Phage display: Potential target proteins are displayed on the phage display and exposed to "immobilized small molecules." Phage is selected on the basis of affinity of displayed protein for the immobilized small molecule. The phage is eluted, amplified, and enriched on the basis of affinity for several rounds. Targets of small molecules can be identified by analyzing the targeted proteins.

cDNA library" consists of randomized cassettes and can be used to develop peptide ligands and to guide the evolution of affinity molecules. It allows for adoption of an iterative selection process whereby sequences with increasing greater specificity and affinity are enriched progressively. The mRNA display may also be based on cDNA libraries from natural organisms. Here, an mRNA-protein fusion molecule is derived from naturally occurring mRNA sequence extracted from a natural system like an organism, tissue, or experimental group, etc. Proteins identified through such cDNA libraries provide a condition or site-specific insight into cellular signaling and enzyme substrate specificity [37].

Small molecules of interest are immobilized to a solid support and incubated with the mRNA display molecule libraries, leading to the formation of protein-nucleic acid complexes. The unbound protein-nucleic acid complexes are washed off, while the bound complexes are eluted and processed further. The cDNA is amplified by PCR, leading to the enrichment of drug-binding proteins. This process may be repeated iteratively, followed by the purification of cDNA, cloning, and identification by sequencing [34].

9. Conclusion and future perspective

The next generation of drugs will need a new generation of drug targets. While the drug screening pipelines have undergone several iterations of improvements, the number of proteins which are targeted have plateaued over the years. Molecular targets of drugs are part of pathways and biological networks that play a role in the mechanism of the drug. Recent regulatory requirements place a premium on elucidating the mechanism of various therapeutic agents, and identifying the targets is the most important step in this process. Computational methods like network biology and machine learning are playing an important role in broadening the elucidation of the mechanism of action of various drugs. The development of databases help collate the drug-protein, protein-protein, as well as drug-drug interactions, thus providing an integrated understanding of the mechanism of various drugs.

References

[1] G. Rodgers, C. Austin, J. Anderson, A. Pawlyk, C. Colvis, R. Margolis, et al., Glimmers in illuminating the druggable genome, Nat. Rev. Drug Discov. 17 (5) (2018) 301–302.
[2] D. Cook, D. Brown, R. Alexander, R. March, P. Morgan, G. Satterthwaite, et al., Lessons learned from the fate of AstraZeneca's drug pipeline: a five-dimensional framework, Nat. Rev. Drug Discov. 13 (6) (2014) 419–431.
[3] S. Drăghici, Statistics and Data Analysis for Microarrays Using R and Bioconductor, second ed., Chapman and Hall/CRC, Boca Raton, FL, 2011. 1036 p.
[4] K. Kubota, M. Funabashi, Y. Ogura, Target deconvolution from phenotype-based drug discovery by using chemical proteomics approaches, Biochim. Biophys. Acta Proteins Proteomics 1867 (1) (2019) 22–27.
[5] E.L. Berg, Phenotypic chemical biology for predicting safety and efficacy, Drug Discov. Today Technol. 23 (2017) 53–60.
[6] J. Lamb, E.D. Crawford, D. Peck, J.W. Modell, I.C. Blat, M.J. Wrobel, et al., The connectivity map: using gene-expression signatures to connect small molecules, genes, and disease, Science 313 (5795) (2006) 1929–1935.
[7] F.E. Faisal, K. Newaz, J.L. Chaney, J. Li, S.J. Emrich, P.L. Clark, et al., GRAFENE: graphlet-based alignment-free network approach integrates 3D structural and sequence (residue order) data to improve protein structural comparison, Sci. Rep. 7 (2017). [cited

2020 Oct 8]. Available from: https://www.ncbi.nlm.nih.gov/pmc/articles/PMC5668259/.
[8] E. Schrodinger, R. Penrose, What is Life?: With Mind and Matter and Autobiographical Sketches, Reprint ed., Cambridge University Press, Cambridge ; New York, 2012. 196 p.
[9] S. Nabirotchkin, A.E. Peluffo, P. Rinaudo, J. Yu, R. Hajj, D. Cohen, Next-generation drug repurposing using human genetics and network biology, Curr. Opin. Pharmacol. (2020). [cited 2020 Jun 15]. Available from: http://www.sciencedirect.com/science/article/pii/S1471489219301237.
[10] P. Csermely, T. Korcsmáros, H.J.M. Kiss, G. London, R. Nussinov, Structure and dynamics of molecular networks: a novel paradigm of drug discovery: a comprehensive review, Pharmacol. Ther. 138 (3) (2013) 333–408.
[11] J. Ferreira da Costa, D. Silva, O. Caamaño, J.M. Brea, M.I. Loza, C.R. Munteanu, et al., Perturbation theory/machine learning model of ChEMBL data for dopamine targets: docking, synthesis, and assay of new l-Prolyl-l-leucyl-glycinamide peptidomimetics, ACS Chem. Nerosci. 9 (11) (2018) 2572–2587.
[12] J.H. Morris, L. Apeltsin, A.M. Newman, J. Baumbach, T. Wittkop, G. Su, et al., clusterMaker: a multi-algorithm clustering plugin for Cytoscape, BMC Bioinf. 12 (2011) 436.
[13] J. Ha, H. Park, J. Park, S.B. Park, Recent advances in identifying protein targets in drug discovery, Cell Chem. Biol. 28 (3) (2021) 394–423.
[14] Z. Shangguan, A review of target identification strategies for drug discovery: from database to machine-based methods, J. Phys. Conf. Ser. (2021) 012013. IOP Publishing.
[15] S. Sharma, A. Prakash, P. Sarma, B. Medhi, Machine learning techniques for development of drugs against coronavirus disease 2019 (COVID-19): a case study protocol, in: K. Roy (Ed.), Silico Modeling of Drugs against Coronaviruses: Computational Tools and Protocols [Internet], Springer US, New York, NY, 2021, pp. 307–325. [Cited 2021 Oct 12]. (Methods in Pharmacology and Toxicology). Available from https://doi.org/10.1007/7653_2020_70.
[16] L. Xu, X. Ru, R. Song, Application of machine learning for drug-target interaction prediction, Front. Genet. 12 (2021) 1077.
[17] L. Cheng, H. Zhao, P. Wang, W. Zhou, M. Luo, T. Li, et al., Computational methods for identifying similar diseases, Mol. Ther.–Nucleic Acids 18 (2019) 590–604.
[18] X. Zeng, S. Zhu, W. Lu, Z. Liu, J. Huang, Y. Zhou, et al., Target identification among known drugs by deep learning from heterogeneous networks, Chem. Sci. 11 (7) (2020) 1775–1797.
[19] S. Korkmaz, G. Zararsiz, D. Goksuluk, Drug/nondrug classification using support vector machines with various feature selection strategies, Comput. Methods Programs Biomed. 117 (2) (2014) 51–60.
[20] J.A. DiMasi, H.G. Grabowski, R.W. Hansen, Innovation in the pharmaceutical industry: new estimates of R&D costs, J. Health Econ. 47 (2016) 20–33.
[21] J. Arrowsmith, P. Miller, Phase II and phase III attrition rates 2011–2012, Nat. Rev. Drug Discov. 12 (8) (2013) 569.
[22] S.K. Wooller, G. Benstead-Hume, X. Chen, Y. Ali, F.M. Pearl, Bioinformatics in translational drug discovery, Biosci. Rep. 37 (4) (2017).
[23] A. Georgios, P. George, Computational approaches in target identification and drug discovery, Comput. Struct. Biotechnol. J. 14 (2016) 177–184.
[24] Y.F. Dai, X.M. Zhao, A survey on the computational approaches to identify drug targets in the postgenomic era, Biomed. Res. Int. 2015 (2015), e239654.
[25] J.O. Sekyere, J. Asante, Emerging mechanisms of antimicrobial resistance in bacteria and fungi: advances in the era of genomics, Future Microbiol. 13 (2) (2018) 241–262.

[26] Z. Zhang, Q. Ren, Why are essential genes essential?—the essentiality of Saccharomyces genes, Microb. Cell 2 (8) (2015) 280–287.
[27] D. Carvalho-Silva, A. Pierleoni, M. Pignatelli, C. Ong, L. Fumis, N. Karamanis, et al., Open targets platform: new developments and updates two years on, Nucleic Acids Res. 47 (D1) (2019) D1056–D1065.
[28] J. Piñero, À. Bravo, N. Queralt-Rosinach, A. Gutiérrez-Sacristán, J. Deu-Pons, E. Centeno, et al., DisGeNET: a comprehensive platform integrating information on human disease-associated genes and variants, Nucleic Acids Res. 45 (D1) (2017) D833–D839.
[29] G. Maggiora, M. Vogt, D. Stumpfe, J. Bajorath, Molecular similarity in medicinal chemistry, J. Med. Chem. 57 (8) (2014) 3186–3204.
[30] K.T. Schomburg, S. Bietz, H. Briem, A.M. Henzler, S. Urbaczek, M. Rarey, Facing the challenges of structure-based target prediction by inverse virtual screening, J. Chem. Inf. Model. 54 (6) (2014) 1676–1686.
[31] G. Wolber, T. Seidel, F. Bendix, T. Langer, Molecule-pharmacophore superpositioning and pattern matching in computational drug design, Drug Discov. Today 13 (1) (2008) 23–29.
[32] L. Wang, C. Ma, P. Wipf, H. Liu, W. Su, X.Q. Xie, TargetHunter: an in silico target identification tool for predicting therapeutic potential of small organic molecules based on chemogenomic database, AAPS J. 15 (2) (2013) 395–406.
[33] M. Raida, Drug target deconvolution by chemical proteomics, Curr. Opin. Chem. Biol. 15 (4) (2011) 570–575.
[34] G.C. Terstappen, C. Schlüpen, R. Raggiaschi, G. Gaviraghi, Target deconvolution strategies in drug discovery, Nat. Rev. Drug Discov. 6 (11) (2007) 891–903.
[35] E.J. Licitra, J.O. Liu, A three-hybrid system for detecting small ligand-protein receptor interactions, Proc. Natl. Acad. Sci. 93 (23) (1996) 12817–12821.
[36] Y. Takakusagi, K. Takakusagi, K. Sakaguchi, F. Sugawara, Phage display technology for target determination of small-molecule therapeutics: an update, Expert Opin. Drug Discovery 15 (10) (2020) 1199–1211.
[37] K. Josephson, A. Ricardo, J.W. Szostak, mRNA display: from basic principles to macrocycle drug discovery, Drug Discov. Today 19 (4) (2014) 388–399.

CHAPTER 7

New drug discovery pipeline

Pooja Mittal[a], Hitesh Chopra[a], Komal Preet Kaur[b], and Rupesh Kumar Gautam[c]
[a]Chitkara College of Pharmacy, Chitkara University, Rajpura, Punjab, India
[b]Northeastern University Toronto, Toronto, ON, Canada
[c]Department of Pharmacology, Indore Institute of Pharmacy, IIST Campus, Indore, Madhya Pradesh, India

1. Introduction

Drug discovery is a multistep and versatile process that can easily take over a decade to simplify and raise questions among the general public. As we know, developing a new idea regarding the expansion of medicines that can benefit the general public often takes a long time and is challenging also. In the recent era, pharmaceutical industries are also trying to develop and custom new methods and technologies to manufacture drugs and medical devices. Moreover, in recent times, to improve the procedures for the development and manufacturing of the medicines, structure-based drug discoveries have been used that define the most recent technological advances that can be used to obtain 3D structures, including the high-profile structural genomics approaches that are being used globally. The utilization of 3D protein structures in the novel and fragment-based drug discovery (FBDD) techniques has also been introduced [1,2].

1.1 Fragment-based drug discovery technique

In the last decade, FBDD has emerged as a powerful technique for finding therapeutic leads. FBDD method begins by identifying beginning points that include very tiny molecules (fragments) roughly half the size of conformist medicines (as shown in Fig. 1). These pieces are then combined or extended to produce pharmacological leads. Although the approach has been around for around 30 years, it was not until the mid-1990s that experimental procedures were sensitive and fast enough for the notion to become viable. Since then, the field has grown exponentially [3]. Additionally, FBDD has developed as a conventional technique for the quick and efficient discovery of building blocks that may be utilized to construct high-affinity ligands against protein targets. According to the practitioners,

Computational Approaches in Drug Discovery, Development and Systems Pharmacology
https://doi.org/10.1016/B978-0-323-99137-7.00003-4

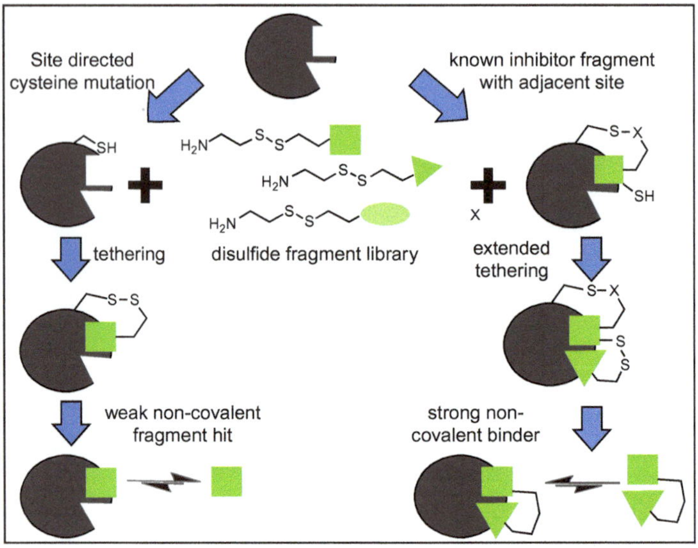

Fig. 1 The ways and means of fragment-based drug design. *(Reproduced with permission from B.C. Doak, R.S. Norton, M.J. Scanlon. The ways and means of fragment-based drug design, Pharmacol. Ther. (2016) 167, https://doi.org/10.1016/j.pharmthera.2016.07.003.)*

FBDD has played a role in developing at least 18 medicines that have entered clinical trials in both academia and business across the world [4].

In the drug discovery pipeline, numerous steps are involved in manufacturing and maintaining the safety and efficacy of drugs. Each of these steps may take many years in and of itself, so it is easy to answer and define why the drug discovery pipeline takes so long. There are initiatives to accelerate this process for potential human volunteers. Apart from this, these steps also help identify medicines or drugs that can easily fight illness without creating difficulties and challenges for the rest of the infected person [1] (Fig. 2).

2. Phases of drug discovery

The phases of the drug discovery pipeline are as follows [1]:

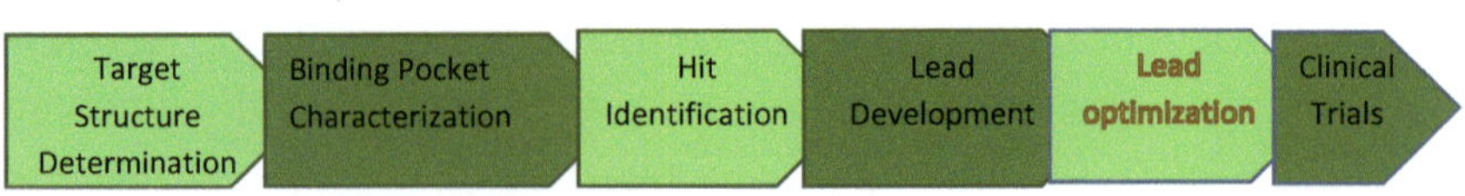

Fig. 2 Schematic of drug discovery pipeline.

2.1 Phase 1

Target identification: Target identification is a preliminary phase of the drug discovery pipeline. In a research trial for the development drug, a clinical investigator needs to be precise with the target thought to drive disease progression to design the drug. Clinical researchers frequently identify drugs that function to battle disease without knowing their target, but if they can act to reverse the disease state, they can be taken forward with minimum molecular workup. Genes, epigenetics, proteins, RNA, and anything else involved in disease pathogenesis might be targets.

2.2 Phase 2

Medicinal Chemistry: Target identification is recognized as an early step of the drug discovery pipeline. In a research study for the development of medicine, a clinical investigator must be specific about the target considered to drive illness progression to build the treatment toward. Clinical researchers routinely find drugs that fight illness without understanding what target they are addressing, but if they can reverse the disease state, they can be moved forward with minimal molecular workup. Targets might include genes, epigenetics, proteins, RNA, and anything else involved in disease etiology.

2.3 Phase 3

In vitro studies are among the most critical phases in the drug development pipeline. In this, the affinity, efficacy, and effectiveness of the drugs are evaluated. In in vitro studies, the target specification of the drug was also estimated. Based on the earlier stages, whatever appears promising must be evaluated in vitro first to determine if it behaves as expected in a cell system, and proof of concept must be demonstrated here before going on to animals. The cell culture, concentration, and frequency of the drug were also investigated.

2.4 Phase 4

In vivo research: In vivo investigations are carried out once the lead complexes have been optimized and characterized to an appropriate degree. This includes the use of animal models of the illness in issue, most commonly mice or rats. This considers a variety of variables such as drug metabolism and clearance, immune response, capacity to enter circulation and reach the target site, and so on and provides the researcher with a plethora of information. It also enables behavioral investigations and functional imaging of both the illness and the chemical itself.

2.5 Phase 5

Clinical Trials: After the in vivo and in vitro research, if the chemical passes the tests necessary for complete clinical trials in people, they can be begun. A medication must go through three phases to be approved: phase I, phase II, and phase III clinical trials, with each having a distinct endpoint aim. If a chemical demonstrates well-being and effectiveness while meeting the required requirements, it may be considered for FDA clearance.

2.6 Phase 6

FDA approval and commercialization: Once a chemical is endorsed for review, pass the examination, and is FDA authorized, it can be utilized clinically by clinicians all across the country. The molecule, or drug, is then commercially accessible for consumption and effectively used in the clinic to enhance the lives and results of patients [1].

Some examples of the drugs in which drug discovery pipelines were used are as follows:

As we all know, the epidemic has increased interest in COVID-19 treatments, often overshadowing other pharmacological discoveries. However, the epidemic has served as a reminder that investing in novel medications may pay off while increasing social respect for the business. A 2019 research published in International Health indicated that medicines introduced after 1981 had resulted in significant increases in life expectancy [5]. The study showed that if drugs had not been introduced between 1981 and 2013, mortality for individuals under the age of 85 would have been 2.16 times more excellent.

There are some pipeline drugs in which effective and safe outcomes were observed while treating patients ranging from cancer to COVID-19 to diabetes.

(1) Deucravacitinib: Deucravacitinib is a selective tyrosine kinase 2 (TYK2) inhibitor with an oral administration route. Also, The POETYK PSO-1 and POETYK PSO-2 trials looked at a daily dosage of 6mg of Deucravacitinib. In comparison to the placebo, both fulfilled both co-primary objectives. According to the reports presented by Bristol-Myers, Squibb Deucravacitinib provided better skin clearance than Amgen's Otezla (apremilast), which it bought from Celgene in 2019 for $13.4 billion [6].

(2) Tirzepatide: This medication is used for the treatment of diabetes and metabolic syndrome. LY3298176 is manufactured and discovered by Eli Lilly and is an investigational drug that outperformed the injectable antidiabetes medication semaglutide in the recent SURPASS clinical study. In the research, tirzepatide outperformed injectable semaglutide in A1C and body weight reductions across three dosages in people with type 2 diabetes. The effects were most evident in those who received the most significant dosage of tirzepatide (15 mg). A1C levels in this subgroup fell by −2.46% from a baseline of 8.28%. In total, 45.7% of individuals who received 15 mg of tirzepatide had normal A1C levels [6]. The results presented by the SURPASS-4 demonstrated that tirzepatide outperformed titrated insulin glargine in improving A1C levels and lowering body weight in people with type 2 diabetes who were at high risk of cardiovascular disease. According to Lilly, the registration package would be submitted to regulatory authorities before the end of the year.

(3) Roflumilast: According to Global Data, the topical phosphodiesterase-4 (PDE4) inhibitor roflumilast for plaque psoriasis might be accessible in various regions by 2022. Arcutis Bio therapeutics' experimental medication performed well in its crucial DERMIS-1 and DERMIS-2 studies."According to the published clinical trial findings, roflumilast cream was usually safe and well tolerated. Ninety per cent of patients in the randomized roflumilast therapy group finished the entire eight weeks," stated Tiffany Chan, immunology analyst at Global Data. While the medication has potential for plaque psoriasis, it would join a crowded therapeutics area as the second PDE4 inhibitor following Amgen's Otezla (Apremilast). On the other hand, Roflumilast is a topical cream, as opposed to the tablet-based Otezla [6].

3. Product lifecycle management

In the drug development phase, product lifecycle management plays a vital role. Product lifecycle management is a platform that manages the entire product lifetime "efficiently" and "cost-effectively," beginning with conception and ending with service disposal. The product life cycle is the most critical aspect of any healthcare product in commercialization. With the help of product life cycle management, pharmaceutical markets can produce healthcare products more effectively and with lower risk, as pharmaceutical industries require more efficient drug development and production in today's era. As a result, product lifecycle management serves as a company's product information backbone, reducing time to market and delaying product removal from the market. Product Life Cycle Management is something that all businesses undertake in order to develop in the market. It is usually done in three stages: the beginning of life (BOL), middle of life (MOL), and end of life (EOL) [7].

Product regulatory compliance plan must include lifecycle management. It is critical to use life cycle management correctly to make the document review process as comfortable for the health authority as feasible by maintaining just the most recent, up-to-date information in the current view of the electronic common technical document (eCTD).

A product's life cycle is typically split into four stages: introduction, growth, maturation, and decline. Every product has a different life cycle, and the time spent at each step varies (as shown in Fig. 3).

3.1 To begin, when a product is released or marketed, it enters the introduction stage. During this time, businesses should aim to enhance customer knowledge of the product and urge them to try it.

3.2 Second, during the growth stage, firms should expound on the product's qualities and values compared to rival items to encourage their consumers to purchase it. Some products, on the other hand, never grow.

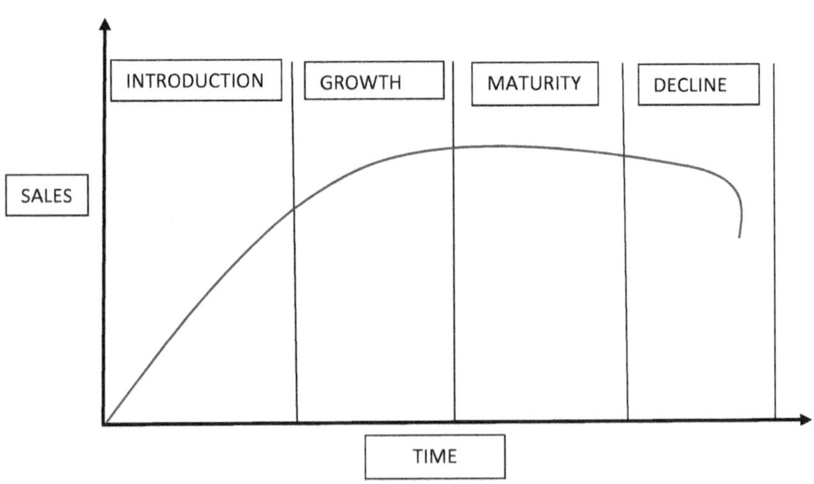

Fig. 3 Graph representing product life cycle.

3.3 Third, the bulk of items are available in the mature stage. At this time, sales are increasing at a constant rate, and market competition is increasing. Following that, the firms modify their market objectives, products, or marketing strategies to extend the mature stage and avoid their product from entering the declining stage. If a product's sales fall, the company should determine whether to maintain it, manufacture it, and cut their investment until all of their product is sold or divest and get rid of it.

If a corporation maintains a firm grip on these four stages of a product's life cycle, their business will optimize profits and recognize when the moment is appropriate to divest them from the product. Furthermore, failure to do so may result in a significant financial loss and a product with a limited life cycle. The use of lifecycle management (LCM) is critical for the pharmaceutical business to minimize time-to-market and postpone product removal from the market. Creating a product and bringing it to market is a collaborative process that involves several teams. Secondary stakeholders such as regulatory authorities impose significant R&D spending, QC, and quality assurance. PLC describes the procedure, processes, and permissions that are necessary and the function of each team member in a pharmaceutical business that enables the seamless development of a product from industry to market.

4. Phases of drug discovery to market

4.1 Phase I

New medicines are developed via drug discovery. For the most part, medications are discovered via experiments that examine active components derived from old remedies or by accident. Afterward, the study of chemical libraries and natural products found therapeutic benefits, which was achieved through traditional pharmacology. Reverse pharmacology has discovered new cures for previously untreatable illnesses by analyzing human DNA (deoxyribonucleic acid).

4.1.1 Target identification and validation

Drug development goes through the following cycles: researchers uncover disease mechanisms, molecular compound testing, current therapies with unexpected effects, and new technology. The process of drug development nowadays begins with finding "hits," followed by medicinal chemistry, and then optimizing those hits to minimize any adverse effects (increasing affinity and selectivity). Further improvements include increased efficacy and potency, better metabolic stability (half-life), and greater oral bioavailability. Being well-versed on the clinical spectrum of disease and the precise role of a target in that illness are critical elements in developing a "good" pharmaceutical. It is considered "druggable" when a biological target's activity may be changed by a therapeutic agent—a small molecule or a biopharmaceutical—in a clinical trial. "Good" drug targets typically have "universal" advantageous properties and can be discovered in a variety of ways, including scouring published scientific literature, searching available databases, or using "practical" methods such as target deconvolution and target discovery. "Good" drug targets are typically those that have "universal" advantageous properties [8–10]. Once a target has been discovered, it must be verified to determine its eligibility for pharmaceutical development before a screening campaign can be launched to find potential "hits".

Research studies and public databases, such as Drug Bank or TTD (Therapeutic Target Database), serve as starting points for identifying potential targets [11,12]. Competition occurs between drug developers when using this technique to discover pharmacological targets. To advance the drug development process, some people are ready to take more scientific risks in the hopes of finding "more established" targets, while others are willing to accept higher competition in order to increase their chances of discovering "more established" targets. There is a multitude of methods for target identification, apart from the literature review. In this example, you begin with a medication that seems compelling and end by identifying the target retroactively. The second method, target discovery, involves looking for targets, after which chemical libraries are searched to identify drugs that target the target and provide the desired effect.

4.1.2 Assay development and screening

An assay is a collection of reagents that generates a detectable signal for measuring a biological process. An assay's quality is determined by the signal's robustness and repeatability without a test substance. To determine the assay quality, one must first determine the kind of signal being measured. Assay quality is determined by reagents, reaction conditions, automation equipment, and statistical models for data processing. The assay and data quality affects the predictive analysis of a compound's biological and pharmacological activity. Assay development is a technique for objectively screening substances for target interaction or alteration. Understanding illness and etiology help researchers create more thorough tests using new techniques and technologies. The design step selects test settings and methods to minimize possible sources [13,14]. Failed hit rates are linked to an assay's selectivity and sensitivity. A *hit* is defined as a molecule's activity in a biochemical or cell-based test represented as a percentage of control substances. The assay development and optimization cycle may be viewed as a way to evaluate many factors and parameters to improve the "reading window." This kind of optimization experiment relies on technology. Increasing the signal-to-noise ratio of positive and negative controls and decreasing inter-well fluctuations owing to pipetting errors and temperature gradients throughout the microtiter plate are critical aspects of optimization. Generally, coefficients of variation under 10% and Z values over 0.5 are ideal. Assay validation certifies that the assay is fit for its purpose. Validation is essential since tests must work reliably for years throughout preclinical research. A robust assay needs a signal that can provide physiologically meaningful data [15,16].

The chemical structure and target-based activity in a biochemical or cell-based test must match to produce a lead from a pool of candidate compounds. A variety of tests are used to evaluate potential drugs. Multiple substances may be identified via high-throughput screening [17]. Testing a compound's absorption, distribution, metabolism, and excretion include cellular and toxicological tests (ADME). Cell-free (biochemical) or cell-based assays are available. The choice of a biochemical or cell-based test, as well as the detection format, is personal. Cell-based assays measure not only chemical potency but also cytotoxicity, permeability, and growth impacts, which may be used to forecast late development. In recent years, cell-based tests have been increasingly successful in discovering novel medication classes. Enzymes are also significant therapeutic targets, and many medicines work by inhibiting enzymes that cause illness. It is essential to understand enzyme biochemistry and kinetics. Plate readouts use colorimetric, fluorescence, bioluminescence, and resonance energy transfer (FRET) assay detection techniques. Fluorescence techniques offer a lower background and a better signal to noise ratio than other methods for screening tiny molecule modulators [18–21]. High-throughput screening is the repeated testing of various chemicals in an experiment. High-throughput screens may test >10,000 assays (wells) each day. High-throughput testing enables researchers to swiftly run millions of experiments to discover essential modifier genes, proteins, or chemicals. These screenings may reveal structure-function connections in minor chemical "hits" and functional clustering inside biological pathways [22]. In vitro and high-throughput screening has significantly improved drug screening efficiency in the current drug development process. Biological activity screening of candidate compounds was a significant barrier in discovering new medicines before current methods.

4.1.3 Hit to lead

The hit to lead (H2L) stage of drug development looks to find compounds of interest (leads) from a pool of compounds (hits) that have therapeutic potential. The H2L process happens after target validation, assay development, and high-throughput screening investigations. A *hit* is a substance that has desirable therapeutic efficacy against a target molecule [23–25]. Various assays are used to assess its activity throughout the hit discovery and confirmation procedures Hits give vital information about the molecular structure, identification, and purity [26,27]. This affects its biological action with the target. After discovering a sequence of hits, researchers may use various tests to validate the hits, depending on the therapeutic target, compound screening scale, and accessible equipment. For example, pharmacological tests discover molecules with the required mechanism of action. During this stage, assay reproducibility, quality, and sensitivity are critical.

High-Throughput Screening (HTS) is the primary method for finding novel drugs. Focused-based screening is another critical component of hit discovery. This requires a detailed study of a chemical library, including subsets of compounds with possible target site activity [28–30]. Fragment-based screening and physiological screening methods may be used to supplement these approaches. Optimizing the characteristics of many hits is a difficult task. It was created to solve these issues and thoroughly investigate hits' chemical and biological components to remove weakly active substances. To be active in primary assay screening, a chemical must fulfill specific criteria. Potency, selectivity, solubility, permeability, metabolic stability, minimal CYP inhibition, and desirable pharmacokinetic characteristics may all be measured. A H2L involves evaluating a new drug's pharmacokinetic and toxicological characteristics, as well as perfecting its efficacy. Optimizing one feature (like absorption) without sacrificing another (like the drug's efficacy) is a frequent problem for medicinal chemists. Because decreasing a drug's molecular weight improves absorption, reducing a compound's molecular weight may negatively affect overall potency. Parallel optimization of potency, selectivity, pharmacokinetics, and physical characteristics in common. Each of the above drug characteristics is measured using multiparametric methods. Thus, researchers may create medicines with more consistent properties, which will help predict their destiny in subsequent preclinical and clinical trials.

4.1.4 Lead optimization

The lead optimization phase's ultimate aim is to retain the characteristics of the drug's most essential ingredients while minimizing any flaws in the structure [31]. Additionally, the lead compounds' chemical structures may be changed if needed to increase their selectivity and specificity for a particular target. An example is the optimization of lead metabolites in drug metabolism investigations. This research will also find any safety issues and see whether more significant throughput trials are needed. During the lead optimization phase, interesting compounds will be judged as having fulfilled the original aims of this stage, after which they will go-ahead to the next step of the programmed, final characterization tests. It is also possible that these last characterization tests will be included in the lead optimization phase of the company. A commonly used way to evaluate the drug in vivo pharmacokinetic data after the lead optimization stage is using DMPK (drug metabolism and pharmacokinetics) in vitro experiments [32,33]. One of the latest innovations in automated screening systems is allowing screening tests to become a standard component of pharmaceutical and biopharmaceutical drug development procedures. For example, in the case of drug candidates, mass spectrometry is often employed to look for and quantify any metabolites in tissues. Additional methods for selecting lead compounds during preclinical screening processes include nuclear magnetic resonance (NMR) fragment-based screening techniques.

4.2 Phase II

Before starting clinical testing, a chemical must go through a series of tests. The first step in treating an illness is finding a possible target for treatment. Multiple compounds are then screened to identify those that have therapeutic promise. If they are safe, they must undergo toxicity testing before going ahead to clinical trials to minimize the risk of damage. Before a new medication may be used, the U.S. Food and Drug Administration (FDA) requires that a set of studies be done. Research to identify a specific illness and then screen for small molecules or biological compounds that demonstrate the ability to treat the disease are done in the first phase.

Before the clinical trials, the second step is referred to as the preclinical research phase, and it includes identifying the possible toxicity of the chemical [34]. In addition to dosage, method, and frequency of administration, variables like dose, delivery mechanism, and dosing interval are also assessed to assist in the following stage, which is clinical research. In this experiment, individuals are used to decide if the chemical can be used to treat the illness that led to the experiment. The most common cause of failure for compounds employed as medicines is that the molecule does not act as a drug or is poisonous. Drug targets should thus be identified during the early stages of preclinical testing [35,36]. Technological advancements in the recent past have led to an exponential rise in the number of potentially applicable targets. Thanks to improved bioinformatic techniques, researchers may mine the existing data to find these prospective drug targets. Many biologically important compounds, including proteins, RNA (Ribonucleic acid), and DNA, are used as targeting ligands. For a chemical to be deemed a potential therapeutic target, it must be "druggable." Various compounds have different classes of targets. Therefore, certain classes of targets are better suited to other classes of compounds. One example of this is the excellent fit that ligand-receptor systems (i.e., G-protein coupled receptors) have for tiny molecules, whereas the best alternative for inhibiting protein-protein interactions is the use of antibodies. Once the treatment goal has been established, the next step is to identify "positive results." These chemicals are expected to affect the illness under consideration. Multiple assays are used here.

A vast pool of compounds is tested against the target to determine whether any seem to be a good candidate for proceeding to the next step. To find possible inhibitors of a protein target, these tools run thousands of computer-aided assays and never assume that any of the assays could detect substances that would bind to the target and reduce its effectiveness [37–39]. Compressed screening examines a few substances but just the most potent ones. Fragment screening and physiological screening are two other preclinical screening techniques used in this phase of preclinical testing. Once an area has been discovered, the chemicals are further studied to refine their effects. This is the early stages of preclinical research in which the substance's structure-activity connection with the target is examined, and then if the compounds interact with the target from another species is examined.

Compounds may be evaluated in an animal model of the illness, which is an essential step in toxicology testing before doing preclinical studies. The final compound is then processed to keep the good qualities while removing or reducing the undesirable characteristics. Preclinical testing should consider the characteristics of the illness and the demographics of the individuals who are affected by it [40]. Alzheimer's is a progressive illness; therefore, the therapy must be long-term. Thus, it is critical to carry out preclinical testing in a manner that emulates long-term use. This shows any chemicals that may be harmful after a prolonged period of exposure.

Research into reproductive toxicity may be performed before testing when neurological disorders are more common in older individuals. However, it may be wise to screen for potential drug interactions during preclinical testing due to the patients' medication use. Other essential factors that should be considered when formulating a treatment regimen for a particular patient demographic include the ease of administration. For example, in neurodegenerative diseases, patients will respond better to treatments administered once or twice a day, such as small tablets or liquids taken every day or less. Something that could be tested in preclinical studies would be a good idea for identifying chemicals that could be given this manner. Much progress has been achieved in developing bioinformatics, virtual reality, and the internet of things in the last several decades. Simulations are used to anticipate the performance of chemical entities both in vivo and in vitro. For the in silico model, SAR and QSAR are typical methods for structural/activity relationship (SAR/activity relationship) assessment. Complex models in silico, which use all available information, are based on statistical, mathematical, bioinformatics, biochemistry, and molecular biology collected into a single file. Typically, the NOAEL (no-observed-adverse-effect-level) has served as the starting point for determining the optimal dosing levels in preclinical and early phase clinical research [41,42]. Despite recommendations in many regulatory guidance documents, the NOAEL continues to be used and followed widely, as specified in the regulatory documents. In the last several years, there have been numerous reports detailing obstacles to the approach, and a collaborative effort has emerged to seek a return to previous advances that would help develop new and innovative approaches. Both BMD (benchmark dose) models and AOPs (adverse outcome pathway), which are both computer-based, are adopted by major regulatory bodies to help maintain human safety [43,44]. Some concerns currently exist for almost all of these ideas, but these concepts may find their complete application and acceptance over the next several decades.

4.3 Phase III

While fundamental concerns about a medication's safety are answered in preclinical research, this does not address how the medicine interacts with the human body. In clinical research, experiments or trials that are done on individuals are called "clinical research." Before doing clinical research, researchers need to do the Investigational New Drug Process (IND). Medical device development has used adaptive clinical trial designs, and learning from that process is now being applied to medication development. The practice of adaptive design decreases the number of patients in a study and generally reduces the number of trials [45]. These findings may be more useful as trials. While the adaptive design may also improve the acceptance of stakeholders, it provides more flexibility. When conducting clinical safety and effectiveness studies that need a high degree of control, adaptive design is beneficial. Early-phase and exploratory studies may benefit from adaptive design. This is particularly relevant for follow-on trials to fulfill post-marketing obligations. Design that adapts in the exploration phase gives the researcher the chance to test a wide variety of dosages, regimens, populations, and so on while also allowing them to terminate testing of poor decisions [45].

Additionally, this method provides greater flexibility while also benefiting those involved by exposing them to fewer inferior therapies. Adaptive design refers to adjusting design elements on the fly as conditions change. The FDA finalized "Adaptive Designs for Clinical Trials of Drugs and Biologics" in November 2019 to provide the answers to this issue [45]." Adaptive design, as defined in the 2019 guideline, is "a clinical trial design that enables the design change depending on data from subjects." Nonadaptive trial designs do not contain features that may be modified in response to market conditions. Early-phase dosage escalation studies provide a typical example of adaptive design. Interim analysis studies use a review committee to conduct prospectively designed interim pharmacokinetic and safety data assessments, using which the committee then decides on the next steps. Committee membership and criteria for whether to halt, repeat the previous dosage, or continue to a higher dose should be specified beforehand in these instances. Planning a preliminary unblinded test midway through the scheduled trial is an adaptive design method to discover whether an efficacy target has been reached. Early achievement of the goal may substantially decrease the trial time and resources. When the endpoint is not reached, the trial proceeds with the next test. With the second example, the number of tests will increase the likelihood of this final analysis being inaccurate. As a result, the statistical validity of the study must be considered while preparing plans for the future [46]. Traditional type 1 and type 2 error control has relied on statistical theory to account for nonadaptive trials. Using a predetermined significance threshold such as 5% is frequently used. Unfortunately, this method cannot be used for designs that utilize many different components.

The use of clinical trial simulators may aid adaptive trial design. An approximation of the error that may occur in hypothetical clinical trials may be produced via a set of assumptions. The data and trial settings in nonadaptive design research are prepared using assumptions and the best available estimations. In addition to all of these, we need to take into consideration population mean and event rates, variation, and dose-response impact size, as well as discontinuation rates. Estimation and assumptions are best if they are correct, but things may go awry if they are inaccurate [46]. In a nonadaptive research design to help deal with the risk associated with uncertainty, there are various factors to consider [46]. As an example, while researching to discover the correct dosage, many randomized fixed-size groups may be included to guarantee the best dosage is found. Since it is assumed that several groups would be underdosed, design choices have to be taken. This approach sacrifices efficiency for a reduced chance of missing the optimum dosage. However, what would happen if you did not have to sacrifice efficiency to guarantee that the optimum dosage is accurately measured? An adaptive design may employ a model-based method to choose Phase 2 dosages compared to traditional research designs. Once interim data is available, the model can be adapted to accommodate the data and inform alterations to the study design. The alterations will likely focus on reducing the number of subjects receiving suboptimal doses and directing the resources toward doses expected to yield positive results [46].

Futility criteria (also known as noneffectiveness criteria) may be used when medication efficacy is questionable. When intermediate research results reveal a failed study, an adaptive design may decide to increase the size of the study population before the final results are known. When the adaptive design is advantageous, for example, in selecting the correct sample size for research, another possible use of it is observed. If estimates of variance and treatment impact are too optimistic, the trial may be underpowered; conversely, if these parameter estimates are too cautious, the research might yield an unnecessarily large population. An underpowered study means that the research data is too limited to be helpful when it comes to statistical findings. Time and money are lost if the research population is too big. To prevent undesired results, the sample size may be changed as research data accumulates adaptively.

While this program has some minor advantages, its most significant feature is its ability to include future planned changes to the research design components and hypotheses based on interim data analyses. Future changes in the procedure should be anticipated, and any intermediate analyses should have a built-in method for controlling statistical bias. Some sources of bias may arise because of changes in the kind of data used in the primary analysis (endpoints and populations). For example, analysis results may be challenging to understand due to this bias. Estimates that may be biased should be found ahead of time and present findings only if adjustments are available. In situations where this approach may not always be accessible, at the very least, the degree of bias must be assessed, as must the impact estimates. Also, results and interpretations must be provided and presented in an accurate, trustworthy manner. Planning should be rigorous and account for all variables that might impact the planned analyses. These variables include, but are not limited to, the anticipated numbers and timings of interim analyses, the types of adaptations, the statistical inferential methods to be used, and the algorithm governing the adaptation decision. Before starting the trial, an investigation strategy that covers all relevant aspects may be created to provide further assurance that adaptive choices were not taken due to cumulative information accumulation in an unintended manner. The accumulation of trial data may influence trial direction and sponsor behavior, as well as participant behavior. Thus, to guard against any conflict of interest, it is highly advised that access to interim comparative findings be restricted to people who are not associated with the trial's conduct or management. It is essential to identify potential causes and implications of trial conduct problems while preparing for an adaptive trial. Several planning strategies have been established to help prevent these problems, including controlling blinding and documenting access throughout the trial. After the data have been gathered, these and related issues may be challenging to change. Additionally, design constraints should be taken into account when using an adaptable design. During an adaptive design (e.g., by removing exploratory research in favor of including exploratory aims inside an adaptive design study), careful assessments after an exploratory study may lead to the discovery of essential insights. If the resulting therapy is incorrect, it may mean that safety concerns are not adequately recognized or other important information about the treatment response, interactions with concurrent treatments or other factors are missing. Thus, such oversights may incur significant financial and development costs [47,48].

In clinical trials, it is not always an adaptive design that should be used. This refers to short-term studies (2–8 weeks) among populations that may be rapidly accessed (3–6 months) [49]. For example, while interim analyses are performed, recruiting is suspended. Instead, an adaptive design may be well suited for a more comprehensive study where interim data from a short-term endpoint (e.g., 6 weeks) is used to predict a long-term endpoint (e.g., 6–12 months). Because this study does not need to stop recruitment, interim data from a short-term endpoint (e.g., at 6 weeks) can be used to predict a long-term endpoint (e.g., 6–12 months). When just a few problems (e.g., dosage, demographic subgroups, outcomes) need to be investigated, adaptive designs perform best and carry lower risk. Programs with considerable ambiguity about numerous parameters may gain valuable insights by performing an exploratory trial before doing the "adequately controlled" experiment. Implementing this method will result in less ambiguity and lead to more efficient and informative use of the technique.

4.4 Phase IV

The first in a series of steps culminating in an authorized product is just giving a marketing application to the FDA. However, the work of the regulators is not the only activity occurring; in addition, sponsors need to be involved. It is critical that no errors with any of these, else we may delay or fail the project. In general, the review process aims to offer a comprehensive, efficient system that enables thorough but efficient evaluation of a product's safety, efficacy, and quality while also moving as quickly as possible through the regulatory process.

The time it takes for an application to go from submission to approval varies. Prescription Drug User Fee Act (PDUFA) rules state that the FDA plans to process 90% of typical NDA and BLA submissions within 10 months of the application date [50]. When it comes to prioritized application evaluation, the deadline is 6 months. The PDUFA goal date is a popular name for this review objective. While the FDA is actively exploring alternate review timeframes (e.g., the Real-Time Oncology Review pilot programmed), it is also testing other mechanisms (i.e., removing the existing time requirement) to ensure that patients have access to safe and effective cancer treatments as quickly as possible. The first barrier in all commercial marketing applications is passing an automated technical evaluation. The application will be rejected if the research data are absent or fails to comply with certain technical specifications.

Assuming the application passes this automated assessment, it will be sent to the relevant review division for further processing and dissemination. In order to verify that the application satisfies preliminary regulatory and user fee criteria, the RPM (regulatory project managers) in the review division will do the job [51].]. A review team is established when these criteria are fulfilled. The FDA has 60 days from the time a marketing application is filed to complete the first evaluation. In this instance, the FDA will examine the submission to see whether it is enough to handle a more substantial examination. Filing determination day is marked as Day 60 post-submission. The review disciplines offer recommendations on the "file-ability" of the application before the filing determination date. The FDA is required to notify the sponsor of any issues they find with the application after the first evaluation. If problems are discovered, they will also send an information request to the company. File designations cannot be made by Day 60 after submission; otherwise, the creator of the submission will be informed of filing review problems by Day 74 in a letter called the 74-Day Letter. When using this document, the sponsors should keep in mind that their response time to deal with any flaws in the 74-Day Letter is short, and they should have enough resources on hand [51].

To plan out timeframes and actions, FDA also begins review planning. By speeding up the whole review process, this phase helps guarantee that the review is up to date and efficient. After they have mapped out the evaluation stages, the FDA will inform the sponsor of any significant milestone deadlines. An in-depth analysis runs from the date of the filing decision to approximately Month 8 post-submission and continues through Month 5 for all priority applications. FDA conducts a thorough examination of the application during this phase. Often requires the input of reviewers from different disciplines and advisors from the various departments within the FDA. Sponsors are expected to receive several follow-up questions from the FDA throughout the whole review process. To be prepared to answer any such inquiries as quickly and thoroughly as possible, the sponsor should be ready [51].

Tasks beyond responding to information requests may be part of the review process. Those are all safety and configuration-related issues that need to be reported as soon as possible and are included in the Safety Update Report, Mid-Cycle Communication, Pre-approval Inspection (PAI), Late-Cycle Meeting, Advisory Committee (AC) Meeting (if necessary), and Labeling Discussions. In addition to 21 CFR 314.50 (d)(5)(vi), sponsors are now obliged to give FDA a 120-Day Safety Update (b). The filing of this update to the FDA must occur 4 months after submitting the first version. The FDA is always the most current about safety information, and this upgrade guarantees that their decision-making process includes the most up-to-date information.

The FDA Mid-Cycle Meeting takes place around month five. It provides management and review teams with an opportunity to discuss the findings, timelines, and risks associated with a REMS (risk evaluation and mitigation strategies) and an additional PMR (post-marketing requirement) and PMC (post-marketing commitment) study. The RPM and other relevant members of the review team will typically contact the sponsor shortly after the mid-cycle meeting to update the review progress. Mid-cycle communication is referred to as this.

One of the most critical milestones alongside the complete CMC quality assessment is the Pre-Approval Inspection (PAI) [52]. FDA will send a team of specialists to the manufacturing site to assess the facility's ability to manufacture the medication and that the data in the marketing application is correct and comprehensive. A PAI slide presentation may be seen on FDA's website. A meeting is conducted in the late cycle with the FDA and the sponsor to address any significant flaws, the need for a REMS, substantial labeling concerns, and further post-marketing studies. For the other applications, an Advisory Committee (AC) meeting is required. Once the FDA chooses to convene an AC meeting, the information will be sent to the sponsor in advance to enable both parties to discuss their respective concerns and prepare their respective presentations. FDA and the sponsor meet to discuss and agree on the contents and language of the prescription information (i.e., product label, package insert). Completing this stage significantly affects the product's advertised usage and how the product is categorized. While this period is passing, all project management committees (PMC), project management review (PMR), and risk management processes are all established. Because of the compressed period, the sponsor is strongly urged to take effective communication with FDA and provide clear and concise responses instead of submitting a significant quantity of new data to support labeling claims. The action phase is the last step in the action package creation process. This is the latter stage of the organization evaluation, namely, the formal notice of the sponsor. A communication formally called an action letter informs the sponsor of the FDA's decision [52].

When the signing authority has rejected the application, RPM prepares a complete response (CR) letter, in which it lists the areas that need attention and provides a proposed plan for correcting the issues. Disciplinary deficiency letters, specifically associated with the sponsor, may also be issued to the sponsor. The RPM writes an approval letter after receiving permission from the customer. The discipline-specific evaluations and the overall summary rationale for approval for approved applications (which may be accessed on FDA's Drugs FDA website) are made public with proper redaction. The post-action phase starts after the FDA decides on approval. It is at this time that both the FDA and the sponsor may act. During this period, the FDA will have the opportunity to discuss parts of the review process that were particularly effective and any issues encountered. This information is being communicated in order to enhance the workflow and guarantee compliance with PDUFA objectives. A post-approval feedback meeting may be provided if a sponsor gets an approval letter (i.e., FDA and sponsor). This gathering is not a PDUFA meeting, but it is used to develop existing procedures further.

A sponsor may seek an End-of-Review Conference after they get a CR letter (d). The meeting's primary goal is to let the sponsor know about the shortcomings in the application and what answers are anticipated. To draw attention to this meeting, we have noted that it serves to increase mutual understanding, and it does not represent an agreement between FDA and sponsor. A Type A meeting if requested within 3 months after the CR action; otherwise, it is a Type B meeting (Type A meetings receive more rapid responses from FDA and earlier scheduling).

4.5 Phase V

Clinical trials help gain a better understanding of the effectiveness and safety of a medication, but their use comes to an end the moment that a drug is approved for sale. Despite going through a long and thorough medication development process, there are limits. An actual image of the safety of a product is in flux and on the move all during the lifespan of a product in the marketplace. The FDA is responsible for inspecting complaints of problems with prescription and over-the-counter medications and decides if warnings and other measures are warranted in the medication dose or use instructions, as well as other severe concerns.

(1) Postmarked monitoring operations need a wide variety of FDA regulations. This approach of post marketed monitoring seeks to actively collect, analyze, and interpret data or other information on a marketed device in order to detect unexpected and unanticipated adverse occurrences, as well as other information required to safeguard public health and safety [53,54]. Requirements that impose severe and irreversible adverse health consequences on a medical device that it is intended to be implanted into the human body for more than 1 year;

(2) Poses a high risk of failure; or
(3) It is expected to be used to sustain or support life, may be imposed on Class II or Class III medical devices.

Postmarket surveillance procedures and obligations are described in 21 CFR 822. Following the release of a new medical device, the FDA places an obligation on the maker of that device to perform postmarket monitoring on it [54,55]. The FDA will identify the devices subject to the order and the reasons for the monitoring requirements in advance or part of the order. To further help create a postmarket monitoring strategy, the FDA will provide the manufacturer with any general or particular advice that is available. Once FDA issues a postmarket surveillance order, the manufacturer's postmarket surveillance plan must be submitted to FDA within 30 days.

The U.S. Food and Drug Administration requires class II and III device manufacturers to undertake postmarket monitoring, even for class II and III devices that "are anticipated to have a substantial usage in juvenile populations [56,57]. However, the FDA is aware that this rule does not apply to devices designated for use on children. To simplify: The direction goes as follows: "Section 522(a)(1)(B) of the Act allows the agency to require postmarket monitoring as a condition of clearance or approval for devices with a substantial usage in pediatric populations." According to section 522 of the FD&C Act, "pediatric population" is not defined. It is also following the statutory definition given under section 520(m)(6)(E)(i) of the FD&C Act.

A company can request an order from the FDA for a surveillance program of up to 36 months (plus/minus any extensions) under section 522(b)(1) of the Act [58]. This order can be issued if a disagreement cannot be resolved or after the conclusion of a dispute resolution procedure established under section 562 of the Act. Despite this, the guideline says that medical devices for use in juvenile populations anticipated to have substantial usage must be under observation for at least 36 months. This assessment looks at the device's effect on overall growth, development, activity level, and other variables related to devising safety or efficacy.

In addition to the clearance/approval or any time after approval or clearance, the FDA may request postmarket monitoring if a recall. Within 15 months after obtaining the order, the producer must commence postmarket monitoring. DEPI, OSB, and CDRH will evaluate whether criteria for 522 orders have been fulfilled once the Agency has found a possible problem with a device. A team will be formed to do a more thorough investigation into the problem. Because this team may be made up of anybody relevant to the assessment, this group might include FDA epidemiologists, physicians, or other specialists. The team will take a close look at different pieces of the data in order to understand it further. The panel will propose a 522 order to the DEPI Division Director and OSB Director after the review's conclusion. The OSB Director will issue an order for postmarket monitoring if a new market presents a risk [53,59]. The premarket submission order identifies the premarket submission (e.g., 510(k), PMA, PDP, or HDE), public health questions, the rationale for the 522 order, and design recommendations postmarket.

5. Why drug development is costly?

The cost of drug research may increase significantly if over nine out of every 10 therapeutic candidates do not get regulatory clearance. However, if drug candidates from the laboratory to the clinic are to be moved from one stage to the next, what motivates failure rates, and how does the pharmaceutical industry increase productivity? The majority of individuals who have ever been associated with the pharmaceutical industry are likely to be able to provide an estimate of the expenses involved in the clinical trials and regulatory approval of a medication candidate. According to the CSDD, the average cost of getting medication to market is now $2.6 billion.

Numerous of these high costs are the result of many causes, such as: Using data from across the industry, Tufts estimated that $1.4 billion in out-of-pocket expenses and $1.1 billion in "time costs"—the investment returns lost while the medication is in development—were incurred for every drug project. However, some opponents from the industry have claimed that this is deceptive since the lost investment from unsuccessful medicines is included in Tufts' total cost estimate. According to MSF, an overinflated medication development bill helps explain pharma company expenses that are inflated similarly. Failure may be the single most significant financial risk in the pharmaceutical industry. Drugs that are effective and have established a sturdy safety profile are likely to be less costly, in terms of cost per effectiveness, than the $2.6 billion touted by Tufts. Although the number of new medicines failing approval has increased from one in 10 to almost 1 in 5, this translates to pharma and biotech firms facing complex challenges in the clinical development process while also managing costs for all of their pipeline assets. Drug failure is almost inevitable for novel medicines treating complicated and poorly understood diseases. The success rate for new medicines designed to treat Alzheimer's disease is about 99.6% between 2002 and 2012. There is a widespread belief that there is a wave of new contemporary biologics that will soon be able to treat Alzheimer's-related dementia, but so far, this has not occurred.

EPOCH was a Phase 3 trial testing verubecestat, a BACE inhibitor, as a potential treatment for Alzheimer's disease. When results showed there was "virtually no chance of finding a positive clinical effect," Merck discontinued the trial and pronounced the field "virtually devoid of promising options." A second unsuccessful Phase 3 study for an Alzheimer's therapy was reported only a few months earlier in the late months of 2016: the antibody solanezumab targeted the amyloid plaques in the brain, which are essential Alzheimer's indicators. Amyloid as a target for dementia therapy was put to the test and found to be ineffective.

6. Conclusion

Overall, the drug discovery pipeline involves crucial, fundamental, and unprecedented steps required for any drug discovery and development. Additionally, in the present situation of COVID-19, with the help of the drug discovery pipeline, several medicines were manufactured for the general public. The safety, efficacy, and effectiveness are continuously maintained with the drug discovery pipeline as the drug is prepared by undergoing several phases (preclinical and clinical phases).

However, to every advantage, there is a corresponding disadvantage as several challenges are involved in the steps of the drug discovery pipeline. Though breakthroughs in fundamental and preclinical research fuel the drug development pipeline, only a tiny percentage of molecules in the pipeline fulfill FDA approval requirements. Because the drug development pipeline is both labor and resource demanding, new techniques that provide early indications and possibly more accurate readouts of toxicity or effectiveness might bring considerable increases in the success rate and related cost savings for this process.

References

[1] Labroots, The Drug Discovery Pipeline | Drug Discovery and Development, 2021, Available online: https://www.labroots.com/trending/drug-discovery-and-development/7724/drug-discovery-pipeline. (Accessed 13 August 2021).

[2] M. Batool, B. Ahmad, S. Choi, A structure-based drug discovery paradigm, Int. J. Mol. Sci. 20 (2019).

[3] D.A. Erlanson, Introduction to fragment-based drug discovery, Top. Curr. Chem. 317 (2012).

[4] B.C. Doak, R.S. Norton, M.J. Scanlon, The ways and means of fragment-based drug design, Pharmacol. Ther. 167 (2016), https://doi.org/10.1016/j.pharmthera.2016.07.003.
[5] HBR, Link Manufacturing Process and Product Life Cycles, 2021, Available online: https://hbr.org/1979/01/link-manufacturing-process-and-product-life-cycles. (Accessed 13 August 2021).
[6] HBR, Exploit the Product Life Cycle, 2021, Available online: https://hbr.org/1965/11/exploit-the-product-life-cycle. (Accessed 13 August 2021).
[7] Open Lib, 7.2 Managing New Products: The Product Life Cycle—Principles of Marketing, 2021, Available online: https://open.lib.umn.edu/principlesmarketing/chapter/7-2-managing-new-products-the-product-life-cycle/. (Accessed 13 August 2021).
[8] G. Koscielny, P. An, D. Carvalho-Silva, J.A. Cham, L. Fumis, R. Gasparyan, S. Hasan, N. Karamanis, M. Maguire, E. Papa, et al., Open targets: a platform for therapeutic target identification and validation, Nucleic Acids Res. 45 (2017), https://doi.org/10.1093/nar/gkw1055.
[9] S. Wang, T.B. Sim, Y.S. Kim, Y.T. Chang, Tools for target identification and validation, Curr. Opin. Chem. Biol. 8 (2004).
[10] K.K. Kopec, D. Bozyczko-Coyne, M. Williams, Target identification and validation in drug discovery: the role of proteomics, Biochem. Pharmacol. 69 (2005).
[11] E. Manchado, C.H. Huang, N. Tasdemir, D.F. Tschaharganeh, J.E. Wilkinson, S.W. Lowe, A pipeline for drug target identification and validation, Cold Spring Harb. Symp. Quant. Biol. 81 (2016), https://doi.org/10.1101/sqb.2016.81.031096.
[12] M. Jayapal, A.J. Melendez, DNA microarray technology for target identification and validation, Clin. Exp. Pharmacol. Physiol. 33 (2006).
[13] J. Inglese, A practical guide to assay development and high-throughput screening in drug discovery, Edited by Taosheng Chen, ChemMedChem 5 (2010), https://doi.org/10.1002/cmdc.201000229.
[14] L.M. Mayr, P. Fuerst, The future of high-throughput screening, J. Biomol. Screen. 13 (2008).
[15] S. Fox, S. Farr-Jones, L. Sopchak, A. Boggs, H.W. Nicely, R. Khoury, M. Biros, High-throughput screening: update on practices and success, J. Biomol. Screen. (2006) 11.
[16] L.M. Mayr, D. Bojanic, Novel trends in high-throughput screening, Curr. Opin. Pharmacol. 9 (2009).
[17] M.W. Lutz, J.A. Menius, T.D. Choi, R.G. Laskody, P.L. Domanico, A.S. Goetz, D.L. Saussy, Experimental design for high-throughput screening, Drug Discov. Today 1 (1996).
[18] S.M. Rodems, B.D. Hamman, C. Lin, J. Zhao, S. Shah, D. Heidary, L. Makings, J.H. Stack, B.A. Pollok, A FRET-based assay platform for ultra-high density drug screening of protein kinases and phosphatases, Assay Drug Dev. Technol. 1 (2002), https://doi.org/10.1089/154065802761001266.
[19] R.P. Hertzberg, A.J. Pope, High-throughput screening: new technology for the 21st century, Curr. Opin. Chem. Biol. 4 (2000).
[20] K.E. Sapsford, L. Berti, I.L. Medintz, Fluorescence resonance energy transfer: concepts, applications and advances, Minerva Biotecnol. 16 (2004).
[21] S.A. Sundberg, High-throughput and ultra-high-throughput screening: solution- and cell-based approaches, Curr. Opin. Biotechnol. 11 (2000).
[22] V. Aguiar-Pulido, M. Gestal, M. Cruz-Monteagudo, J. Rabunal, J. Dorado, C. Munteanu, Evolutionary computation and QSAR research, Curr. Comput. Aided Drug Des. 9 (2013), https://doi.org/10.2174/1573409911309020006.
[23] B. Deprez, Trends in hit-to-lead: an update, in: Frontiers in Medicinal Chemistry, 3, 2006.

[24] R. Deprez-Poulain, B. Deprez, Facts, figures and trends in lead generation, Curr. Top. Med. Chem. 4 (2005), https://doi.org/10.2174/1568026043451168.
[25] X. Lu, H. Yang, Y. Chen, Q. Li, S. He, X. Jiang, F. Feng, W. Qu, H. Sun, The development of pharmacophore modeling: generation and recent applications in drug discovery, Curr. Pharm. Des. 24 (2018), https://doi.org/10.2174/1381612824666180810162944.
[26] J.L. Dahlin, M.A. Walters, The essential roles of chemistry in high-throughput screening triage, Future Med. Chem. 6 (2014).
[27] G.M. Keseru, G.M. Makara, Hit discovery and hit-to-lead approaches, Drug Discov. Today 11 (2006).
[28] D.A. Pereira, J.A. Williams, Origin and evolution of high throughput screening, Br. J. Pharmacol. 152 (2007).
[29] S.P. Leelananda, S. Lindert, Computational methods in drug discovery, Beilstein J. Org. Chem. 12 (2016).
[30] S. Paricharak, A.P. Ijzerman, A. Bender, F. Nigsch, Analysis of iterative screening with stepwise compound selection based on Novartis in-house HTS data, ACS Chem. Biol. 11 (2016), https://doi.org/10.1021/acschembio.6b00029.
[31] S. Liu, Y. Wu, T. Lin, R. Abel, J.P. Redmann, C.M. Summa, V.R. Jaber, N.M. Lim, D.L. Mobley, Lead optimization mapper: automating free energy calculations for lead optimization, J. Comput. Aided Mol. Des. 27 (2013), https://doi.org/10.1007/s10822-013-9678-y.
[32] K.C. Cheng, C. Li, A.S. Uss, Prediction of oral drug absorption in humans—from cultured cell lines and experimental animals, Expert Opin. Drug Metab. Toxicol. 4 (2008).
[33] W. Korfmacher, Advances in the integration of drug metabolism into the lead optimization paradigm, Mini Rev. Med. Chem. 9 (2009), https://doi.org/10.2174/138955709788452694.
[34] J.M. Collins, C.K. Grieshaber, B.A. Chabner, Pharmacologically guided phase I clinical trials based upon preclinical drug development, J. Natl. Cancer Inst. 82 (1990).
[35] S. Parsi, P.Y. Smith, C. Goupil, V. Dorval, S.S. Hébert, Preclinical evaluation of miR-15/107 family members as multifactorial drug targets for Alzheimer's disease, Mol. Ther.–Nucleic Acids 4 (2015), https://doi.org/10.1038/mtna.2015.33.
[36] E.H. Rubin, D.G. Gilliland, Drug development and clinical trials—the path to an approved cancer drug, Nat. Rev. Clin. Oncol. 9 (2012).
[37] P. Szymański, M. Markowicz, E. Mikiciuk-Olasik, Adaptation of high-throughput screening in drug discovery-toxicological screening tests, Int. J. Mol. Sci. 13 (2012).
[38] M.A. de Brito, Computational drug design—a guide for computational and medicinal chemists, J. Pharm. Pharm. Sci. 14 (2011), https://doi.org/10.18433/j3k59c.
[39] T. Farhadi, S.M.R. Hashemian, Computer-aided design of amino acid-based therapeutics: a review, Drug Des. Devel. Ther. 12 (2018).
[40] J. Saxton, O.L. Lopez, G. Ratcliff, C. Dulberg, L.P. Fried, M.C. Carlson, A.B. Newman, L. Kuller, Preclinical Alzheimer disease: neuropsychological test performance 1.5 to 8 years prior to onset, Neurology 63 (2004), https://doi.org/10.1212/01.WNL.0000147470.58328.50.
[41] B.G. Reigner, K. Blesch, Estimating the starting dose for entry into humans: principles and practice, Eur. J. Clin. Pharmacol. 57 (2002).
[42] J. Shen, B. Swift, R. Mamelok, S. Pine, J. Sinclair, M. Attar, Design and conduct considerations for first-in-human trials, Clin. Transl. Sci. 12 (2019), https://doi.org/10.1111/cts.12582.
[43] R.P. Wheeldon, D.T. Bernacki, S.D. Dertinger, S.M. Bryce, J.C. Bemis, G.E. Johnson, Benchmark dose analysis of DNA damage biomarker responses provides compound potency and adverse outcome pathway information for the topoisomerase II inhibitor class of compounds, Environ. Mol. Mutagen. 61 (2020), https://doi.org/10.1002/em.22360.

[44] S. Halappanavar, S. Van Den Brule, P. Nymark, L. Gaté, C. Seidel, S. Valentino, V. Zhernovkov, P. Høgh Danielsen, A. De Vizcaya, H. Wolff, et al., Adverse outcome pathways as a tool for the design of testing strategies to support the safety assessment of emerging advanced materials at the nanoscale, Part. Fibre Toxicol. 17 (2020).
[45] P. Pallmann, A.W. Bedding, B. Choodari-Oskooei, M. Dimairo, L. Flight, L.V. Hampson, J. Holmes, A.P. Mander, L. Odondi, M.R. Sydes, et al., Adaptive designs in clinical trials: why use them, and how to run and report them, BMC Med. 16 (2018).
[46] FDA, Adaptive Design Clinical Trials for Drugs and Biologics Guidance for Industry, FDA, 2021. Available online: https://www.fda.gov/regulatory-information/search-fda-guidance-documents/adaptive-design-clinical-trials-drugs-and-biologics-guidance-industry. (Accessed 4 August 2021).
[47] FDA, FDA in Brief: FDA Modernizes Clinical Trial Designs and Approaches for Drug Development, Proposing New Guidance on the Use of Adaptive Designs and Master Protocols, FDA, 2021. Available online: https://www.fda.gov/news-events/fda-brief/fda-brief-fda-modernizes-clinical-trial-designs-and-approaches-drug-development-proposing-new. (Accessed 4 August 2021).
[48] FDA, Interacting with the FDA on Complex Innovative Trial Designs for Drugs and Biological Products, FDA, 2021. Available online: https://www.fda.gov/regulatory-information/search-fda-guidance-documents/interacting-fda-complex-innovative-trial-designs-drugs-and-biological-products. (Accessed 4 August 2021).
[49] FDA, Adaptive Designs for Medical Device Clinical Studies, FDA, 2021. Available online: https://www.fda.gov/regulatory-information/search-fda-guidance-documents/adaptive-designs-medical-device-clinical-studies. (Accessed 4 August 2021).
[50] FDA, Prescription Drug User Fee Amendments, FDA, 2021. Available online: https://www.fda.gov/industry/fda-user-fee-programs/prescription-drug-user-fee-amendments. (Accessed 4 August 2021).
[51] FDA, Best Practices for Communication Between IND Sponsors and FDA During Drug Development, FDA, 2021. Available online: https://www.fda.gov/regulatory-information/search-fda-guidance-documents/best-practices-communication-between-ind-sponsors-and-fda-during-drug-development. (Accessed 4 August 2021).
[52] C. Denise DiGIulio, FDA's Pre-Approval Inspection (PAI) Program and How to Prepare for a Successful Outcome, 2019.
[53] N. Raj, S. Fernandes, N.R. Charyulu, A. Dubey, R. GS, S. Hebbar, Postmarket surveillance: a review on key aspects and measures on the effective functioning in the context of the United Kingdom and Canada, Ther. Adv. Drug Saf. 10 (2019), https://doi.org/10.1177/2042098619865413.
[54] Us Guidance for Industry and Investigators Safety Reporting Requirements for INDs and BA/BE Studies, 2012.
[55] D.B. Kramer, S. Xu, A.S. Kesselheim, Regulation of medical devices in the United States and European union, in: The Ethical Challenges of Emerging Medical Technologies, 2020.
[56] FDA, Overview of Device Regulation, FDA, 2021. Available online: https://www.fda.gov/medical-devices/device-advice-comprehensive-regulatory-assistance/overview-device-regulation. (Accessed 4 August 2021).
[57] G.A. Van Norman, Drugs, Devices, and the FDA: part 2: an overview of approval processes: FDA approval of medical devices, JACC Basic Transl. Sci. 1 (2016), https://doi.org/10.1016/j.jacbts.2016.03.009.
[58] US Food and Drug Administration, Medical Device Exemptions 510(k) and GMP Requirements, 2010.
[59] H. Randall, Post-marketing surveillance and vigilance for medical devices: the European approach, Drug Saf. 24 (2001) 869–872, https://doi.org/10.2165/00002018-200124120-00001.

CHAPTER 8

Virtual screening

Ashwani K. Dhingra[a], Bhawna Chopra[a], Sakshi Bhardwaj[b], Ajmer Singh Grewal[a], and Kumar Guarve[a]
[a]Guru Gobind Singh College of Pharmacy, Yamuna Nagar, Haryana, India
[b]Krupanidhi College of Pharmacy, Bangalore, Karnataka, India

1. Introduction

Drug designing creates molecules complementary in shape and charge to the molecular targets they interact and bind. Virtual screening (VS) is a computational technique widely used to identify the hit molecule from the chemical compound data to develop novel potent lead compounds with desired pharmacological activity. It involves a cascade of consecutive filters to characterize the small set of hits molecules from many compounds against a specific drug target with potential pharmacological action. The term "virtual screening" was first given in the late 1990s [1,2], and so far, numerous techniques and tools have been established for VS [3–5]. It is now a valuable approach for drug discovery and development used widely in various pharmaceutical and biotechnology R&D industries and academic labs. VS is categorized into two classes, i.e., structure-based VS and ligand-based VS [6,7].

Ligand-based VS involves the identification of lead molecules for the experimental evaluation based on the structure-activity relationship (SAR) database from a known set of active compounds through quantitative structure-activity relationship (QSAR) and structural similarity searching studies along with pharmacophore, or 3-dimensions (3D) shape matching [8,9]. Besides this, structure-based VS involves ranking candidate compounds based on complementarity scores and/or predicted binding affinity obtained by the docking by utilizing the 3D structure of the biological target into the binding site. In this review, we briefly discussed how to set up and run the VS workflow along with recent developments and applications of VS.

2. Structure-based VS

Structure-based VS has involved three parameters, i.e., receptor 3D structure, molecular docking, and chemical compound library. It starts with the

Computational Approaches in Drug Discovery, Development and Systems Pharmacology
https://doi.org/10.1016/B978-0-323-99137-7.00007-1

preparation of the chemical library and 3D receptor structure, followed by molecular docking, which predicts the potential of the individual compound based on the obtained docking score against the receptor. The combinations with good binding and/or complementarity scores will use for further pharmacological evaluation. However, additional filters may be incorporated in the workflow based on the specific requirements to enhance the success rate.

3. Molecular docking

Its goal is to forecast the molecular orientation of the intermolecular complex formed by two or more constituent analogs and a protein target [10]. Docking workflow involves amalgamating two complementary mechanisms, i.e., a scoring function and a search algorithm. Search algorithm involves the exploration of the conformational space of the ligand and/or the receptor [11], whereas scoring functions involve the evaluation of each of the "sampled" binding modes [12,13]. Many docking tools and approaches, such as DOCK [14,15], AutoDock [16], AutoDock Vina [17], Glide [18], and GOLD [19,20], are now accessible. Apart from the availability of these computational techniques, there will be a great challenge behind molecular docking. However, none of these single tools can reliably predict the correct bioactive compounds [1,3,21].

4. Receptor 3D structures

The Protein Data Bank (PDB), the most significant structural database of big biological compounds characterized by either NMR spectroscopy or X-ray crystallography [22], is used to obtain the receptor's 3D structures. At the time of writing, the PDB has about 150,000 physical macromolecular structures, with the number growing every year. As a result of current structural biology and structural genomics research, 3D structures of crucial biological macromolecules and possible therapeutic targets have been generated, providing an unmatched possibility for structure-based VS and drug discovery.

5. Chemical compound library

It is a group of chemical compounds/analogs that are employed in structure-based VS. PubChem [23,24], ChEMBL [25], ZINC [26], ChemSpider [27], and other commercial and public databases are currently available. These resources potentially reduce entry barriers into the drug development process for small pharma and biotech firms and academic researchers.

6. Denovo design

De novo or rational drug design can be thought of as an optimization process for determining the optimal amalgamation of the molecular fragments that can be well located in the energetic site and constituted into an entire ligand. The synthesized ligand should meet the stated pharmacophoric properties during the optimization process, which reflect the critical receptor-ligand interaction locations. Various de novo design protocols used in drug design is illustrated in Table 1. Most used approaches were developed before 2000, except TOPAS and LEA, reviewed literature [47].

7. Ligand-based virtual screening

Drug design, often known as rational drug design, is the creative process of developing novel treatments and compounds based on a biological target's understanding [48]. The basic principle behind drug designing is the assumption that similar molecules should exhibit similar binding properties concerning a given target [4]. Ligand-based virtual screening (LBVS) starts with either a single compound or a series of compounds known to be potent against a target. Potency and other critical qualities are increased by building appropriate analogs based on structure-activity correlations (SAR) knowledge.

These diverse compounds could potentially be utilized to create a pharmacophore model, which specifies the structural features that a molecule must possess to bind to the target. Once a large data set with a wide variety of potencies is available, QSAR models can be tried and used if robust enough for prediction. Hence, e can state that "The SAR is the link between structure and activity, and ligand-based drug design is the iterative process of altering chemical structures to boost their biological activity (LBDD)." The advantage of LBVS is that it does not require understanding the drug's particular molecular mechanism of action [49].

Indeed, LBVS was the only approach to rational drug design before introducing structural models of protein crystallography and molecular modeling. In the last years, significant advances in molecular biology have shifted the focus of drug research away from symptom-based evaluation

Table 1 Examples of several de novo drug design techniques.

Sr. No.	Method	Description	Reference
1	CAVEAT	Fragment-based, fragment-based 3D database search	[28]
2	TOPAS	Fragment-based, evolutionary algorithm	[29]
3	CAVITY, DBMAKER, SPLICE, FOUNDATION	Fragment-based, production of ligand by 3D database search	[30,31]
4	SMOG	Fragment-based, sequential growth	[32]
5	CONCEPTS	Atom-based, MD optimization, stochastic search	[33]
6	CONCERTS	Fragment-based, stochastic search	[34]
7	PRO_LIGAND	Fragment-based, combinatorial search, sequential growth	[35]
8	DLD	Atom-based, structural sampling	[36]
9	MCDNLG	Atom-based, stochastic search	[37]
10	LUDI	Fragment-based, sequential growth, combinatorial search	[38,39]
11	LEGEND	Atom-based, sequential growth	[40,41]
12	HOOK	Fragment-based linker search	[42]
13	GROW	Peptide design, sequential growth	[43]
14	GenStar	Atom-based, sequential growth	[44]
15	Leapfrog	Fragment-based, combinatorial search	[45]
16	GrowMol	Fragment-based, sequential grow	[46]

of medication activity and targeted targeting of verified biological components. With the advanced approaches now, drugs are developed directly to target proteins. The same concepts apply to the development of medications that bind to enzymes, nucleic acids, lipids, and structural proteins, among other biological targets [49].

Molecular similarities are based on molecular descriptors and similarity measures. Ligand-based VS involves the determination of lead and hit compounds. The two requirements for the optimization and characterization of hit and lead compounds are given below:

8. A suitable biological assay that can be used to determine the efficacy of a drug

It is vital to have a relevant way of assessing chemical activity in an appropriate biological assay to optimize a pharmacological structure. Adams, for example, used a UV light-induced erythema model in guinea pigs to screen compounds for anti-inflammatory properties while developing ibuprofen. However, in recent years, in vitro models based on isolated enzymes have replaced mainly in vivo techniques. Furthermore, in vitro procedures have the advantage of being automated and being far less expensive [50].

9. The "Lead" compound in the assay

To examine the SAR, LBDD requires a starting point. Suitable lead compounds can be found in various origins, including natural products and drug company chemical libraries. Actuality, finding an initial "hit" chemical can be a game of chance. Hit compounds that show activity in the assay are graded in terms of potency and their potential to be transformed into drug-like molecules. When choosing a starting point for drug development, the medicinal chemist will evaluate synthetic tractability so that analogs and potential bioavailability and intrinsic toxicity [51,52].

10. The pharmacophore

The pharmacophore is the bare minimum needed structural framework to elicit the desired biological action, and it can be extrapolated from a variety of active structures. The pharmacophore model is an arrangement of structural elements derived from what traits might complement the lead compound's functional groups. As additional SAR data becomes available, the pharmacophore model is refined, and more active compounds are generated in the process to validate and fit the model [51,52].

11. Increasing drug affinity for protein targets

The chemist's imagination and, perhaps more importantly, the simplicity of synthesis are the sole constraints on the design of analogs given a lead chemical. Drug modification is based on a set of common guiding concepts, and increasing the binding affinity of the leading chemical is a primary goal of medication design. It is worth studying the thermodynamics of drug binding to optimize the changes made to a lead structure. We can say, binding affinity is proportional to the drug's free energy of binding to the target receptor, provided the medication binds in a precise way that causes the therapeutic effect [51,52]. As a result, the equilibrium binding constant (K_{eq}) is proportional to the binding free energy:

$$\Delta G_{bind} = -RT \ \ln \ K_{eq}$$

Here,

$$\Delta G_{bind=} \ \Delta H_{bind} - T\Delta S_{bind}$$

The above equation gives the Gibbs-free energy of a binding event, G_{bind}.

Whereas ΔH_{bind} is an enthalpy word that refers to the sum of all favorable and unfavorable molecular contacts created or broken due to the binding event. To create a potent medicine, the synthetic chemist must maximize these favorable interactions. ΔS_{bind} is an entropy word that defines the change in disorder during the binding event. This phrase refers to entropy changes. It can be observed that both enthalpy and entropy can contribute significantly to the binding free energy. As a result, any LBDD study should seek to address both ΔG_{bind} components. While considering binding affinity, solubility, pharmacokinetics, metabolic susceptibility, and toxicity are all other factors that must be considered. Drug design is a multiparameter optimization process, generally try to create the most active chemical feasible, then refine the drug profile while keeping the target biological activity [51,52].

12. Pharmacophore mapping

The three-dimensional preparation of essential structural properties of a collection of recognized ligands is known as a pharmacophore [53]. Two processes in pharmacophore-based VS are identifying a pharmacophore prototype and the 3D search grounded on specified constraints [54,55].

To begin, a variety of active compounds are being studied to characterize their pharmacophoric properties. A pharmacophore model can be built from the 3D structure using a set of active ligands. The receptor or receptor/ligand composite structure reveals potential and critical communications between ligand and receptor. The 3D structure's data can be processed to characterize the binding site's interaction sites as a pharmacophore model, which can then be utilized in a 3D database screening query. One of numerous commercially available applications for identifying pharmacophore representations is Catalyst [56], Discotech [57], and GASP [58,59]. However, it is occasionally necessary to identify the fundamental structural properties for pharmacophore definition due to the structural complexity. For 3D database search, the most generally used programmes are Catalyst, Unity [57], MDL Information Systems [60], Chem-X, and others [61].

13. Target-based virtual screening

Target-based VS is suitable for reducing inactive molecules [4]. The 3D structural information of the target biomolecules, their binding pockets' type, shape, size, and interactions with ligands, inhibitors, and/or modulators are the target-based VS inputs for all practical purposes. The TBD methods can be thought of as a collection of computational procedures, including visualization tools, that are put together to construct decision support systems for the drug design/discovery process. They are classified as direct approaches since they use the target protein structure inputs in the drug design/discovery process. A therapeutic target, a gene, a genetic product, or a chemical connected to a precise molecular mechanism can be identified using target-based VS. The benefit of performing target-based VS rather than ligand-based through similarity searches is that it allows for the discovery of wholly new scaffolds based on docking score without being influenced by previously identified ligands. Literature survey reveals an array of experimental studies where receptor modeling, receptor model improvement, and docking protocols are introduced and evaluated [62–71]. Several studies report numerous pragmatic workflows based on the automated protocols to produce moderate enrichments with low effort [70–72].

However, it may be cheaper and faster to utilized a crude nonvalidated receptor model, which results in modest enrichments. In this procedure, no mutants are produced; thus, the saved time and money may be utilized to acquire additional compounds and their testing. Most of the published applications involve a compromise, where some efforts are put to improve the receptor model, but relatively lesser mutagenesis experiments are performed for model validation. However, the automated modeling crude model selection methodology can achieve enrichments more considerably than a random selection protocol, which is extremely remarkable [73].

VS approaches based on targets are valuable tools for finding tiny hit compounds for proteins, especially G-protein-coupled receptors (GPCRs). The biological target's 3D structure is at the heart of the approaches used in this research. However, it is a complex technique to apply due to the absence of 3D structural information on GPCRs. As a result, target-based VS can only be achieved by creating a structural model of the GPCR that can be used for docking. GPCR structural modeling, on the other hand, is a time-consuming approach that is not always warranted if the model can't explain all experimental results. As a result, a fully automated procedure is needed in which a large number of GPCR models are prepared and the optimal model for docking is chosen. With a minimum of effort, the complete workflow leads to reasonable enrichments. The targeted GPCR sequence, reference ligand with experimental data, and the small molecules database to be used for docking are all required inputs [73].

14. Data visualization

As advanced strategies to drug design and development are discovered in the current time, pioneering approaches for the technology that supports those methodologies, particularly in the sector of data visualization, are becoming crucial [74]. Information visualization represents the technologies of visually presenting composite statistics sets to attain goals such as showing numerous information magnitudes simultaneously, linking associated information facts from information sets, or displaying statistics dispersal patterns. These tools are worth significance for data processing, investigation, and appearance actions [75]. There has been a pattern swing from seeing information as still graphs to lively three-dimensional picturing, which allows more profound perceptions into the relationship of diverse constraints. The arena of drug discovery stresses this type of visualization software not solitary for the complete and robust illustration of information but also for investigation resulting in novel intuitions and findings [76]. Particularly, structural information at the core of the drug discovery course relating to the description of medicine targets, possible leading compounds, and their interactions. The accessibility of innovative techniques like immersive visualization, coupled with artificial intelligence (AI) founded and deep learning systems for in silico modeling and simulations, would undoubtedly be a vital factor for drug discovery in the coming years. Current software systems comprise web-based algorithms such as ProViz, employed for detailed seeing and manipulating manifold sequence orientations while studying proteins [77]. JalView is a tool that displays the alignment of both the protein sequence from the UniProt database and the coding sequence from The European Molecular Biology Laboratory database [78]. STRAP-NT is a program that enables the structural interpretation of mutations and single nucleotide polymorphisms [79]. The market is gradually being flooded by artificial intelligence-driven data visualization applications that support drug discovery. Like next-generation data discovery software platforms, diverse AI-based drug discovery visualization tools are based on metadata-driven AI technology. These tools are often complemented by data management task automation features enabling semantic searches and tracking data lineage [80]. Leading pharmaceutical companies have used virtual reality to visualize protein targets and small molecules and explore their interactions in a three-dimensional visual mode. Virtual reality-based drug discovery solutions may prove helpful across multiple platforms [77].

15. Recent developments and applications of virtual screening

VS is a supplementary technique to experimental HTS that involves using high-performance computation to examine extensive data of chemical compounds and identify potential drug candidates [81–83]. VS is a knowledge-driven strategy in which the lead molecule is characterized based on existing information about the nature of the receptor-binding pocket, the ligand type that is expected to bind effectively, or both. Furthermore, VS has a variety of computational screens ranging from simple to complex, allowing it to leverage a wide range of information about the receptor successfully. The type of methods employed in VS, on the other hand, is generally determined by the data available as an input or the output result type [84,85].

Molecular docking is a CADD technique in which the favored positioning of a small molecule concerning its binding potential is adjusted to the target, leading to a stable complex. Docking procedures can be used to identify potential ligands in a library, predict the binding process and affinity of the novel or known ligands, and more.

Despite the usefulness of docking procedures, pharmacophore modeling is more typically used. It takes less time, but pharmacophore identification can occur due to docking research on rare occasions. To identify and improve novel bioactive hit and lead compounds, VS uses computer models and algorithms. VS is seen as a supplement to HTS, which provides valuable beginning points for drug research and development in the pharmaceutical sector from massive compound collections. On the other hand, these strategies could be helpful in tiny biotechnology businesses that do not use HTS for hit and lead discovery. Several VS methods and procedures have demonstrated their utility; however, the exact potential of VS has been grilled due to the employment of a vast number of apparently disparate ways. As a result, significant techniques in VS necessitate a thorough understanding of protein folding and macromolecular complex formation dynamics. Furthermore, VS appears to be more suited when considering a problem-centric rather than a method-centric approach.

16. Conclusion and future prospective

Different sets of procedures and VS methods are preferred based on the target's information and ligands. However, VS approaches may be too early or insufficiently accurate at times. Furthermore, the apparent success or failure of the hit identification process is highly dependent on the knowledge and manner of integration used. As a result, progress on advanced VS techniques that improve prediction accuracy and dependability is stalled. VS requires a profound grasp of the forces regulating protein folding, the dynamics involved in complex macromolecular assembly, and the allosteric effects of target activity and ligand-target interactions for significant evolution. In this way, technological progress will permit the practical implementation and use of VS methodologies for hit and lead compound optimization from enormous combinatorial chemistry techniques which are synthetically reachable and directed by pharmacophoric agreement. As a result, VS and intelligent drug design algorithms will help theoretical/medical chemists, and scientists plan, set up, and control robotic synthesis protocols and testing gear, allowing VS to reach its full potential.

References

[1] G. Schneider, Virtual screening: an endless staircase? Nat. Rev. Drug Discov. 9 (2010) 273–276.
[2] A. Lavecchia, C. Di Giovanni, Virtual screening strategies in drug discovery: a critical review, Curr. Med. Chem. 20 (2013) 2839–2860.

[3] G. Klebe, Virtual ligand screening: strategies, perspectives and limitations, Drug Discov. Today 11 (2006) 580–594.
[4] H. Koppen, Virtual screening—what does it give us? Curr. Opin. Drug Discov. Devel. 12 (2009) 397–407.
[5] C.M. Song, S.J. Lim, J.C. Tong, Recent advances in computer-aided drug design, Brief. Bioinform. 10 (2009) 579–591.
[6] K. Heikamp, J. Bajorath, The future of virtual compound screening, Chem. Biol. Drug Des. 81 (2013) 33–40.
[7] I. Muegge, S. Oloff, Advances in virtual screening, Drug Discov. Today Technol. 3 (2006) 405–411.
[8] H. Geppert, M. Vogt, J. Bajorath, Current trends in ligand-based virtual screening: molecular representations, data mining methods, new application areas, and performance evaluation, J. Chem. Inf. Model. 50 (2010) 205–216.
[9] F.L. Stahura, J. Bajorath, New methodologies for ligand-based virtual screening, Curr. Pharm. Des. 11 (2005) 1189–1202.
[10] S.F. Sousa, P.A. Fernandes, M.J. Ramos, Protein-ligand docking: current status and future challenges, Proteins 65 (2006) 15–26.
[11] N. Moitessier, P. Englebienne, D. Lee, J. Lawandi, C.R. Corbeil, Towards the development of universal, fast and highly accurate docking/scoring methods: a long way to go, Br. J. Pharmacol. 153 (Suppl 1) (2008) S7–S26.
[12] S.Y. Huang, S.Z. Grinter, X. Zou, Scoring functions and their evaluation methods for protein-ligand docking: recent advances and future directions, Phys. Chem. Chem. Phys. 12 (2010) 12899–12908.
[13] I.D. Kuntz, J.M. Blaney, S.J. Oatley, R. Langridge, T.E. Ferrin, A geometric approach to macromolecule-ligand interactions, J. Mol. Biol. 161 (1982) 269–288.
[14] T.J. Ewing, S. Makino, A.G. Skillman, I.D. Kuntz, DOCK 4.0: search strategies for automated molecular docking of flexible molecule databases, J. Comput. Aided Mol. Des. 15 (2001) 411–428.
[15] D.T. Moustakas, P.T. Lang, S. Pegg, E. Pettersen, I.D. Kuntz, N. Brooijmans, R.C. Rizzo, Development and validation of a modular, extensible docking program: DOCK 5, J. Comput. Aided Mol. Des. 20 (2006) 601–619.
[16] G.M. Morris, D.S. Goodsell, R. Huey, A.J. Olson, Distributed automated docking of flexible ligands to proteins: parallel applications of AutoDock 2.4, J. Comput. Aided Mol. Des. 10 (1996) 293–304.
[17] O. Trott, A.J. Olson, AutoDock Vina: improving the speed and accuracy of docking with a new scoring function, efficient optimization, and multithreading, J. Comput. Chem. 31 (2010) 455–461.
[18] R.A. Friesner, J.L. Banks, R.B. Murphy, T.A. Halgren, J.J. Klicic, D.T. Mainz, M.P. Repasky, E.H. Knoll, M. Shelley, J.K. Perry, D.E. Shaw, P. Francis, P.S. Shenkin, Glide: a new approach for rapid, accurate docking and scoring. 1. Method and assessment of docking accuracy, J. Med. Chem. 47 (2004) 1739–1749.
[19] G. Jones, P. Willett, R.C. Glen, A.R. Leach, R. Taylor, Development and validation of a genetic algorithm for flexible docking, J. Mol. Biol. 267 (1997) 727–748.
[20] G. Jones, P. Willett, R.C. Glen, Molecular recognition of receptor sites using a genetic algorithm with a description of desolvation, J. Mol. Biol. 245 (1995) 43–53.
[21] T. Cheng, Q. Li, Z. Zhou, Y. Wang, H.S.H. Bryant, Structure-based virtual screening for drug discovery: a problem-centric review, AAPS J. 14 (2012) 133–141.
[22] H.M. Berman, J. Westbrook, Z. Feng, G. Gilliland, T.N. Bhat, H. Weissig, I.N. Shindyalov, P.E. Bourne, The protein data bank, Nucleic Acids Res. 28 (2000) 235–242.
[23] Q. Li, T. Cheng, Y. Wang, S.H. Bryant, PubChem as a public resource for drug discovery, Drug Discov. Today 15 (23–24) (2010) 1052–1057.

[24] Y. Wang, J. Xiao, T.O. Suzek, J. Zhang, J. Wang, S.H. Bryant, PubChem: a public information system for analyzing bioactivities of small molecules, Nucleic Acids Res. 37 (2009) W623–W633.
[25] A. Gaulton, L.J. Bellis, A.P. Bento, J. Chambers, M. Davies, A. Hersey, Y. Light, S. McGlinchey, D. Michalovich, B. Al-Lazikani, J.P. Overington, ChEMBL: a large-scale bioactivity database for drug discovery, Nucleic Acids Res. 40 (2012) D1100–D1107.
[26] J.J. Irwin, B.K. Shoichet, ZINC—a free database of commercially available compounds for virtual screening, J. Chem. Inf. Model. 45 (2005) 177–182.
[27] H.E. Pence, A. Williams, ChemSpider: an online chemical information resource, J. Chem. Educ. 87 (2010) 1123–1124.
[28] G. Lauri, P.A. Barlett, CAVEAT: a program to facilitate the design of organic molecules, J. Comput. Aided Mol. Des. 8 (1994) 51–66.
[29] G. Schneider, M.L. Lee, M. Stahl, P. Schneider, De novo design of molecular architectures by evolutionary assembly of drug-derived building blocks, J. Comput. Aided Mol. Des. 14 (2000) 487–494.
[30] C.M.W. Ho, G.R. Marshall, FOUNDATION: a program to retrieve all possible structures containing a user-defined minimum number of matching query elements from three-dimensional databases, J. Comput. Aided Mol. Des. 7 (1993) 3–22.
[31] C.M. Ho, G.R. Marshall, DBMAKER: a set of programs designed to generate three-dimensional databases based upon user-specific criteria, J. Comput. Aided Mol. Des. 9 (1995) 65–86.
[32] R. DeWitte, SMOG, de novo design method based on simple, fast, and accurate free energy estimates 2 case studies in molecular design, J. Am. Chem. Soc. 119 (1997) 4608–4617.
[33] D.A. Pearlman, M.A. Murcko, CONCEPTS: new dynamics algorithm for de novo drug suggestions, J. Comput. Aided Mol. Des. 14 (1993) 1184–1193.
[34] D.A. Pearlman, M.A. Murcko, CONCERTS: dynamics connection of fragments as an approach to de novo ligand design, J. Comput. Aided Mol. Des. 39 (1996) 1651–1663.
[35] D.E. Clark, D. Frenkel, S.A. Levy, J. Li, C.W. Murray, B. Robson, B. Waszkowycz, D.R. Westhead, PRO_LIGAND: an approach to de novo drug design, J. Comput. Aided Mol. Des. 9 (1995) 13–32.
[36] A. Miranker, M. Karplus, An automated-method for dynamic ligand design, Proteins Struct. Funct. Genet. 23 (1995) 472–490.
[37] D.K. Gehlaar, De novo design of enzyme inhibitors by Monte Carlo ligand generation, J. Med. Chem. 38 (1995) 466–472.
[38] H.J. Bohm, The computer program LUDI: a new method for the de novo design of enzyme inhibitors, J. Comp. Aided Mol. Des. 6 (1992) 61–79.
[39] H.J. Bohm, LUDI: rule based automatic design of new substituents for enzyme inhibitor leads, J. Comp. Aided Mol. Des. 6 (1992) 593–606.
[40] Y. Nishibata, A. Itai, Automatic creation of drug candidate structures based on receptor structure-starting point for artificial lead generation, Tetrahedron 47 (1991) 8985–8990.
[41] Y. Nishibata, A. Itai, Confirmation of usefulness of a structure construction program based on three-dimensional receptor structure for rational lead generation, J. Med. Chem. 36 (1993) 2921–2928.
[42] M.B. Eisen, D.C. Wiley, M. Karplus, R.E. Hubbard, HOOK: a program for finding novel molecular architectures that satisfy the chemical and steric requirements of a macromolecule binding site, Proteins 19 (1994) 199–221.
[43] J. Moon, W. Howe, Computer design of bioactive molecules: a method for receptor-based de novo ligand design, Proteins 11 (1991) 314–328.
[44] S.H. Rotstein, M.A. Murcko, GenStar: a method for de novo drug design, J. Comput. Aided Mol. Des. 7 (1993) 23–43.
[45] LUDI is available from Accelrys, 9685 Scranton Road, San Diego, CA 92121, USA.

[46] R.S. Bohacek, C. McMartin, Multiple highly diverse structures complementary to enzyme binding sites: results of extensive application of a de novo design method incorporating combinatorial growth, J. Am. Chem. Soc. 116 (1994) 5560–5571.
[47] M. Murcko, Recent advances in ligand design methods, in: K.B. Lipkowitz, D.B. Boyd (Eds.), Reviews in Computational Chemistry, vol. 11, Wiley-VCH Inc., 1997, pp. 1–66.
[48] M. Ulf, K.L. Povl, L. Tommy, Textbook of Drug Design and Discovery, Taylor & Francis, Washington, DC, 2002.
[49] S. Vidushi, W. Sharad, K. Hirdesh, Structure and ligand-based drug design: concepts, approaches, and challenges, in: Chemoinformatics and Bioinformatics in the Pharmaceutical Sciences, Elsevier, 2021, pp. 27–53.
[50] A. Hemant, S.M. Coumar, Lead identification and optimization, in: T. Bhatt, S. Nimesh (Eds.), The Design & Development of Novel Drugs and Vaccines, vol. 1, Academic Press, 2021, pp. 31–63.
[51] W.L. Gregory, L.A. Markus, Integrating structure-based and ligand-based approaches for computational drug design, Future Med. Chem. 3 (6) (2011) 735–750.
[52] K.C. Aman, K. Ajay, B. Shiv, C. Ravi, S. Shakti, Ligand-based approach for in-silico drug designing, in: Bioinformatics Techniques for Drug Discovery, 2018, pp. 11–19.
[53] P. Gund, Three-dimensional pharmacophore pattern searching, Prog. Mol. Subcell. Biol. 5 (1977) 117–143.
[54] Y. Kurogi, O.F. Guner, Pharmacophore modeling and three dimensional database searching for drug design using catalyst, Curr. Med. Chem. 8 (2001) 1035–1055.
[55] T. Langer, R.D. Hoffmanne, Virtual screening: an effective tool for lead structure discovery? Curr. Pharm. Design 7 (2001) 509–527.
[56] CATALYST is available from Accelrys, 9685 Scranton Road, San Diego, CA 92121, USA.
[57] DISCO is available from Tripos Inc 1699 South Hanley Road, St Louis, MO 63144-2913, USA.
[58] GASP is available from Tripos Inc 1699 South Hanley Road, St Louis, MO 63144-2913, USA.
[59] G. Jones, P. Willett, R.C. Glen, A genetic algorithm for flexible molecular overlay and pharmacophore elucidation, J. Comput. Aided Mol. Des. 9 (1995) 532–549.
[60] M.J. McGregor, P.V. Pallai, Clustering of large databases of compounds: using the MDL "Keys" as structural descriptors, J. Chem. Inf. Comput. Sci. 37 (1997) 443–448.
[61] Y.C. Martin, 3D database searching in drug design, J. Med. Chem. 35 (1992) 2145–2154.
[62] A. Evers, G. Klebe, Successful virtual screening for a submicromolar antagonist of the neurokinin-1 receptor based on a ligand supported homology model, J. Med. Chem. 47 (2004) 5381–5392.
[63] O.M. Becker, Y. Marantz, S. Shacham, B. Inbal, A. Heifetz, O. Kalid, B.H. Shay, D. Warshaviak, M. Fichman, S. Noiman, G protein-coupled receptors: in silico drug discovery in 3D, Proc. Natl. Acad. Sci. U. S. A. 101 (2004) 11304–11309.
[64] C. Bissantz, P. Bernard, M. Hibert, D. Rognan, Protein-based virtual screening of chemical databases. II. Are homology models of G-protein coupled receptors suitable targets? Proteins 50 (2003) 5–25.
[65] J.Z. Chen, J. Wang, X.Q. Xie, GPCR structure-based virtual screening approach for CB2 antagonist search, J. Chem. Inf. Model. 47 (2007) 1626–1637.
[66] A. Evers, G. Hessler, H. Matter, T. Klabunde, Virtual screening of biogenic amine-binding G-protein coupled receptors: comparative evaluation of protein- and ligand-based virtual screening protocols, J. Med. Chem. 48 (2005) 5448–5465.
[67] A. Evers, T. Klabunde, Structure-based drug discovery using GPCR homology modeling: successful virtual screening for antagonists of the alpha1A adrenergic receptor, J. Med. Chem. 48 (2005) 1088–1097.
[68] T. Klabunde, C. Giegerich, A. Evers, Sequence-derived three-dimensional pharmacophore models for G-protein-coupled receptors and their application in virtual screening, J. Med. Chem. 52 (2009) 2923–2932.

[69] F.M. McRobb, B. Capuano, I.T. Crosby, D.K. Chalmers, E. Yuriev, Homology modeling and docking evaluation of aminergic G protein-coupled receptors, J. Chem. Inf. Model. 50 (2010) 626–637.
[70] M. Nowak, M. Kolaczkowski, M. Pawlowski, A.J. Bojarski, Homology modeling of the serotonin 5-HT1A receptor using automated docking of bioactive compounds with defined geometry, J. Med. Chem. 49 (2006) 205–214.
[71] I.G. Tikhonova, C.S. Sum, S. Neumann, S. Engel, B.M. Raaka, S. Costanzi, C.G. Marvin, Discovery of novel agonists and antagonists of the free fatty acid receptor 1 (FFAR1) using virtual screening, J. Med. Chem. 51 (2008) 625–633.
[72] B. Kneissl, B. Leonhardt, A. Hildebrandt, C.S. Tautermann, Revisiting automated G-protein coupled receptor modeling: the benefit of additional template structures for a neurokinin-1 receptor model, J. Med. Chem. 52 (2009) 3166–3173.
[73] S.T. Christofer, Target based virtual screening by docking into automatically generated GPCR models, in: V. Nagarajan, K.S. Judith (Eds.), Membrane Protein Structure and Dynamics: Methods and Protocols, Methods in Molecular Biology, vol. 914, Springer Science, LLC, 2012.
[74] T. Silva, Information visualization—important IT considerations, in: W.T. Loging (Ed.), Bioinformatics and Computational Biology in Drug Discovery and Development, Cambridge University Press, 2016, pp. 137–154.
[75] K. Xu, Data visualization and the DDP process, in: W.T. Loging (Ed.), Bioinformatics and Computational Biology in Drug Discovery and Development, Cambridge University Press, 2016, pp. 114–136.
[76] D.M. Maniyar, I.T. Nabney, B.S. Williams, A. Sewing, Data visualization during the early stages of drug discovery, Chem. Inf. Model. 46 (2006) 1806–1818.
[77] P. Jehl, J. Manguy, D.C. Shields, D.G. Higgins, N.E. Davey, ProViz-a web-based visualization tool to investigate the functional and evolutionary features of protein sequences, Nucleic Acids Res. 44 (W1) (2016) W11–W15.
[78] A.M. Waterhouse, J.B. Procter, D.M. Martin, M. Clamp, G.J. Barton, Jalview Version 2—a multiple sequence alignment editor and analysis workbench, Bioinformatics 25 (9) (2009) 1189–1191.
[79] C. Gille, C. Frommel, Strap: editor for structural alignments of proteins, Bioinformatics 17 (2001) 377–378.
[80] L. Brynne, A. Bresell, N. Sjögren, Effective visualization of integrated knowledge and data to enable informed decisions in drug development and translational medicine, J. Transl. Med. 11 (2013) 250.
[81] W.P. Walters, M.T. Stahl, M.A. Murcko, Virtual screening—an overview, Drug Discov. Today 3 (1998) 160–178.
[82] P.D. Lyne, Structure-based virtual screening: an overview, Drug Discov. Today 7 (2002) 1047–1055.
[83] G. Schneider, H.J. Bohm, Virtual screening and fast automated docking methods, Drug Discov. Today 7 (2002) 63–70.
[84] H. Mauser, W. Guba, Recent developments in de novo design and scaffold hopping, Curr. Opin. Drug Discov. Devel. 11 (2008) 365–374.
[85] W.L. Jorgensen, Efficient drug lead discovery and optimization, Acc. Chem. Res. 42 (2009) 724–733.

Further reading

Structure Based Focusing is available from Accelrys, 9685 Scranton Road, San Diego, CA 92121, USA.

CHAPTER 9

Success stories in computer-aided drug design

Christos Tsagkaris[a], Anna Chiara Corriero[b], Rehab A. Rayan[c], Dimitrios V. Moysidis[d], Andreas S. Papazoglou[d], and Athanasios Alexiou[a,e]

[a]Novel Global Community Educational Foundation, Hebersham, NSW, Australia
[b]Anglia Ruskin University—Rivermead Campus, Chelmsford, United Kingdom
[c]Department of Epidemiology, High Institute of Public Health, Alexandria University, Alexandria, Egypt
[d]Faculty of Medicine, Aristotle University of Thessaloniki, Thessaloniki, Greece
[e]AFNP Med, Wien, Austria

1. Introduction: Definition of CADD and systems pharmacology, the concept of "success stories"

Computer-aided drug discovery (CADD) is a multidisciplinary field of scientific inquiry in the intersection of informatics and pharmacology. CADD employs computational methods to discover, develop, and analyze pharmaceutical agents and physiologically active molecules. The main asset of CADD consists of the analysis of potentially beneficial and harmful interactions between the 2D and 3D structures of the analyzed compounds and other medicines or biological substances. Such an analysis simulates the biological effect of given pharmaceutical agents, providing valuable insights about its effectiveness and safety in the context of particular biological systems and health conditions [1]. An overview of CADD is provided in Fig. 1.

Such an approach can only be accomplished in the context of systems pharmacology. This field is based on applying the computational and mathematical modeling of biological systems (cardiovascular, nervous system, etc.) to pharmacology. It consists of a fusion of systems biology, pharmacokinetics, and pharmacodynamics seeking to interpret the effect of medicines on human physiology and pathophysiology. Systems biology, systems pharmacology, and subsequently CADD have emerged to fill the knowledge gaps created by the reductionist approach to biology, an approach delving into the cellular and molecular interactions of biomolecules but often missing the larger picture [2].

A thorough and just assessment of the contribution of CADD to contemporary biomedical sciences can only be achieved through a

Computational Approaches in Drug Discovery, Development and Systems Pharmacology
https://doi.org/10.1016/B978-0-323-99137-7.00001-0

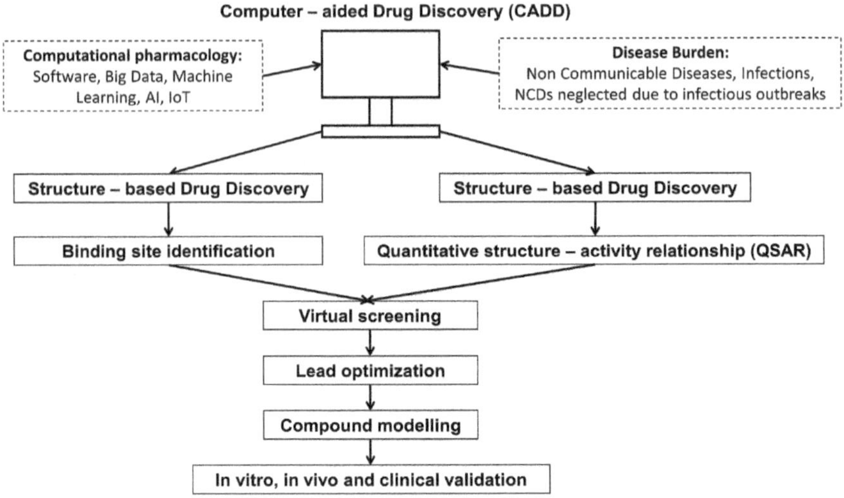

Fig. 1 An overview of computer-aided drug discovery; advances in computational pharmacology in combination with a rapidly increasing burden of communicable and noncommunicable diseases create the need for computational drug design to develop novel regimens or improve the effectiveness or safety profile of existing drugs.

comprehensive overview of the relevant literature combined—possible—with a cost-benefit analysis of the funding and labor dedicated to the field and its output in clinical practice and the market. "Success—stories" represent a qualitative, yet partial, assessment of the field's contribution, highlighting its successful applications and attempting to dissect them and highlight the components that spearheaded its particular success. In this sense, success stories can be perceived as an opportunity for researchers to contemplate their approach, get informed about good practices, and adapt them to their work.

The main objective of this chapter is to provide an overview of success stories in CADD and critically discuss their key components.

2. Methods

The authors performed a thorough search of the literature in the PubMed/Medline, Scopus, Embase, and Web of Science biomedical databases. In addition, gray literature in the form of reports published by the industry, stakeholders, policymakers, and concerned health bodies and agencies were also screened. Success stories were perceived as so and included as long as they contained information about CADD-based scientific (academic or entrepreneurial) projects that led to concrete results, which could be verified in peer-reviewed literature or other credible sources (pharmaceutical agencies, health organizations, and patent authorization bodies). No time limitation was set. Potential success stories were excluded if they were not verified through the aforementioned sources or if relevant information was not accessible in English.

3. History and development of CADD

The inception of CADD can be traced back to 1981 when CADD methodology was first applied to characterize a number of pharmaceutical compounds [3]. Indeed, computer-aided design (CAD), as an umbrella concept for CADD, has preceded. CAD first appeared in 1957, in the form of PRONTO, a commercially available numerical-control programming system. The creation of SKETCHPAD in an MIT laboratory in 1960 showcased the fundamentals of computer technical design. CAD initially served as a 2D digital alternative to drawing boards, depicting 2D wire-frame primitives (line, arc, B spline, etc.). 3D features of CAD a few years after 1960, leading to the release of Syntha Vision, a solid modeler program, in 1969. However, CAD was limited to technical drawing until 1974 because of the complexity and the limited availability of computers. This limitation would be waived in the following years [4].

Subsequently, CADD was introduced in pharmacology as a potential solution to a significant stalemate, namely, the fact that drug development from the bench to the market and the clinic is quite lengthy and costly. In most cases, the cost exceeds US$ 800 million, and the time required can reach up to 15 years. Experimentation with candidate agents who fail to yield the expected results beyond the cellular and tissue level results in a significant loss of time and funding. The possibility to accelerate the process while ruling out compounds incapable of inducing the desired biochemical and physiological outcomes would become the vision of CADD research [1].

4. CADD success stories in systems pharmacology

A quick search in major biomedical databases such as PubMed and Scopus reveals more than 8000 publications, including CADD or related terms in their title and abstract. Relevant research has exponentially increased since 2001, reaching an annual average of 500 publications from 2018 onwards.

The majority of the CADD research output consists of original in silico studies. There are fewer in vitro and in vivo studies and a quite low number of clinical trials. The latter reflects that CADD still faces obstacles in translating its results into clinically effective and market-wise competitive drugs. Although the disparity between the enormous amount of candidate drugs and the limited amount of eventually authorized drugs is a common pattern in all branches of pharmacological research, discussing promising CADD cases can help identify the elements of their success.

4.1 Benzoylpropionic acid derivatives as an alternative to ibuprofen

A 2019 study by Bittencourt and colleagues [5] has evaluated the potential of the anti-inflammatories MBPA and DHBPA, two benzoylpropionic acid derivatives, and compared it with the anti-inflammatory Ibuprofen.

Ibuprofen, a nonselective nonsteroidal anti-inflammatory drug (NSAID), has analgesic, antipyretic, and anti-inflammatory activities and has been shown to slow the development of tumors in mice [6]. Ibuprofen also has lighter side effects than compounds used in similar ways, such as acetylsalicylic acid and indomethacin, and is therefore, more tolerated by patients as an analgesic [7].

However, as there have been many concerns with the efficacy and toxicity of the drug, scientists have been working on researching and trialing other compounds that could be more efficacious and less toxic; therefore, this study compared the efficacy and toxicity of Ibuprofen with MBPA and DHBPA.

The investigators used molecular docking and molecular dynamics prediction techniques to calculate the oral bioavailability, bioactivity, and toxicity of all compounds.

The GOLD program was used to compare the mechanism of action of all the compounds. Moreover, the thermodynamic profiles by molecular dynamics of the compounds were studied using the MMPSA routine via GROMACS, whereas oral bioavailability and bioactivity predictions were made using the Molinspiration server. Lastly, toxicity analysis was performed using the server Protox.

The study concluded that, due to having the same ability to inhibit COX-2 as Ibuprofen, both benzoylpropionic acid derivatives were effective anti-inflammatories. However, as the literature suggests, the study also confirmed the predictions of Ibuprofen's hepatotoxicity and gastrointestinal tract irritation.

Furthermore, the study showed that the benzoylpropionic acid derivatives MBPA and DHBPA have good oral bioavailability and low toxicity (LD50 < 700 mg/kg). Overall, they were safe when compared to commercially available products. The study suggested that future research will have to evaluate the efficacy of these compounds further. Future projects could also use similar theories to evaluate other COX inhibitors to improve efficacy and limit side effects.

4.2 CADD research into repurposing a previously withdrawn COX-2 inhibitor

Leão et al. studied the new Rofecoxib-based cyclooxygenase-2 (COX-2) inhibitors with a bioinformatic approach [8]. The study started with an analysis of Rofecoxib, a COX inhibitor approved for use in 1999 and later withdrawn in 2004 due to its side-effect profile [9,10]. The side effects of the drug included the NSAIDs side effects such as GI toxicity, but also a significantly higher risk of serious cardiovascular events. Therefore, this study focused on analyzing compounds similar to Rofecoxib in efficacy but had a safer side-effect profile and was cost effective in development and manufacturing.

The study searched for similarly shaped ROCS (rapid overlay of chemical structures) and electrostatic compounds and later used pharmacokinetic and toxicological parameters to identify the best compound. This was done by using the software Qikprop and Derek. The serve Swiss was used for biological target prediction, and Molinspiration was used as in the study mentioned above by Bittencourt et al. to evaluate bioactivity. Finally, molecular dynamics were used to analyze the interaction over time of the chosen compounds.

After a process of selection and virtual screening of molecules coming from six commercial molecular databases, looking for chemical similarity, pharmacokinetic properties, and toxicological properties, three structures were identified: LMQC72, LMQC36, and LMQC50.

These three molecules showed good pharmacokinetic predictions, comparable to those of the products available in commerce, and good oral bioavailability; in particular, human oral absorption was found to be 100% for all three molecules, compared to an 82.40% value for Rofecoxib.

The three studied compounds also showed better octanol/water permeability than Rofecoxib, thus showing better cellular absorption and easy overcoming of the phospholipid bilayer of biological membranes. In addition, a more favorable intestinal absorption compared to Rofecoxib was also shown, with values consistently above 900 nm/s, 400 nm/s above the limit of 500 nm/S (value above which prediction of passive transport is considered good).

However, the three compounds showed low permeability of the CNS and no CNS side effects in humans. Overall, the study concluded that these three molecules can be considered adequate COX inhibitors and should be further studied and evaluated as potential anti-inflammatory drugs.

4.3 Molecular modeling of μ opioid receptor ligands

A 2020 study by Podlewska et al. focused on the molecular modeling of μ opioid receptor ligands with various functional properties; the study involved two G protein-based μ opioid receptor agonists (PZM21 and SE-17′18), alongside unbiased morphine and fentanyl (β-arrestin-2-biased agonist). This was done using LigPrep and the Protein Preparation Wizard from the Schrödinger Suite, the PDB database, Glide, and Desmond software. Lastly, the interactions between ligands were analyzed with the Simulation Interaction Diagram from the Schrödinger Suite [11].

The rationale behind the study was that, while opioids are effective analgesics and their use is nowadays approved and widespread worldwide, their side effects can limit their utilization [12]. Furthermore, in western countries and developing countries alike, many patients tend to abuse these painkillers—and unfortunately, many lose their lives due to the side effects of these drugs, including respiratory depression [13].

The mentioned side effects pose a concern in orthopedics, while opioids are effective in managing musculoskeletal pain, their potency comes with high morbidity and mortality; therefore, the literature has suggested that in case of prescription of opioids, these should be prescribed alongside other analgesic drugs. Furthermore, patients should be warned about the careful use of these drugs and their side effects [14].

Recently, the WHO declared that worldwide, 500,000 deaths are dependent on drug use, of which 70% depend on opioids. Moreover, overdoses account for 30% of these deaths [15]. Therefore, there has been pressure to find analgesics with similar potency to the approved opioids but with less addictive characteristics and less dangerous side effects.

For the above reason, the study by Podlewska et al. [11] analyzed the simulations of molecular docking and dynamics as well as statistics regarding the ligand-protein contacts. Furthermore, there have been approaches based on the observation of signaling pathways, which thought the μ opioid receptor would activate intercellular pathways with different potencies. Thus, it is suggested that some opioids can activate the G protein signal pathway, thus two G protein-based μ opioid receptor agonists (PZM21 and SE-17′18) were analyzed in the study, alongside other two G protein receptors, namely unbiased morphine and fentanyl—as these compounds avoid activating β-arrestin-2 pathway, which is taught to be responsible for the side effects of opioids (respiratory depression, constipation, and addiction).

Furthermore, the study also investigated the interaction between the compounds and the residues of proteins. It correlated this with the in vitro and in vivo tests, thus generating high values of Pearson coefficients (above 0.94).

In this type of study, due to the variety of obtained results, it is necessary to analyze a great breadth of structural data rather than choosing one type of structure or receptor to focus on. The study also concluded that three proteins should be taken into special consideration when designing new ligands with computer-aided technology in the field of analgesia, namely the amino acids W133, $I144^{3\times29}$, and $I322^{7\times38}$.

Overall, this analysis can help in the CAD of new G protein-biased ligands of the μ opioid receptor and provide new frontiers in the challenge against the opioid overdose pandemic.

5. CADD market analysis

The growth of CADD-related market is an additional indicator of the field's success. According to a recent analysis, the global CADD market accounted for $2741.1 million in 2020 and is expected to reach a value of $7914.2 million by 2028. This is the equivalent of a compound annual growth rate (CAGR) of 15%. Ligand-based drug design is the core component of CADD achieving the largest market growth. In particular, it is expected to rise from $1175.3 million in 2020 to more than $3366.4 million by 2028. The therapeutic areas expected to attain the highest benefits of CADD are cardiovascular disease (CVD), oncology, diabetes, neurology, and respiratory diseases. Cardiometabolic diseases constitute the most rapidly growing segment in the global market, generating a revenue of $1368.6 within 2028. Indeed their market size is estimated to grow from $93,494.41 million in 2021 to $121,804.49 million in 2028 with a CAGR of 3.8%.

In this context, the growth of CADD seems mainly associated with the burden of noncommunicable diseases (NCDs), and particularly CVDs, which currently account for the highest morbidity and mortality burden in the western world [16]. The emergence of NCDs burden associated with infectious diseases has been documented since 2017 [17] and is an additional factor increasing the need for therapeutic tools in the field, including those produced utilizing CADD. The COVID-19 pandemic is a novel and potentially crucial driver of the latter. The burden of poorly managed or nondiagnosed NCDs during the COVID-19 pandemic appears as a key concern for the future [18]. Combining this with the use of CADD for the development of treatments against COVID-19, it appears that COVID-19 will also become a key driver for the economic growth of CADD in the foreseeable future. Nevertheless, the need for highly confident personnel with a combined background in informatics and biomedicine has been regarded as a restrictive factor for CADD's market growth.

Overall, the financial success of CADD will depend on the ability of relevant research to provide marketable products in the coming years and on the ability of educational institutions to educate a sufficient number of researchers with relevant expertise. The contemporary landscape of disease burden, including both NCDs and infectious diseases, provides favorable opportunities for extended use of CADD in the coming years. The principal lessons from the financial success of CADD until now include the adaptability of CADD in many diseases' contexts. So far, CADD has been adapted to well-established health challenges, such as cardiometabolic diseases and emerging health challenges such as COVID-19.

6. Discussion

So far, it seems that CADD has significant potential in the field of musculoskeletal and pain medicine. The existing efforts focus on identifying novel molecules with a more favorable profile of side effects to produce alternative regimens to currently used or withdrawn pain medication. In this sense, CADD emerges as a contributor in mitigating pain medication side effects [19]. The latter represents a significant concern given that opioids' side effects have been associated with higher in-hospital treatment costs and increased healthcare resources utilization [20], especially when administered to elderly patients with active diseases, history of major surgical interventions, and concurrent use of benzodiazepines [21]. On the other hand, Ibuprofen has a favorable profile in cost-benefit analyses, making it preferable to opioids or other NSAIDs in patients with osteoarthritis [22]. Nevertheless, several older studies have set the alarm for the cost of side effects related to NSAIDs; therefore, research on regimens with equal effectiveness and fewer side effects remains relevant [23,24].

6.1 CADD opportunities and limitations

Nowadays, the methods used in drug development are costly and time consuming, regardless of the extensive scientific progress in drug discovery methods. Since the uphill force of trimming time and price for risk-free and efficacious drugs, the direction has gone to the first stages of drug discovery and development [25,26]. CADD was a developing subject about 30 years ago with minor techniques. However, it has evolved into a mature subject with a comprehensive combination of techniques available now. A vital research trade is being applied in rationally drawing compounds involving broad groups of virtual flow charts [27].

For over three decades, CADD methods have been used vastly in distinct phases of drug discovery, further with efficiency and quality. The cost of discovery and development of drugs could be decreased by 50% with the utility of CADD. Some CADD methods have been regulated and are being routinely used, still various coming into court CADD methods that are similarly adopted at various drug discovery stages. A lot of the marketed drugs discovered so far have been developed applying CADD methods. Moreover, CADD assists in anticipating the new curative usages of the FDA (Food and Drug Administration) authorized drugs; this scheme is called "drug repurposing" [28,29].

CADD is a potent means in modern drug discovery for the hunt of possible medicinal drug compounds. Today, it has become the most desirable option for high-throughput screening that is applied habitually in drug discovery and development. The approaches utilized in CADD are employed in every phase of the drug discovery pipeline since it can fasten the procedure of hit finding, hit to lead, and lead optimization. Recently, advances in the computational drug designing protocol and computational power have enabled scientists to bring forth illness-directed fast and trustworthy results at reduced expenditure in controllable time space [30,31].

Because all the CADD techniques are intended to be user-friendly, knowledgeable scientists in fundamental sciences could expeditiously utilize them. However, CADD techniques might seem plain, and it is crucial to recognize the basic science behind the technique for better utilization. Yet, CADD techniques do not give conclusive solutions; they simply render developed lucidity to the logical design of drugs [29].

Lately, with the progress in IT, computational power, and accessibility to big data, novel techniques have been used in CADD that involve ML, DL, AI, and data mining to foster the rate and quality of drug discovery. It is expected that drug discovery approaches would use such innovative technologies, facilitating choosing drug and receptor properties, processing images, clustering of compounds, among other applications. The value of ML in CADD is well acknowledged, and there are numerous studies on its booming uses [32,33]. In the ML-derived technique, big data sets are trained using a mathematical model, which is then used to forecast or analyze a different data set [34]. Progress in the diverse computational methods assisted in CADD, like ML techniques, aid in complicated patterning systems that give perceptiveness into a compound's structure and prior knowledge. Nevertheless, DL methods assist in rapidly choosing compounds via pattern recognition, and they could be applied in the early discovery of illness and management of them [35,36].

The circulating pandemic arose since the coronavirus could be interpreted as the optimal illustration of such a kind where more studies have appeared worldwide against various coronavirus target proteins [37,38]. Contemporary computational methods have assisted in reaching molecular-level perception and foretelling the inhibitors. Aside from the progress in rational drug designing techniques, large-scale production of the big biologic data has grown more the ML/DL/AI-driven framework evolution that has exhibited better anticipation quality compared to conventional methods. However, such data-determined frameworks are extremely hooked upon the quality and quantity of the data. As much data evolves, the forecasting quality will evolve as well. Meanwhile, there is a constant demand for more advances in forecasting algorithms to detect promising novel drugs and foretell brand new uses for present ones [39].

This chapter offered a glance at well-consented and developing CADD methods through success stories in this field. Although much research is being done via applying CADD techniques, it has not gone exhaustively through all the drug discovery arena. This is because of the reality that several of such techniques necessitate a careful reading of the subject area related to them. The number of novel methods being presented to execute pharmacy informatics research is tremendous. Such a realism could be seen as an asset and a liability—since each of these and many more are needed, too numerous are being presented, holding course is getting hard. Ultimately, we cannot neglect the efforts in pharmacy informatics that shall come in every area for experts in pharmaceutical disciplines; merely at the same time, the present gaps call for further research [40].

6.2 CADD limitations and challenges

Despite its potential and contribution, CADD is subject to certain limitations and challenges (Fig. 2). First, it requires a solid background in both

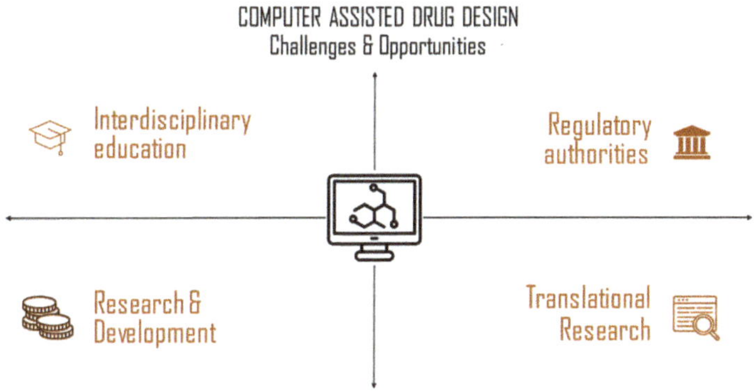

Fig. 2 Schematic representation of the main challenges and opportunities for CADD.

pharmacology and informatics. Researchers trained exclusively in either of the fields can face difficulties in immersing themselves in CADD research or even comprehending its results and using them in their non-CADD research. This limitation should be addressed by integrating CADD and computational pharmacology in biomedical educational curricula. Moreover, as a form of in-silico research, CADD research needs to be validated by in vitro, in vivo, and clinical research. Tracing the discrepancies in CADD research outputs that were not validated in clinical settings can help researchers optimize CADD approaches. The latter requires establishing a feedback loop between CADD and conventional pharmacological research and enhancing CADD-associated pharmacovigilance [41].

In addition to these, CADD is subject to legislative and regulatory impediments. The harmonization of regional and national regulatory frameworks with advances in the field of in silico pharmacological research can provide researchers with more liberty to conduct studies that will build upon the current perception of CADD as a tool for biomedical research. This process can be accelerated through initiatives implemented at international level, which will put pressure on national governments to adopt CADD favorable provisions in the national research frameworks. An overview of agencies capable of supporting this goal is provided in Table 1. [42–44] From this, it becomes evident that agencies serving as one-stop-shop regulatory authorities currently operate only in North America, Europe and Africa. Developments related to CADD in these regions can be conveniently adopted in all the concerned countries and territories. Nevertheless, it appears that there is no such capacity in South America and Asia. To date, the FDA is represented in 44 countries and territories in this region, however, multiple stakeholders call for the establishment of a separate regional

Table 1 Regional and International Medicines Agency with regulatory responsibility over multiple countries and territories.

Agency	Region	Year of establishment	Capacity
US Food and Drug Administration (FDA)	United States of America	1906	Oversees drug development and authorization in the United States of America, has on—site presence in the 44 countries and territories of the Latin America
European Medicines Organization (EMA)	European Union	1995	Oversees drug development and authorization within the European Union (EU), works closely with the European Institutions and the national medicines agencies of the EU member states
African Medicines Agency (AMA)	Africa	2018	The African Union (AU) and its New Partnership for Africa's Development (NEPAD) in cooperation with the World Health Organization have integrated national medicines regulatory authorities (NMRAs) in Africa, in order to establish an African Medicines Agency (AMA). AMA resembles the EMA serving as the one-stop-shop regulator for the entire continent

medicines agency, namely the Latin American Medicines Agency [44,45]. In Africa, the effort of putting together a regional medicines agency was supported by the WHO [46]. Similarly, the regional representations of the WHO in the Americas and Asia can help establish capable medicines regulatory authorities.

It is essential that such initiatives will go beyond calling for authorization of CADD or CADD – related methodologies and tools. This means that they should strengthen digital innovation in healthcare as a whole, creating a framework where CADD findings will have the chance to be integrated in a wider research ecosystem. The European Health Data Space (EHDS), which was launched on May 3, 2022, constitutes a representative example of this paradigm. In this context, multifaceted healthcare innovation including CADD is integrated in the broader goal of harnessing data so that healthcare systems become more resilient and efficient [47].

Putting CADD in the broader cadre of research and development (R&D) in the industry and the entrepreneurial sphere is a notable consideration as well. Academic funding is oftentimes scarce and cannot support innovative ventures at full scale. On the other hand, the industrial ecosystem of in-silico pharmacology, where CADD belongs, accounts for more than 2129 million steadily increasing to more than 6500 million by 2030 [48]. What is more challenging is integrating relevant innovation in low – resources settings. In Spring 2022, a correspondence to Nature highlighted the need for jobs related to bioinformatics and digital health in Africa, as a means to encourage local experts not to migrate while contributing to the development of their national economies [49]. In this sense, harnessing CADD for R&D in low- and middle-income countries should be considered.

7. Conclusion

CADD represents a shift from conventional to computational pharmacological research. Given the high costs and time consumption associated with candidate drug failure in conventional pharmacology, this is a necessary step. Furthermore, CADD can contribute to selecting candidate drugs with favorable bioactivity and side-effect profiles. This is applicable in both designing novel drugs or replacing existing ones. So far, CADD research has led to promising outputs in medication for pain and inflammation associated with musculoskeletal conditions. Nevertheless, its results still have a long way to go through validation in vivo and clinical research. Thus, in the future, on top of increasing funding and infrastructure for CADD-related research, it is also necessary to invest in the education of a generation of researchers and clinicians who can comprehend CADD research outputs and appropriately use them in their research and practice.

References

[1] V.T. Sabe, T. Ntombela, L.A. Jhamba, G. Maguire, T. Govender, T. Naicker, H.G. Kruger, Current trends in computer aided drug design and a highlight of drugs discovered via computational techniques: a review, Eur. J. Med. Chem. 224 (2021), 113705, https://doi.org/10.1016/j.ejmech.2021.113705.

[2] W. Yu, A.D. MacKerell Jr., Computer-aided drug design methods, Methods Mol. Biol. 1520 (2017) 85–106, https://doi.org/10.1007/978-1-4939-6634-9_5.

[3] O. Osakwe, The Significance of Discovery Screening and Structure Optimization Studies, 2016, https://doi.org/10.1016/B978-0-12-802220-7.00005-3.

[4] D. Geddes, The Historyof Computer-Aided Design and Computer-Aided Manufacturing (CAD/CAM), Technical Foam Services, 2020.

[5] J. Bittencourt, M. Neto, P.S. Lacerda, R. Bittencourt, R.C. Silva, C.C. Lobato, L.B. Silva, F. Leite, J.P. Zuliani, J. Rosa, R.S. Borges, C. Santos, In silico evaluation of ibuprofen and two benzoylpropionic acid derivatives with potential anti-inflammatory activity, Molecules 24 (8) (2019) 1476, https://doi.org/10.3390/molecules24081476.

[6] G. Xie, Y. Sun, T. Nie, G.G. Mackenzie, L. Huang, L. Kopelovich, D. Komninou, B. Rigas, Phospho-ibuprofen (MDC-917) is a novel agent against colon cancer: efficacy, metabolism, and pharmacokinetics in mouse models, J. Pharmacol. Exp. Ther. 337 (3) (2011) 876–886, https://doi.org/10.1124/jpet.111.180224.

[7] M. Ershad, M.A. Ameer, D. Vearrier, Ibuprofen toxicity, in: StatPearls, StatPearls Publishing, 2021.

[8] R.P. Leão, J.V. Cruz, G.V. da Costa, J.N. Cruz, E. Ferreira, R.C. Silva, L.R. de Lima, R.S. Borges, G.B. Dos Santos, C. Santos, Identification of new rofecoxib-based cyclooxygenase-2 inhibitors: a bioinformatics approach, Pharmaceuticals 13 (9) (2020) 209, https://doi.org/10.3390/ph13090209.

[9] B. Sibbald, Rofecoxib (Vioxx) voluntarily withdrawn from market, CMAJ 171 (9) (2004) 1027–1028, https://doi.org/10.1503/cmaj.1041606.

[10] E.J. Topol, Failing the public health—rofecoxib, Merck, and the FDA, N. Engl. J. Med. 351 (17) (2004) 1707–1709, https://doi.org/10.1056/NEJMp048286.

[11] S. Podlewska, R. Bugno, L. Kudla, A.J. Bojarski, R. Przewlocki, Molecular modeling of μ opioid receptor ligands with various functional properties: PZM21, SR-17018, morphine, and fentanyl—simulated interaction patterns confronted with experimental data, Molecules 25 (20) (2020) 4636, https://doi.org/10.3390/molecules25204636.

[12] R. Benyamin, A.M. Trescot, S. Datta, R. Buenaventura, R. Adlaka, N. Sehgal, S.E. Glaser, R. Vallejo, Opioid complications and side effects, Pain Physician 11 (2 Suppl) (2008) S105–S120.

[13] N.P. Coussens, G.S. Sittampalam, S.G. Jonson, M.D. Hall, H.E. Gorby, A.P. Tamiz, O.B. McManus, C.C. Felder, K. Rasmussen, The opioid crisis and the future of addiction and pain therapeutics, J. Pharmacol. Exp. Ther. 371 (2) (2019) 396–408, https://doi.org/10.1124/jpet.119.259408.

[14] L.D. Delaney, D.J. Clauw, J.F. Waljee, The management of acute pain for musculoskeletal conditions, J. Bone Joint Surg. 102 (Suppl 1) (2020) 3–9, https://doi.org/10.2106/JBJS.20.00228.

[15] L. Degenhardt, M. Glantz, S. Evans-Lacko, et al., Estimating treatment coverage for people with substance use disorders: an analysis of data from the World Mental Health Surveys, World Psychiatry 16 (3) (2017) 299–307, https://doi.org/10.1002/wps.2045.
[16] A. Boutayeb, S. Boutayeb, The burden of non communicable diseases in developing countries, Int. J. Equity Health 4 (1) (2005) 2, https://doi.org/10.1186/1475-9276-4-2.
[17] M.M. Coates, A. Kintu, N. Gupta, E.B. Wroe, A.J. Adler, G.F. Kwan, P.H. Park, R. Rajbhandari, A.L. Byrne, D.C. Casey, G. Bukhman, Burden of non-communicable diseases from infectious causes in 2017: a modelling study, Lancet Glob. Health 8 (12) (2020) e1489–e1498, https://doi.org/10.1016/S2214-109X(20)30358-2.
[18] X.F. Pan, J. Yang, Y. Wen, N. Li, S. Chen, A. Pan, Non-communicable diseases during the COVID-19 pandemic and beyond, Engineering 7 (7) (2021) 899–902, https://doi.org/10.1016/j.eng.2021.02.013.
[19] M.O. Martel, P.H. Finan, A.J. Dolman, S. Subramanian, R.R. Edwards, A.D. Wasan, R.N. Jamison, Self-reports of medication side effects and pain-related activity interference in patients with chronic pain: a longitudinal cohort study, Pain 156 (6) (2015) 1092–1100, https://doi.org/10.1097/j.pain.0000000000000154.
[20] S.L. Kane-Gill, E.C. Rubin, P.L. Smithburger, M.S. Buckley, J.F. Dasta, The cost of opioid-related adverse drug events, J. Pain Palliat. Care Pharmacother. 28 (3) (2014) 282–293, https://doi.org/10.3109/15360288.2014.938889.
[21] R.D. Urman, D.L. Seger, J.M. Fiskio, B.A. Neville, E.M. Harry, S.G. Weiner, B. Lovelace, R. Fain, J. Cirillo, J.L. Schnipper, The burden of opioid-related adverse drug events on hospitalized previously opioid-free surgical patients, J. Patient Saf. 17 (2) (2021) e76–e83, https://doi.org/10.1097/PTS.0000000000000566.
[22] J.N. Katz, S.R. Smith, J.E. Collins, D.H. Solomon, J.M. Jordan, D.J. Hunter, L.G. Suter, E. Yelin, A.D. Paltiel, E. Losina, Cost-effectiveness of nonsteroidal anti-inflammatory drugs and opioids in the treatment of knee osteoarthritis in older patients with multiple comorbidities, Osteoarthr. Cartil. 24 (3) (2016) 409–418, https://doi.org/10.1016/j.joca.2015.10.006.
[23] R. Andrew Moore, C.J. Phillips, Cost of NSAID adverse effects to the UK National Health Service, J. Med. Econ. 2 (1–4) (1999) 45–55, https://doi.org/10.3111/199902045055.
[24] S.E. Gabriel, J.L. Wagner, Costs and effectiveness of nonsteroidal anti-inflammatory drugs: the importance of reducing side effects, Arthritis Care Res. 10 (1) (1997) 56–63, https://doi.org/10.1002/art.1790100109.
[25] R. Collier, Drug development cost estimates hard to swallow, CMAJ 180 (3) (2009) 279–280, https://doi.org/10.1503/cmaj.082040.
[26] M. Schlander, K. Hernandez-Villafuerte, C.Y. Cheng, et al., How much does it cost to research and develop a new drug? A systematic review and assessment, Pharmacoeconomics 39 (2021) 1243–1269, https://doi.org/10.1007/s40273-021-01065-y.
[27] X. Mingli, C. Yu, F. Wenjie, C. Lijuan, M. Yirong, Computer-aided drug design:lead discovery and optimization, Comb. Chem. High Throughput Screen. 15 (4) (2012), https://doi.org/10.2174/138620712799361825.
[28] G. Sliwoski, S. Kothiwale, J. Meiler, E.W. Lowe Jr., Computational methods in drug discovery, Pharmacol. Rev. 66 (1) (2013) 334–395, https://doi.org/10.1124/pr.112.007336.
[29] S.J. Macalino, V. Gosu, S. Hong, S. Choi, Role of computer-aided drug design in modern drug discovery, Arch. Pharm. Res. 38 (9) (2015) 1686–1701, https://doi.org/10.1007/s12272-015-0640-5.
[30] N. Schaduangrat, S. Lampa, S. Simeon, et al., Towards reproducible computational drug discovery, J. Cheminform. 12 (2020) 9, https://doi.org/10.1186/s13321-020-0408-x.

[31] P. Jamkhande, M. Ghante, B. Ajgunde, Software based approaches for drug designing and development: a systematic review on commonly used software and its applications, Bull. Fac. Pharm. Cairo Univ. 55 (2017), https://doi.org/10.1016/j.bfopcu.2017.10.001.
[32] J. Vamathevan, D. Clark, P. Czodrowski, et al., Applications of machine learning in drug discovery and development, Nat. Rev. Drug Discov. 18 (2019) 463–477, https://doi.org/10.1038/s41573-019-0024-5.
[33] M. Khamis, W. Gomaa, Comparative assessment of machine-learning scoring functions on PDBbind 2013, Eng. Appl. Artif. Intel. (2015), https://doi.org/10.1016/j.engappai.2015.06.021.
[34] R.C. Deo, Machine learning in medicine, Circulation 132 (20) (2015) 1920–1930, https://doi.org/10.1161/CIRCULATIONAHA.115.001593.
[35] R. Gupta, D. Srivastava, M. Sahu, et al., Artificial intelligence to deep learning: machine intelligence approach for drug discovery, Mol. Divers. 25 (2021) 1315–1360, https://doi.org/10.1007/s11030-021-10217-3.
[36] H. Chen, O. Engkvist, Y. Wang, M. Olivecrona, T. Blaschke, The rise of deep learning in drug discovery, Drug Discov. Today 23 (6) (2018) 1241–1250, https://doi.org/10.1016/j.drudis.2018.01.039.
[37] R. Patil, R. Chikhale, P. Khanal, N. Gurav, M. Ayyanar, S. Sinha, S. Prasad, Y.N. Dey, M. Wanjari, S.S. Gurav, Computational and network pharmacology analysis of bioflavonoids as possible natural antiviral compounds in COVID-19, Inform. Med. Unlocked 22 (2021), 100504, https://doi.org/10.1016/j.imu.2020.100504.
[38] F. Napolitano, X. Xu, X. Gao, Impact of computational approaches in the fight against COVID-19: an AI guided review of 17 000 studies, Brief. Bioinform. (2021), bbab456, https://doi.org/10.1093/bib/bbab456.
[39] T. Anwar, P. Kumar, A.U. Khan, Chapter 1—Modern tools and techniques in computer-aided drug design, in: M.S. Coumar (Ed.), Molecular Docking for Computer-Aided Drug Design, vol. 2021, Academic Press, 2021, pp. 1–30, ISBN: 9780128223123, https://doi.org/10.1016/B978-0-12-822312-3.00011-4.
[40] P.V. Bharatam, Computer-aided drug design, in: R. Poduri (Ed.), Drug Discovery and Development, Springer, Singapore, 2021, https://doi.org/10.1007/978-981-15-5534-3_6.
[41] P. Natsiavas, A. Malousi, C. Bousquet, M.-C. Jaulent, V. Koutkias, Computational advances in drug safety: systematic and mapping review of knowledge engineering based approaches, Front. Pharmacol. 10 (2019) 415, https://doi.org/10.3389/fphar.2019.00415.
[42] Is the Time Right for a Latin American Medicines Agency after the African Medicines Agency?, International Alliance of Patients Organizations, 2017. Accessed 30 May 2022, Available at: https://www.iapo.org.uk/news/2017/jul/3/time-right-latin-american-medicines-agency-after-african-medicines-agency.
[43] History of EMA, European Medicines Organization, 2015. Accessed 30 May 2022, Available at: https://www.ema.europa.eu/en/about-us/history-ema.
[44] FDA History, US Food and Drug Administration, 2018. Accessed 30 May 2022, Available at: https://www.fda.gov/about-fda/fda-history.
[45] Latin America Office, US Food and Drug Administration, 2022. Accessed May 30 2022, Available at: https://www.fda.gov/about-fda/office-global-operations/latin-america-office.
[46] International Federation of Pharmaceutical Manufacturers and Associations, Towards an African Medicines Agency, 2019, Accessed 30 May 2022, Available at: https://www.ifpma.org/subtopics/african-medicines-agency/.

[47] Questions and Answers—EU Health: European Health Data Space (EHDS), European Commission, 2022. Accessed 30 May 2022, Available at: https://ec.europa.eu/commission/presscorner/detail/en/QANDA_22_2712.

[48] Global In-Silico Drug Discovery Market Analysis and Forecast, 2021–2031: Massive Scope for Adoption of In-Silico Drug Discovery in Developing Nations & Adoption of AI in In-Silico Drug Discovery, CISION, Research and Markets, 2022. Accessed 30 May 2022, Available at: https://www.prnewswire.com/news-releases/global-in-silico-drug-discovery-market-analysis-and-forecast-2021-2031-massive-scope-for-adoption-of-in-silico-drug-discovery-in-developing-nations- -adoption-of-ai-in-in-silico-drug-discovery-301515645.html.

[49] A.A. Akintola, U.W. Hwang, A.T. Aborode, Africa needs more bioinformaticians for population studies, Nature 605 (7911) (2022) 619, https://doi.org/10.1038/d41586-022-01378-8.

CHAPTER 10

Computer-aided drug design-based system pharmacology applications for the treatment of diabetes mellitus

Shabana Bibi[a,b], Mohammad Mehedi Hasan[c,d], Md. Shahadat Hossain[c,e], Muhammad Saad Khan[f], Qudsia Yousafi[f], Fahadul Islam[g], Hitesh Chopra[h], and Mohammad Amjad Kamal[g,i,j,k,l]
[a]Department of Biosciences, Shifa Tameer-e-Millat University, Islamabad, Pakistan
[b]Yunnan Herbal Laboratory, College of Ecology and Environmental Sciences, Yunnan University, Kunming, China
[c]Department of Biochemistry and Molecular Biology, Faculty of Life Science, Mawlana Bhashani Science and Technology University, Tangail, Bangladesh
[d]Division of Computer-Aided Drug Design, The Red-Green Research Centre, BICCB, Dhaka, Bangladesh
[e]Department of Pharmacy, Faculty of Life Science, Mawlana Bhashani Science and Technology University, Tangail, Bangladesh
[f]Department of Biosciences, Faculty of Sciences, COMSATS University Islamabad, Sahiwal, Pakistan
[g]Department of Pharmacy, Faculty of Allied Health Sciences, Daffodil International University, Dhaka, Bangladesh
[h]Chitkara College of Pharmacy, Chitkara University, Rajpura, Punjab, India
[i]Institutes for Systems Genetics, Frontiers Science Center for Disease-related Molecular Network, West China Hospital, Sichuan University, China
[j]King Fahd Medical Research Center, King Abdulaziz University, Jeddah, Saudi Arabia
[k]Enzymoics, Hebersham, NSW, Australia
[l]Novel Global Community Educational Foundation, Hebersham, NSW, Australia

1. Current statistics of diabetes mellitus and major factor involved in its prevalence

Diabetes mellitus (DM) is noncommunicable disease (N-CD) that include cardiovascular disease (CVD), malignancies, and chronic respiratory ailments, which together account for 63% of N-CD fatalities globally [1,2]. The number of persons suffering from DM worldwide increased from 108 million to 442 million between 1980 and 2014 [3,4]. About two-thirds of persons with DM are of working age; in 2017, 425 million people worldwide were projected to have the disease, with that proportion expected to climb to 629 million by 2045. DM claimed the lives of 4 million people aged 20 to 79 years old every 8 seconds in 2017 [5]. Both patients suffering from DM and the dying from DM are expected to rise if present DM growth continues. Low-income nations are forecasted to see the dramatic rise in DM prevalence that accounts

Computational Approaches in Drug Discovery, Development and Systems Pharmacology
https://doi.org/10.1016/B978-0-323-99137-7.00002-2

92%, distinct by subordinate-income-related nations accounts for 57%, highest-income related nations accounts for 46%, and advanced countries account for 25% [3,4,6]. DM cases that go undiagnosed community health issues with considerable financial consequences. Unmedicated DM is common all over the world. Undiagnosed DM was estimated to affect 50% of adults aged 20 to 79 globally [5]. Undiagnosed diabetics are more prone to develop issues even before diagnosis [5]. This can result in higher costs for households [6] and already overwhelmed health systems, necessitating a global escalation in testing efforts to avoid DM development [7].

HbA1c, blood pressure (BP), and the management of serum cholesterol levels are clinically important factors that are widely targeted to reduce CVD risk in diabetics [8,9] since statins are the immediate therapeutic options for lipid control, and management of low-density lipoprotein (LDL) cholesterol was chosen for cholesterol management. Personalized HbA1c targets for glycemic control have been emphasized, and they were indicated as, less than 6.5 percent in the people over 18 to 44 years without health problems, less than 7.0 percent in the people with health problems and people in the range of 45 to 64 years noticed without DM complications, and less than 8.0 percent for both middle-aged people and people with 65 years age or above having health problems, and less than 7.5 percent for people of 65 years age or above having health problems [8,9]. Self-reported CVDs issues damaging heart badly, retinopathy damaging eyes, a urine albumin to creatinine ratio of 30 mg/g or over it, or a predicted glomerular filtration rate of less than 60 mL/min/1.73 m^2 were all considered complications. BP control in DM should be smaller than 130/80 or 140/90 mmHg, according to 13 recommendations [10]. A systolic BP of 130 mmHg or less has been linked to a lower risk of CVD [11]. In DM, lipid therapy has evolved from lowering LDL-cholesterol levels to smaller than 100 mg/dL to providing statins of varying intensities based on age, the existence of atherosclerotic CVD and risk factors, and without a defined LDL-cholesterol target [8].

2. Status of computational system pharmacology (CSP) for different diseases

CADD basically relies on the computer modeling and predicting applications, such as computational system pharmacology (CSP) is one of the important methods of CADD that helps to understand and predict the behavior of selected compound or drug with respect to biological systems, and highly significant later for the drug optimization phase, so that unwanted or adverse effects of drugs can be reduced in drug design and development phases [12]. It reveals the solutions for the complex disease drug discovery and understands the molecular target-drug interactions and explains their mechanism of action [13,14]. CSP explains the calculation of effectiveness and toxicological protocols for the identification of chemicals during CADD pipelines [15]. The human system is very complicated and has an integrated system explaining different functional pathways that can be associated with the study of biological networks and toxicology in the advanced CSP [16]. The pathogenesis of multifaceted disease and their systems with respect to proteins, genes, other small therapeutic options and pathways is still a very big challenge for the disease identification and then treatment [13,17].

In society, as we are facing the burden of metabolic diseases, DM is a very crucial disease to handle, so there is a need for modern pharmacological methods to discover novel therapeutics against different metabolic diseases so that many companies and scientists are continuously working on the improved and advance computational system pharmacology (CSP) techniques [18,19]. These advanced methods would be highly significant in decreasing the pharmaceutical issues, that is a major cause of decreased productivity of novel therapeutics development, and increase the hit's number of upcoming better drugs, and also improving the situation of persistent gaps between many medicinal requirements urgently needed to treat the several metabolic diseases for example, obesity, DM, and CVDs [20]. These CADD approaches are significant in screening and identification of new biomolecular targets that can significantly inhibit or enhance the signaling pathways and reduce the experimental cost to minimum level in the drug identification and early developing research pipelines [18].

As the maximum USD for launching a novel chemical compound /medicine in market for any disease is probably 1.8 billion USD [21,22]. In the report of 2013, out of 50 drugs approved drugs, 17 drugs were identified by the computational application of computer-aided drug design (CADD) methods [23]. It suggested that experimental libraries are making the CADD approaches a standard and taking place of conventional pharmacological laboratory methods in the next coming times, as the previous traditional drug discovery methodologies are not sufficient and need the implementation of CADD and CSP applications along with the authentications [18,24].

CADD delivers benefits for experimental outcomes, defines the repurposed drugs mechanisms of action, and adds innovative ideas for novel drug synthesis and development procedures, and it can benefit in creating profitable conclusions over earlier the expensive procedure of drug synthesis as followed in previous times [25]. Several synthetic and natural bioactive metabolites were discovered and/or optimized with the help of advanced methods of CSP and finally these metabolites could reach in the clinical stages of drug development and approved by FDA [19,26].

CSP application can upsurge the hit's rate for the treatment of DM and therefore explains the enormous chemical search space to discover an appropriate molecular target and can compare with outmoded high-throughput screening procedures. Virtual screening assisted the outcomes and increase the CADD-based identified hit-rate tenfold to 1700-fold [27,28].

CSP is now obligatory in medicinal study since the amount of biological records has improved and labor-intensive screening in contradiction of such data entails a lot of time and human efforts [29]. CSP methods are significant for the discovery of therapeutics for DM for past three decades [30]. The increased usage of these approach is revealed in the number of latest publications. Publications on CSP for 4 utmost crucial ailments are shown in Fig. 1. DM has the second most papers published on CSP until first week of January 2022, but published papers for cancer with CSP studies are more and have shown that the research of DM, HIV, and Coronavirus can be improved by adding this method with the conventional drug discovery approaches.

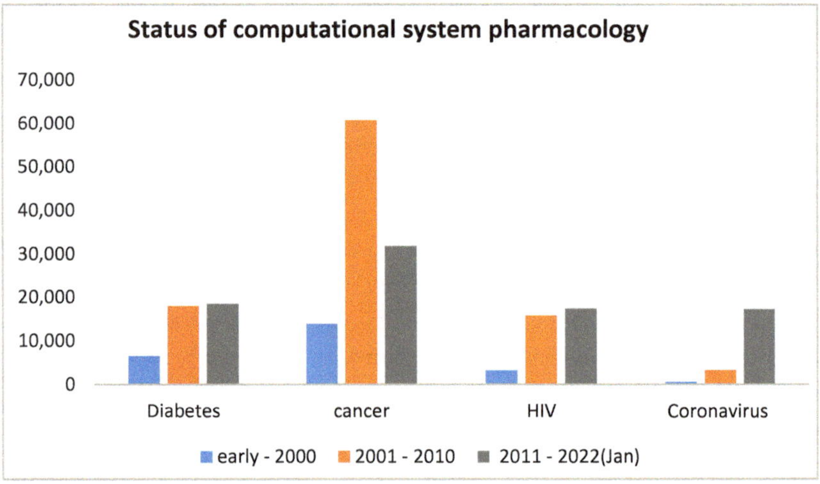

Fig. 1 Publications for the computational system pharmacology (CSP) and ailments. Keywords applied in "Google Scholar" search bar were as: computational system pharmacology and ailment, such as diabetes.

3. Modern computer-aided drug design-based system pharmacology techniques

There are ligand-based or receptor/structure-based CADD strategies to discover novel drugs against DM by screening the large data sets or libraries followed by the ADMET profile estimations to reduce the adverse effects of identified virtual hits [31] (Fig. 2). These procedures are cost-effective, reliable, and time-saving and take place of old traditional drug discovery approaches [32]. These methods are helpful in hit identification followed by hit-to-lead optimization [30]. Macromolecules (protein/enzymes) structures are useful in the lead identification with the assistance of computer modeling of protein-ligand complex [33].

There are modern CADD-based system pharmacology techniques that assisted the single or multiple target drugs discoveries and development pipelines, multitarget drugs have fascinated the audience in the last decades, as prospective therapeutics solutions of intricate etiology and healthiness associated to drug resistance and toxicological concerns [12]. With respect to the single drug-single target molecule strategy, extremely important and explicit managements would be better endured due to lack of off-target toxicological issues. Hence, weak correlation between the experimental studies of an identified drug while in vivo and in vivo effectiveness is usually due to target-driven calculations [34]. These days more focused technique is multiple-target based drug design and discovery, in the past decades, many identified therapeutics are based on the multitarget drugs pipelines [20],

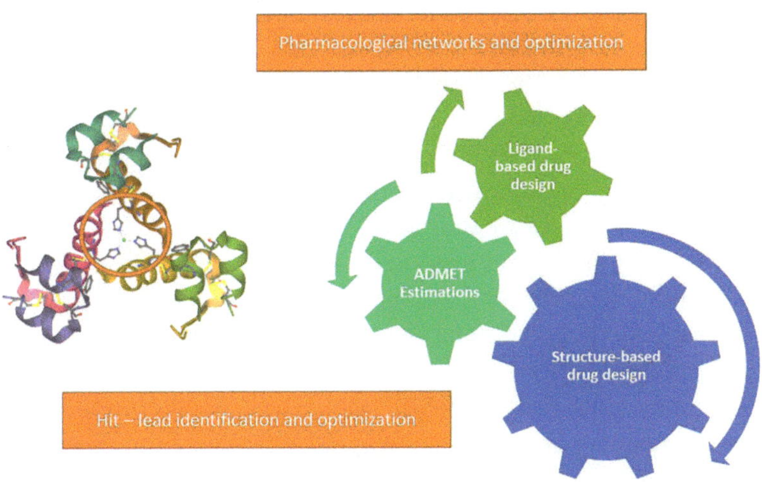

Fig. 2 Modern computer-aided drug design-based system pharmacology approaches.

which is particularly correct for those drugs that were identified by serendipity, phenotypic screening, and from nature as traditional medicine [35]. It is noteworthy that all these reported studies adds the knowledge on the pharmacological effect and mechanism of action [20].

4. Case studies of computational systems pharmacology for diabetes mellitus

Responses to tissues of insulin, such as muscle, adipose tissue, and liver, are the root mechanism of resistance to insulin in nonsufficient control. Glucose homeostasis control from the brain, hormonal effect of incretin on insulin has been explored in detail by mathematical modeling and CSP approaches [36,37] (Fig. 3). To calculate the incretin consequence, models were developed, i.e., to study the dissimilarities among intravenously and orally administered glucose aimed at various states of glucose tolerance.

For numerous decades, different mathematical models have been extensively used in medicine and biology and in definite areas, previously gained prevalent recognition. The initial and utmost known model is established by Hodgkin and Huxley in early 1952 [38]. After that mathematical modeling is considered as a needed component of the research process for field involved in electrical activity in cells. Models have demonstrated to be of favorable outcomes within the ground of DM research, for certain insulin treatments for testing animals US Food and Drug Administration has approved regulatory acceptance for glucose homeostasis model as a viable replacement, together with closed-loop algorithms, and controlled revolution in the field of device production for insulin dosage [39,40].

To understand the phenomenon like reduction in cellular reaction to insulin that rises from some regions of the intracellular protein interaction network, reason of spread on this resistance to the other areas of the network and in which manner other organs being affected by this resistance in case of DM has been helped out by multilevel models [41,42].

Many models have been proposed to understand the response in case of DM at different levels, e.g., longer-term dynamics of a meal or therapeutic drug treatment, due to over-eating increase in weight, disease development, and progression with the passage of time and longer term improvements of a drug [43,44]. Model unfolding immediate drug effects—so-called pharmacodynamics and pharmacokinetic models are considered as a typical approach in the forecasting of drug authorization reports [45]. Use of fluorescent proteins in pancreatic beta cells has been

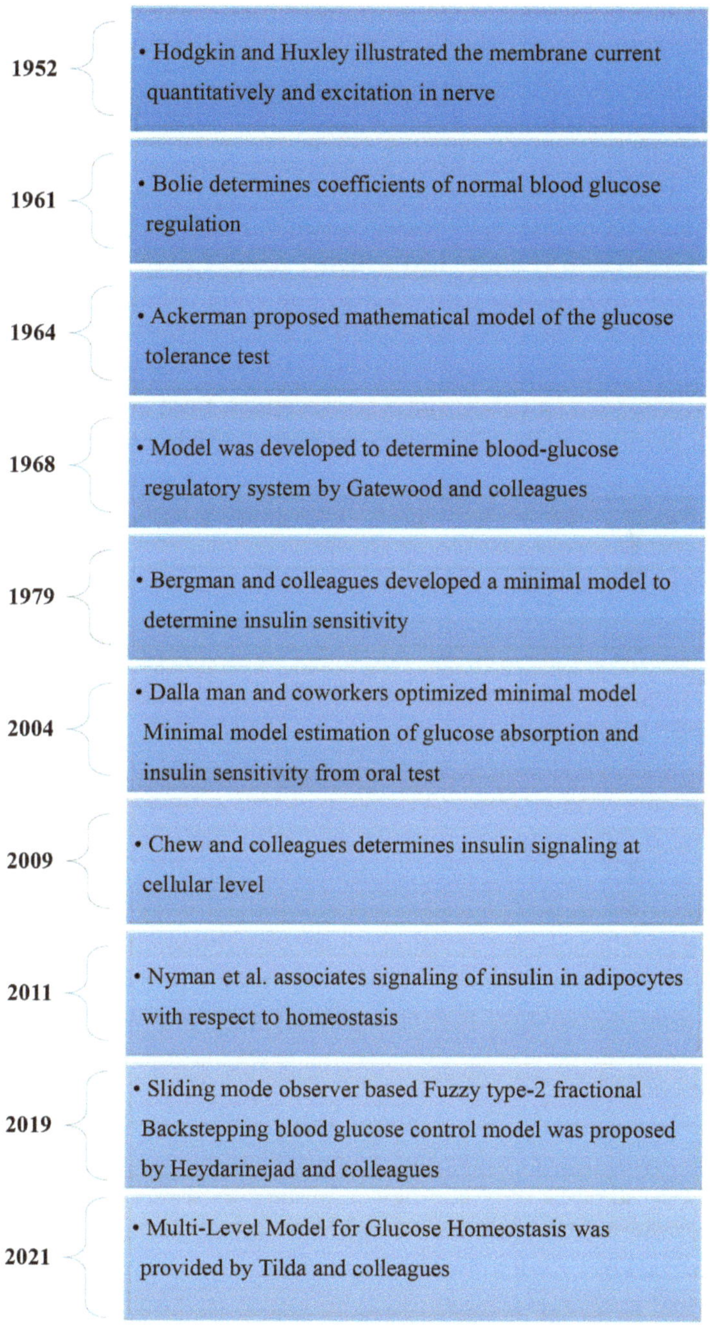

Fig. 3 Different mathematical models used in medicinal research of diabetes mellitus.

investigated for Insulin granule trafficking that are subjected to be secretory granules in recent years that helps to understand the imaging of granules in living cells in real time [46]. To simulate the insulin granules movement in an ideal beta-cell a three-dimensional based model on random walk process was used by Shibasaki et al. [47]. Second-phase response was produced by the introduction of a bias, which involves the granules recruitment to plasma membrane. By supposing that the arbitrarily dispersed granules had a higher density near the plasma membrane, the first phase was generated by the computational model [47].

In the sixties, primary linear models of glucose-insulin homeostasis, by the use of the intravenous glucose tolerance test (IVGTT), have been validated [37,48–50]. However, in the late seventies, Berg man and coworkers developed a model that is called minimal model (MM), which is considered to be the most well known and until now significantly prevalent model used in clinical estimations, for example, to approximate the sensitivity index of insulin [51].

For the oral test, the basic proposed model for the IVGTT was extended as the oral glucose minimal model [52], with the alteration that glucose management in the initial condition does not extensively seem as a bolus dose D in the kinetics equation of glucose [53,54].

A model proposed by Brubaker et al. incorporates numerous factors like the effect of incretins that perform a major action in observed reaction to the orally administrated glucose load [54]. In 1979, a model was proposed for examining and quantifying resistance of insulin euglycemic hyperinsulinemic clamp (EHC) [55]. For the determination of insulin sensitivity, experimentally it is the most widely used model. Model that takes account of detail regarding insulin signaling at cellular level was proposed by Chew and colleagues [56,57]. In this study, two self-determining publications of whole-body glucose homeostasis [58] and insulin signaling [59] are merged in a manner that keeps reliability with the fundamental data at both levels in reaction to glucose.

A model proposed by Nyman et al. that associates signaling of insulin in adipocytes with respect to the homeostasis of whole-body glucose is might be the very suitable methodology published to date (2011) [60]. With respect to the whole-body level to govern glucose homeostasis at the top physiological level, numerous important organs (muscle, pancreas, liver, gastrointestinal tract, and adipose tissue) cooperate by insulin and glucose. In 2019, Heydarinejad and coworkers proposed a sliding mode observer model, which is an enhancement to Bergman minimal model by incorporating estimation of nonmeasurable states variables data generated by glucose monitoring sensor, which plays an important role to prevent failure and control law design [61]. An updated glucose homeostasis multilevel model was provided by Tilda and colleagues, which accurately determines glucose uptake by the different organs quantitatively [62]. For the understanding of the mechanism of the DM development patients are followed for decades. Still physiology-based number of rational, hypotheses can be developed to understand the mechanisms, inferring from the existing experimental limited-time data. Variation of the beta-cell mass in a given individual is of particular interest considering its sensitivity to glucose toxicity, and its likely reaction to therapeutic involvements is among such hypotheses [63] (Fig. 3).

5. Identification of antidiabetic potential target and lead compounds by computational pharmacology

Biological targets or drug targets are the proteins along with some other macromolecules and biological processes linked with a particular disease process [18]. These molecules are addressed to prevent, manage, and finally cure the disease [64]. Nowadays, DM is a common disease experienced all age's people that occurs either insufficient insulin production from the pancreas (T1DM) or the body fails to utilize the insulin that produces (T2DM) [13]. In the biological system, many natural processes and& molecular functions are associated with DM pathogenesis and development that would be suitable drug targets [65]. Distribution of these targets is summarized in Table 1.

To design an appropriate therapeutic drug, the selection of target molecules is crucial. The study of target molecules is a prerequisite for better selection as well as better therapeutic drug design for a particular disease [66,67]. DM has numerous drug targets already mentioned earlier. Some common drug targets and their mechanism are summarized in Table 2.

Although many therapeutic drugs have been introduced in the market in the last few years, effective treatment is still insufficient for DM patients. As DM damages most body parts, it is challenging to manage a DM patient. Many alternative approaches are developed for better insulin action and sufficient secretion of insulin from β-cells. Some orally active lead compounds discovered to control blood sugar level of T2DM that is summarized in Table 3.

Table 1 Commonly studied therapeutic drug targets for drug discovery of diabetes mellitus.

Target	Number of reported targets	Mechanism of action in body	Number of reported targets
Kinases and transferase	7	Protein metabolism	5
G-protein-coupled receptor	5	Other metabolism-related targets	5
Hydrolases and proteases	4	Targets of cytokine	5
Transcriptional factors	4	Signal transduction	4
Interleukin receptor	3	Insulin release	3
Signaling molecule	3	Fatty acid oxidation	2
Oxidoreductase	2	Transport and uptake	2
Transfer carrier protein	2	Dehydrogenase	1
Insulin resistance	2	Growth factor	1
Homeostasis	2	Lipid metabolism	1
Ligase	2	Phosphorylation	1
Tyrosine kinase	1	Transport	2
Serine and/or threonine kinases	2		

Table 2 Common targets and their mechanism.

Target molecules	Mechanism
SGLT2 inhibitors	Inhibit the sodium/glucose cotransporter and manage the blood glucose
GLP agonist	DM drugs that could improve the blood sugar, secretion of insulin, lower secretion of glucagon levels in both alpha and beta cells, and also shakes the weight
DPP-4 inhibitors	FDA-approved DM drugs that suppress incretin, increase insulin production, and decrease the glucagon secretion in both alpha and beta cells
GPR119 agonist	DM drugs that enhance the insulin production in glucose-dependent way and encourage the induction of glucose-dependent insulinotropic peptide and GLP-1
GPR40 and GPR120	GPR40 potentiates insulin secretion and GPR120 encourages GLP-1 and cholecystokinin secretion
DGAT-1 protein	DGAT-1catalyses triglyceride synthesis inhibitors and block the activity and assist in the treatment of DM
11β-HSD1 enzymes	Suppress NADPH-facilitated decline; convert cortisone to cortisol that improves glucose homeostasis in the body
PPAR transcription elements	DM drugs that works for nonesterified fats endorsement and its consumption, also triggered the genes by PPAR elements and shakes the uptake of lipid profile and assist adipogenesis. PON1 activated by PPAR-gamma that releases paraoxonase 1 from the liver

Table 3 Available therapeutics for type 2 diabetes mellitus.

Class	Mechanism	Agents
Oral hypoglycemic		
Sulphonylureas	Stimulate insulin secretion	Glibenclamide
Meglitinides	Stimulate insulin secretion	Repaglinide
Biguanides	Decrease hepatic gluconeogenesis	Metformin
Glucosidase inhibitors	Decrease glucose absorption	Miglitol and Acarbose
DPP4 inhibitors	Prolong GLP-1 action	Gliptins
Thiazolidinediones	Decrease insulin resistance	Pioglitazone
Parenteral hypoglycemic		
Insulin	Glucose utilization	Human insulins
GLP 1 receptor agonist	Stimulate insulin, suppress glucagon	Ezenatide, Liraglutide
Amylin agonist	Slow gastric emptying	Praminitide

These are the most ancient and first medicine used to treat type two DM, which decreases the absorption rate of carbohydrates from GI tract. They are mainly two types (sulfonylureas and nonsulfonylureas). Sulfonylureas stimulate insulin secretion from pancreatic β-cell and also have an action for glucagon inhibition [66,67]. Sulfonylureas (stimulate the pancreatic β-cell) are chlorpropamide, glipizide, glibenclamide (glyburide), tolbutamide, and glimepiride [18]. These agents increase the Ca^{2+} permeability from voltage-gated Ca^{2+} channels and increase the production of insulin from pancreatic β-cell, which have a unique receptor to bind sulfonylurea in its membrane called sulfonylurea receptor (SUR) [66,67]. Insulin secretagogue work on in six possible sites, such as encouragement of β-cell metabolic rate, upsurge of β-cell $[Ca^{2+}]i$ by obstruction of KATP channels, upsurge of $[Ca^{2+}]i$ by achievement at these sites other than KATP channels, promotion of amplification pathways of insulin in β-cells, a significant achievement of β-cell membrane and nuclear receptors [66,67].

Alpha-glucosidase inhibitors are taken orally that inhibit the absorption of glucose in the upper GI tract. Alpha-glucosidase is an enzyme found in the gut membrane that converts starch residue to oligosaccharides and disaccharides, thus releasing glucose in GI tract from upper polysaccharide units [68]. They do not affect blood glucose levels; they maintain hypoglycemia by reducing the absorption of glucose. Inhibition of alpha-glucosidase enzyme reduces or delays the conversion that decreases the absorption as well as acts as a hypoglycemic agent. Mostly used agents are acarbose, voglibose, and miglitol [18]. DPP-4 inhibitors are the most recent agents used to treat DM but are not suitable for initial therapy of T2DM. They inhibit DPP-4 enzyme that involves incretion increment which subsequently increases production of insulin in pancreas and lower the level of glucagon [69,70]. The most common agents are sitagliptin, linagliptin, saxagliptin, alogliptin, vildagliptin, etc. In a recent study, patients with severe renal disease might improve after DPP-4 inhibitors [69,70].

Glucagon-like peptide-1 receptor also known as GLP-1 receptor; agonist of this receptor also known as incretin analog or incretin mimetic [71]. These agents bind with the GLP-1 receptor as an agonist, and they also have action on the pancreas like DPP-4 inhibitors. Currently approved agonists are albiglutide, dulaglutide, exenatide, liraglutide, and lixisenatide. Nowadays, these agonists are appealing as a combinatory therapy with metformin for patients with uncontrollable T2DM [71]. Generally, sodium-glucose transporter-2 inhibitor (SGLT2) is designed to treat T2DM, and they are highly effective in decreasing blood sugar levels, patients with insulin resistance. These membrane proteins reabsorb about 90% of glucose after glomerular filtration of glucose; thus, they inhibit glucose reabsorption and facilitate excretion of glucose through urine as well as decrease blood glucose levels [67,71]. Some recently developed inhibitors are canagliflozin, dapagliflozin, and empagliflozin [67,71]. Peroxisome proliferator-activated receptor-gamma (PPAR-γ) is a nuclear receptor, primarily found in adipose tissue. It has three isoforms. Among them, PPAR-gamma-2 and PPAR-gamma-3 are mainly found in adipose and skeletal tissues and become highly expressive there and promote insulin resistance [72]. Few classes of drugs like thiazolidinedione or other ligands activated the PPAR-γ receptor, which promote insulin sensitivity and helps to endorse the maximum glucose in these muscles [72].

11β-hydroxysteroid dehydrogenase has two isoforms (11β HSD1, 11β HSD2) highly expressed in adipose tissue, liver, and central nervous system [73,74]. For metabolic tissues, 11β HSD1 activates cortisone to form cortisol, which subsequently triggers the glucocorticoid receptors and a few others. In this way, 11β HSD enzyme plays a key role in DM, especially for T2DM [73,74]. The 17β-HSD1 enzyme helps in the interconversion of the following hormones [75].

$$17\beta - \text{estradiol} + \text{NADP}^{+} \rightleftharpoons \text{estrone} + \text{NADPH} + \text{H}^{+}$$

$$\text{testosterone} + \text{NADP}^{+} \rightleftharpoons \text{androstenedione} + \text{NADPH} + \text{H}^{+}$$

This conversion is a characteristic marker for diagnosing the patient with breast cancer and T2DM. Suppression of these enzymes is promising treatment for breast cancer and T2DM prevention [75]. Glutamine: fructose-6-phosphate aminotransferase enzyme (GFAT) is a crucial macromolecule assists the regulation of hexosamine synthesis pathway that involves glucose toxicity and insulin resistance. HPB utilizes only a tiny portion of glucose, and most of them are handled by glycolysis [76]. GFAT has four isoforms (GFAT1, GFAT2, GFAT3, and GFAT4); among them, GFAT1 is mainly expressed in the liver and other fatty tissues, that is why it has an interest as a drug target for DM and obesity [76].

G-protein coupled receptor (GPR), such as GPR120, is a membrane protein articulated in the intestinal tract and adipose tissue and that is triggered by fatty acid. Activated GPR120 stimulates the secretion of GLP-1 and subsequently promotes insulin production from pancreatic cells and declines the level of glucagon production [77,78]. It also has two isoforms:

(1) GPR40: Activated GPR40 stimulates the release of calcium that stimulates insulin release.

(2) GPR119: Activated GPR119 increases the intracellular cAMP level that stimulates GLP1 and insulin secretion.

Targeting the GPR may be a new approach for DM as it stimulates insulin secretion as well as inhibits glucagon secretion [77,78].

Protein tyrosine phosphatase 1B (PTP1B) is an enzyme that regulates tyrosine phosphorylation and regulates many biological processes in the cell system [13]. In a recent study, it is reported that PTP1B is an essential and negative regulator for insulin signaling pathways. Very little data have been reported yet so there is room for this new target to be studied for T2DM and as well as obesity [79]. Glucose transporter type 4 (GLUT4) is involved in insulin regulation and principally expressed in adipose tissue, skeletal, and cardiac muscle that transport glucose molecules across the cell membrane into the muscle and fat cells. Many transporters carry the glucose molecules outward direction and maintain low glucose levels. Likewise, only GLUT4 transports glucose hormone inward in reaction to insulin and plays a crucial role in insulin resistance. For this reason, GLUT4 may be a promising drug target for T2DM. Synthetic molecules are so much toxic as compared to natural products that is why this approach might be novel for targets identification for the treatment of DM [64,67]. Few widely used medicinal plants are as follows *Momordica charantia, Catharanthus roseus, Anacardium occidental, Syzygium cumini, Eucalyptus globulus, and Lupinus albus*, etc. [64,67]. These plants and their chemical products are the significant natural targets for the discovery of therapeutics against DM (Fig. 4).

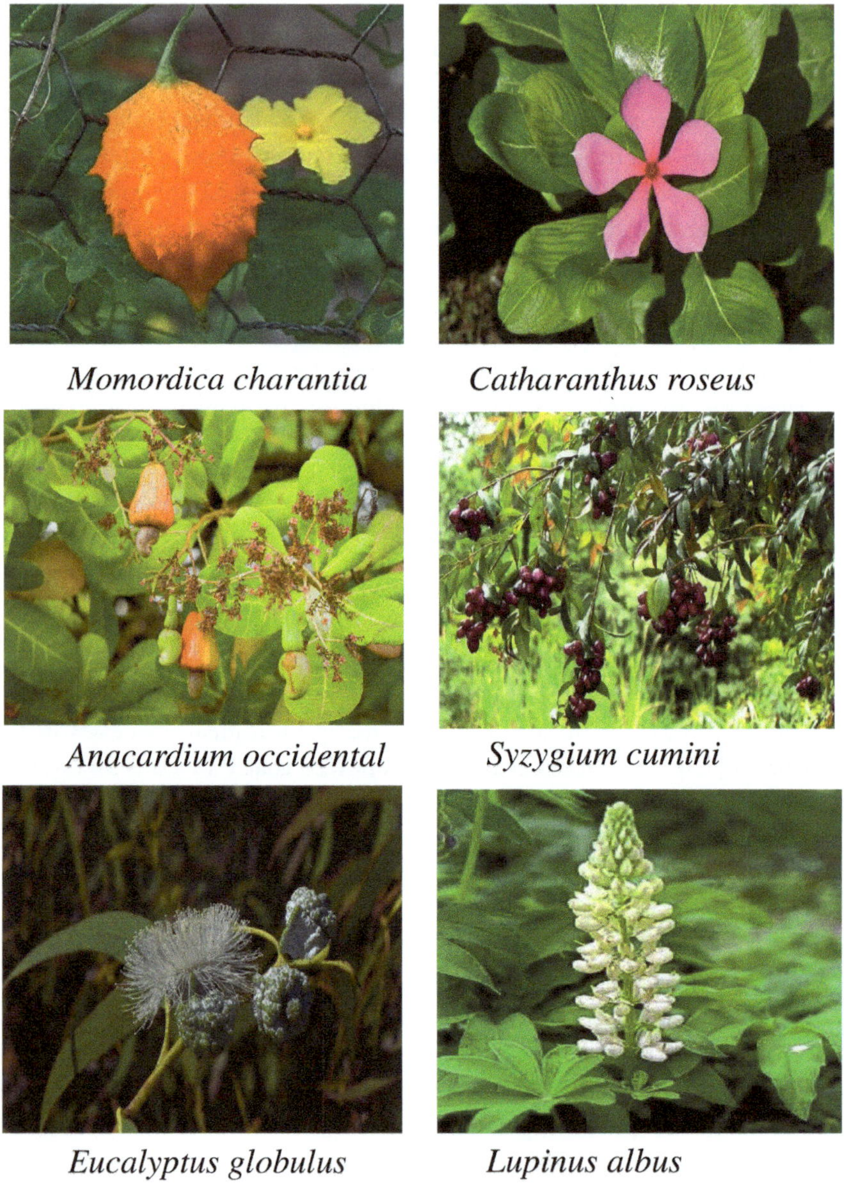

Fig. 4 Natural therapeutic targets for treatment of diabetes mellitus.

6. Investigation of drug-target-disease pharmacological networks

There is a rapidly increasing volume of data available about the chemicals, protein, and disease interactions. This big data available about the disease, drugs, and targets are available separately. Integration of all these data sets to find out appropriate interactions is the need of time for developing new effective drugs [15] [80]. Along with the construction of a drug-target network, other types of networks, such as drug with disease networks, drug with (toxicological aspects) side effect networks, and drugs with molecular fragment networks, have been developed by various researchers [81]. Similar to these categories of graphs are drugs with drug networks. For instance, the use of quantitative structure-activity relationship models to construct drug-drug networks of antiviral drugs and antifungal compounds [82]. The links in these networks connect drug-drug pairs, and the information contained in the link is related to the activity of the drug for different targets [83]. These networks can be used for the following: (1) to find new drug targets; (2) to construct the whole network by inferring missing links from the information of known links; (3) to reposition existing drugs; (4) to conclude possible side effects from the network; (5) to infer potential side effects from network; (6) to design an effective drug combination that can maximize the efficacy of targeting disease; and (7) to find new relationships among disease, treatment, patients, and targets [83] [84]. Drug-target networks and other drug-related networks can be built from the interaction data (Fig. 5). A single or multiple drugs interact with appropriate single or multiple target protein(s); thus, as a result, disease can be modulated. Based upon these steps of drug action, it is clear that not only information on individual biological components (such as drugs, genes, proteins, cell types, and diseases) but also information on the component relationships is essential to understand the whole process [85].

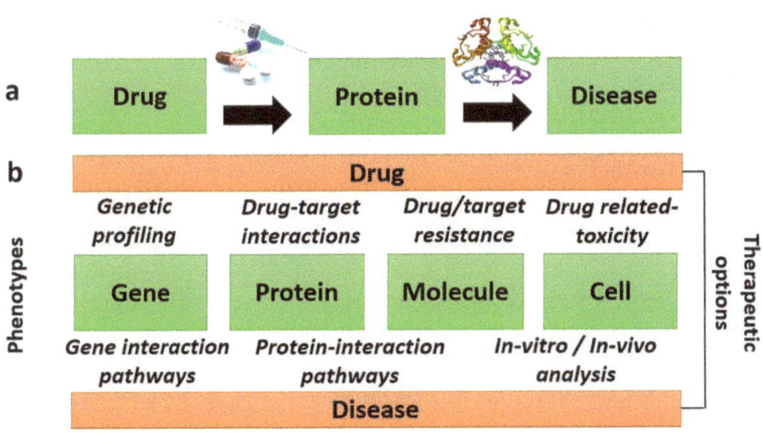

Fig. 5 Relationships among drugs, disease, and phenotypic contexts. The central dogma of drug action (A). The drug-disease relationship with phenotypic context that includes genomic, proteomic, and cellular states (B).

7. Databases to construct drug-target-disease-related networks

With the definition, a network consists of nodes and links. To create drug-related networks, it is necessary to collect information on drugs, genes, protein targets, and diseases as nodes and their interactions as links [86]. There are freely available databases for retrieval of three-dimensional structural information of chemicals/drugs, and protein targets, also have information for genes and their interactions in human signaling pathways (Table 4).

Table 4 Databases for retrievals of chemicals/drugs, protein target, genome and their interactions information.

Database	Description	Web-Link
DrugBank	Contains 7759 drugs and their related 15199 protein-target interaction information	https://go.drugbank.com/
PubChem	Contains chemical structures, literature and their activities related information's	https://pubchem.ncbi.nlm.nih.gov/
KEGG Ligand	Have information of compounds/ligand structures, biopolymers, and their reactions with respect to biological system	https://www.genome.jp/kegg/compound/
ChEMBL	Contains functional information of protein, chemicals, and ADMET-related properties for drug-like compounds. Also contains 5.4 million bioactive measurements for the novel drug discovery and development	https://www.ebi.ac.uk/chembl/
Integrity	Contains drugs and protein target information with associated diseases and clinical phase information's of drugs	https://www.drugpatentwatch.com/index.php?utm_source=thomson-pharmacom
PDB	Contains millions of three-dimensional structures of protein/receptors, nucleic acid and drugs interactions information	https://www.rcsb.org/
UniProtKB/Swiss-Prot	Contains protein sequence, structures, and its functions	https://www.expasy.org/resources/uniprotkb-swiss-prot

Table 4 Databases for retrievals of chemicals/drugs, protein target, genome and their interactions information—cont'd

Database	Description	Web-Link
Therapeutic Target Database (TTD)	Contains significant macromolecules, receptors, proteins and nucleic acid target, disease, pathways, and drug data. Also contains 1755 biomarkers for 365 different diseases situations and 210 chemical scaffolds for the date of 714 drugs	http://db.idrblab.net/ttd/
TDR targets database	Contains pathogen genomes information', chemical compounds and protein target structures and bioactivities information	https://tdrtargets.org/
TargetDB/ Protein Structure Initiative (PSI)	Target registration and identification of chemical structures	http://targetdb.pdb.org/
SuperTarget	Contain information of drug targets, metabolization, and pathways	http://bioinf-apache.charite.de/supertarget_v2/
Target protein database (TPDB)	Contains extensive information of protein target interactions with reactive metabolites and details of toxicity information	http://tpdb.medchem.ku.edu/tpdb.html
Drug-induced toxicity-related proteins (DITOP)	Contains information of protein that is significant to mediate the adverse drug reactions and drug resistance creating toxicity by interacting drugs. 529 drugs, and 418 toxicity measurements data is stored	http://bioinf.xmu.edu.cn/databases/ADR/index.html.
STITCH	Contains predicted molecular interactions with the evidence of experimental data and literature	http://stitch.embl.de/
MATADOR	Contain information of chemical-target interaction models	http://matador.embl.de
BindingDB	Contains experimentally identified 489,416 chemical ligands and 7020 associated target proteins information	http://www.bindingdb.org/bind

8. Databases for diseases drugs, phenotypes, and proteins

Information for chemical compounds can be obtained from various free online sources. The representative databases such as PubChem [87], Drug Bank [88], and Protein Databank [89] are widely significant for the CADD studies. Because these PubChem and Drug Bank are the largest information sources having chemical structures and their biological activities [87] [88]. Molecular drug targets/receptors are typically proteins whose activities are modulated by specific chemicals or drugs. The Protein Data Bank (PDB) [89] and the SWISS-PROT [90] are the most widely used databases for three-dimensional structures and sequences of protein molecules, respectively. Table 4 has enlisted different important databases that contain the chemical compounds and proteins information.

9. Databases for the interactions among drugs, proteins, and diseases

In a drug-target network, biological components (i.e., drugs, proteins, genes, and diseases) are represented by nodes; it is necessary to link nodes by edges based on the relationships between them [91]. Several databases offer information on these interactions on a large scale. DrugBank [88] and therapeutic target database (TTD) [92] provide a list of drugs targeting proteins with information on related diseases. SuperTarget and Matador provide a list of target proteins found by searching the database with the information of a query drug (i.e., adverse drug effect and structural similarity) [93] [94]. STITCH is a freely available database to discover known and estimated interactions of drugs/compounds with macromolecules such as proteins and is popular for the study of interaction networks and CSP [95].

10. Computational system pharmacological analysis of drug and selected target networks

10.1 Drug target network

Global mapping of pharmacological entitles by integrating several sources of medicinal chemistry structure-activity relationship data has been performed [17]. They built a CSP-interaction network representing the correlation between protein molecules in chemical space by using binding data from Pfizer. In addition, they built a human disease network, from OMIM-based complaints with diseased gene relatives [83].

10.2 Drug-ADR target networks

Campillos et al. developed an identifier of drug targets using toxicological affect comparison [96]. Xie et al. applied their computational tool of identification of receptor and chemical entities interactions profiles to build an off-target binding network of CETP inhibitors [97].

10.3 Disease and treatment networks

Instead of focusing on the target and off-target proteins, many researchers have attempted to build networks related to drugs and treatment. Yildirim et al. also built a human disease network produced from OMIM-based complaints with the disease gene relatives [98].

11. Network pharmacology (NP) for understanding mechanism of diabetes

DM offers number of other chronic ailments and severe complications of body organs [18]. NPS method is introduced for DM research that uses multidrugs, target proteins molecules, and disease information for generation of beneficial networks, so that infer the information of drug and target and disease networks [98]. NP was immensely studied previously for the analysis of bioactive secondary metabolites involved in the control of DM associated with multiple mechanisms, multiple macrotargets, and subordinates of the toxicological effects [16].

NP is functional for the study of several complicated diseases mechanisms, such as Alzheimer's disease, CVDs, cardiocerebral ischemic diseases, DM, pancreatitis, obesity, cancer, gout, and other metabolic syndrome [99] [100]. For DM treatment, NP has been extensively applied in the mechanism-based analysis [67]. Scientists composed of 287 accessible chemical ingredients, with 42 of them originating in Ge-Gen, 57 of them originating in Huang-Qin, 22 of them originate in Huang-Lian, and 166 of them originating in Gan-Cao. NP examination has explained the associations among natural metabolites and their biological activities. NP method also subsidized to improve the understanding of mechanisms of action of selected GQD formula. 4-Hydroxymephenytoin, a novel secondary metabolite from a herb known as "*Puerariae Lobatae radix*" (Ge-Gen), could upsurge the production of insulin levels and help to maintain insulin resistance [101]. NP approach had effectively overtaken the traditional approaches of herbal drugs identification for DM, and the bioactive compounds with multiple medicinal properties can be discovered and mechanisms of multiple targets can be interpreted [16,102].

Most favorites drink after water is black and green tea extracted from the plant "*Camellia sinensis L.*" has been approved as an anti-DM therapeutic in the literature of folk medicine [103]. Tea polyphenols are the important ingredients of tea, mainly comprising of active metabolites. Study of NP method on tea polyphenols identified function in the three significant pathways, (1) p53 network of genes, (2) neurotrophin related, and (3) insulin signaling pathway and also linked with 147 other networks of genes and established a DM-related NP by mixing these three pathways [104].

Potential inhibitors obtained from Chinese medicine are beneficial T2DM targets, an integrated approach has been generated that combined CADD methods, such as molecular docking (protein-ligand interaction analysis), pharmacophore mapping, and model generation, and created important drug and target interaction network for the advanced anti-DM study. Totally, 2479 nonduplicated chemicals from thirty-two Chinese herbal extracts of fifty-two conventional Chinese medicine formulas were searched from two public databases. The Bayesian classifiers with acceptable refinement potential for 15 molecular targets were engaged for the virtual screening of 2479 chemicals. The outcomes presented that protein-ligand interaction and pharmacophore mapped entities could give acceptable results for most frequently used anti-DM molecular targets and that showed some herbal constituents could bind with T2DM-related molecular targets, hence few constituents reassured T2DM with respect to antioxidant potential or additional medicinal bioactivities [105].

Male Zucker diabetic fatty rats were treated by JCU, an important Chinese medicine that consists of three herbs and also berberine. The report presented that JCU has the ability to manage insulin production and insulin resistance, normalize important organs and skeletal muscles, and also manage liver-related enzyme [106]. For the processing of miRNA level, protein level, and mRNA level, the report clarified mechanisms of JCU, modifying the complicated cytokines in the connected NP results and enlightening the value of cell survival, upgrading the glucose uptake, and upgrading insulin production and sensitivity [16] [106]. In detail, CSP methods were validated and presented that it is of great significance in multi-ingredient study based on Chinese medicine for the identification of drugs for DM.

References

[1] J. Kazibwe, P.B. Tran, K.S. Annerstedt, The household financial burden of non-communicable diseases in low-and middle-income countries: a systematic review, Health Res. Policy Syst. 19 (1) (2021) 1–15.

[2] A. Afshin, P.J. Sur, K.A. Fay, L. Cornaby, G. Ferrara, J.S. Salama, et al., Health effects of dietary risks in 195 countries, 1990–2017: a systematic analysis for the Global Burden of Disease Study 2017, Lancet 393 (10184) (2019) 1958–1972.
[3] A.R.M. Hazaveh, M.H. Panahi, E. Yousefi, S. Yarahmdi, Some facts on the diabetes surveillance in rural regions of Iran, Iran. J. Public Health 47 (12) (2018) 1967–1968.
[4] World Health Organization, WHO Global Report on Traditional and Complementary Medicine 2019, World Health Organization, 2019.
[5] M.C. Nwadiugwu, D.R. Bastola, C. Haas, D. Russell, Identifying glycemic variability in diabetes patient cohorts and evaluating disease outcomes, J. Clin. Med. 10 (7) (2021) 1477.
[6] T. Tönnies, W. Rathmann, A. Hoyer, R. Brinks, O. Kuss, Quantifying the underestimation of projected global diabetes prevalence by the International Diabetes Federation (IDF) Diabetes Atlas, BMJ Open Diabetes Res. Care 9 (1) (2021), e002122.
[7] World Health Organization, et al., Primary Health Care on the Road to Universal Health Coverage: 2019 Global Monitoring Report, 2021.
[8] L. Wang, X. Li, Z. Wang, M.P. Bancks, M.R. Carnethon, P. Greenland, et al., Trends in prevalence of diabetes and control of risk factors in diabetes among US adults, 1999-2018, JAMA 326 (8) (2021) 704–716.
[9] A.D. Association, 10. Cardiovascular disease and risk management: Standards of Medical Care in Diabetes—2021, Diabetes Care 44 (Suppl_1) (2021) S125–S150.
[10] R.M. Carey, P.K. Whelton, Prevention, detection, evaluation, and management of high blood pressure in adults: synopsis of the 2017 American College of Cardiology/American Heart Association Hypertension Guideline, Ann. Intern. Med. 168 (5) (2018) 351–358.
[11] A. Zanchetti, G. Grassi, G. Mancia, When should antihypertensive drug treatment be initiated and to what levels should systolic blood pressure be lowered? A critical reappraisal, J. Hypertens. 27 (5) (2009) 923–934.
[12] A. Talevi, Multi-target pharmacology: possibilities and limitations of the "skeleton key approach" from a medicinal chemist perspective, Front. Pharmacol. 6 (2015) 205.
[13] S. Bibi, K. Sakata, An integrated computational approach for plant-based protein tyrosine phosphatase non-receptor type 1 inhibitors, Curr. Comput. Aided Drug Des. 13 (4) (2017) 319–335.
[14] S. Bibi, M.M. Hasan, Y.-B. Wang, S.P. Papadakos, H. Yu, Cordycepin as a promising inhibitor of SARS-CoV-2 RNA dependent RNA polymerase (RdRp), Curr. Med. Chem. 29 (2021).
[15] L. Zhao, H.L. Ciallella, L.M. Aleksunes, H. Zhu, Advancing computer-aided drug discovery (CADD) by big data and data-driven machine learning modeling, Drug Discov. Today 25 (2020).
[16] W. Li, G. Yuan, Y. Pan, C. Wang, H. Chen, Network pharmacology studies on the bioactive compounds and action mechanisms of natural products for the treatment of diabetes mellitus: a review, Front. Pharmacol. 8 (2017) 74.
[17] G.V. Paolini, R.H.B. Shapland, W.P. van Hoorn, J.S. Mason, A.L. Hopkins, Global mapping of pharmacological space, Nat. Biotechnol. 24 (7) (2006) 805–815.
[18] S. Bibi, K. Sakata, Current status of computer-aided drug design for type 2 diabetes, Curr. Comput. Aided Drug Des. 12 (2) (2016) 167–177.
[19] D.E. Clark, What has computer-aided molecular design ever done for drug discovery? Expert Opin. Drug Discovery 1 (2) (2006) 103–110.
[20] A. Anighoro, J. Bajorath, G. Rastelli, Polypharmacology: challenges and opportunities in drug discovery: miniperspective, J. Med. Chem. 57 (19) (2014) 7874–7887.
[21] J.A. DiMasi, H.G. Grabowski, R.W. Hansen, Innovation in the pharmaceutical industry: new estimates of R&D costs, J. Health Econ. 47 (2016) 20–33.

[22] S.M. Paul, D.S. Mytelka, C.T. Dunwiddie, C.C. Persinger, B.H. Munos, S.R. Lindborg, et al., How to improve R&D productivity: the pharmaceutical industry's grand challenge, Nat. Rev. Drug Discov. 9 (3) (2010) 203–214.
[23] M.R. Hurle, L. Yang, Q. Xie, D.K. Rajpal, P. Sanseau, P. Agarwal, Computational drug repositioning: from data to therapeutics, Clin. Pharmacol. Ther. 93 (4) (2013) 335–341.
[24] S.R. Martha, G. Panda, M. Patri, Energy-based virtual screening of drugs documented for schizophrenia against DRD2 and HTR2A, Int. J. Comput. Vis. Robot. 12 (1) (2022) 53–65.
[25] A.C. Kaushik, S. Sahi, D.-Q. Wei, Computational methods for structure-based drug design through system biology, in: Computational Methods for Estimating the Kinetic Parameters of Biological Systems, Springer, 2022, pp. 161–174.
[26] T.T. Talele, S.A. Khedkar, A.C. Rigby, Successful applications of computer aided drug discovery: moving drugs from concept to the clinic, Curr. Top. Med. Chem. 10 (1) (2010) 127–141.
[27] T.N. Doman, S.L. McGovern, B.J. Witherbee, T.P. Kasten, R. Kurumbail, W.C. Stallings, et al., Molecular docking and high-throughput screening for novel inhibitors of protein tyrosine phosphatase-1B, J. Med. Chem. 45 (11) (2002) 2213–2221.
[28] P.C. Wyss, P. Gerber, P.G. Hartman, C. Hubschwerlen, H. Locher, H.-P. Marty, et al., Novel dihydrofolate reductase inhibitors. Structure-based versus diversity-based library design and high-throughput synthesis and screening, J. Med. Chem. 46 (12) (2003) 2304–2312.
[29] S.J. Trenfield, A. Awad, L.E. McCoubrey, M. Elbadawi, A. Goyanes, S. Gaisford, et al., Advancing pharmacy and healthcare with virtual digital technologies, Adv. Drug Deliv. Rev. 114098 (2022).
[30] S. Verma, R.K. Pathak, Discovery and optimization of lead molecules in drug designing, in: Bioinformatics, Elsevier, 2022, pp. 253–267.
[31] B. Shaker, S. Ahmad, J. Lee, C. Jung, D. Na, In silico methods and tools for drug discovery, Comput. Biol. Med. 137 (2021), 104851.
[32] N. Jabalia, A. Kumar, V. Kumar, R. Rani, In silico approach in drug design and drug discovery: an update, in: Innovations and Implementations of Computer Aided Drug Discovery Strategies in Rational Drug Design, Springer, 2021, pp. 245–271.
[33] J. Greer, J.W. Erickson, J.J. Baldwin, M.D. Varney, Application of the three-dimensional structures of protein target molecules in structure-based drug design, J. Med. Chem. 37 (8) (1994) 1035–1054.
[34] N. Kamaly, Z. Xiao, P.M. Valencia, A.F. Radovic-Moreno, O.C. Farokhzad, Targeted polymeric therapeutic nanoparticles: design, development and clinical translation, Chem. Soc. Rev. 41 (7) (2012) 2971–3010.
[35] E. Proschak, H. Stark, D. Merk, Polypharmacology by design: a medicinal chemist's perspective on multitargeting compounds, J. Med. Chem. 62 (2) (2018) 420–444.
[36] A. Tura, E. Muscelli, A. Gastaldelli, E. Ferrannini, A. Mari, Altered pattern of the incretin effect as assessed by modelling in individuals with glucose tolerance ranging from normal to diabetic, Diabetologia 57 (6) (2014) 1199–1203.
[37] P.L. Brubaker, E.L. Ohayon, L.M. D'Alessandro, K.H. Norwich, A mathematical model of the oral glucose tolerance test illustrating the effects of the incretins, Ann. Biomed. Eng. 35 (7) (2007) 1286–1300.
[38] A.L. Hodgkin, A.F. Huxley, A quantitative description of membrane current and its application to conduction and excitation in nerve, J. Physiol. 117 (4) (1952) 500–544.
[39] B.P. Kovatchev, M.D. Breton, C. Dalla Man, C. Cobelli, In silico model and computer simulation environment approximating the human glucose/insulin utilization, Food Drug Adm. Master File MAF. 1521 (2008) 338–346.

[40] C.D. Man, F. Micheletto, D. Lv, M. Breton, B. Kovatchev, C. Cobelli, The UVA/PADOVA type 1 diabetes simulator: new features, J. Diabetes Sci. Technol. 8 (1) (2014) 26–34.
[41] C. Brännmark, E. Nyman, S. Fagerholm, L. Bergenholm, E.-M. Ekstrand, G. Cedersund, et al., Insulin signaling in type 2 diabetes: experimental and modeling analyses reveal mechanisms of insulin resistance in human adipocytes, J. Biol. Chem. 288 (14) (2013) 9867–9880.
[42] E. Nyman, M.R. Rajan, S. Fagerholm, C. Brännmark, G. Cedersund, P. Strålfors, A single mechanism can explain network-wide insulin resistance in adipocytes from obese patients with type 2 diabetes, J. Biol. Chem. 289 (48) (2014) 33215–33230.
[43] I. Ajmera, M. Swat, C. Laibe, N. Le Novere, V. Chelliah, The impact of mathematical modeling on the understanding of diabetes and related complications, CPT Pharmacometrics Syst. Pharmacol. 2 (7) (2013) 1–14.
[44] G. Cedersund, P. Strålfors, Putting the pieces together in diabetes research: towards a hierarchical model of whole-body glucose homeostasis, Eur. J. Pharm. Sci. 36 (1) (2009) 91–104.
[45] P.H. der Graaf, N. Benson, Systems pharmacology: bridging systems biology and pharmacokinetics-pharmacodynamics (PKPD) in drug discovery and development, Pharm. Res. 28 (7) (2011) 1460–1464.
[46] P. Rorsman, E. Renström, Insulin granule dynamics in pancreatic beta cells, Diabetologia 46 (8) (2003) 1029–1045.
[47] T. Shibasaki, H. Takahashi, T. Miki, Y. Sunaga, K. Matsumura, M. Yamanaka, et al., Essential role of Epac2/Rap1 signaling in regulation of insulin granule dynamics by cAMP, Proc. Natl. Acad. Sci. 104 (49) (2007) 19333–19338.
[48] V.W. Bolie, Coefficients of normal blood glucose regulation, J. Appl. Physiol. 16 (5) (1961) 783–788.
[49] E. Ackerman, L.C. Gatewood, J.W. Rosevear, G.D. Molnar, Model studies of blood-glucose regulation, Bull. Math. Biophys. 27 (1) (1965) 21–37.
[50] L.C. Gatewood, E. Ackerman, J.W. Rosevear, G.D. Molnar, T.W. Burns, Tests of a mathematical model of the blood-glucose regulatory system, Comput. Biomed. Res. 2 (1) (1968) 1–14.
[51] R.N. Bergman, Y.Z. Ider, C.R. Bowden, C. Cobelli, Quantitative estimation of insulin sensitivity, Am. J. Physiol. Metab. 236 (6) (1979) E667.
[52] A. Caumo, R.N. Bergman, C. Cobelli, Insulin sensitivity from meal tolerance tests in normal subjects: a minimal model index, J. Clin. Endocrinol. Metab. 85 (11) (2000) 4396–4402.
[53] C. Della Man, A. Caumo, C. Cobelli, The oral glucose minimal model: estimation of insulin sensitivity from a meal test, IEEE Trans. Biomed. Eng. 49 (5) (2002) 419–429.
[54] C. Dalla Man, A. Caumo, R. Basu, R. Rizza, G. Toffolo, C. Cobelli, Minimal model estimation of glucose absorption and insulin sensitivity from oral test: validation with a tracer method, Am. J. Physiol. Metab. 287 (4) (2004) E637–E643.
[55] R.A. DeFronzo, J.D. Tobin, R. Andres, Glucose clamp technique: a method for quantifying insulin secretion and resistance, Am. J. Physiol. Metab. 237 (3) (1979) E214.
[56] Y.H. Chew, Y.L. Shia, C.T. Lee, F.A.A. Majid, L.S. Chua, M.R. Sarmidi, et al., Modeling of oscillatory bursting activity of pancreatic beta-cells under regulated glucose stimulation, Mol. Cell. Endocrinol. 307 (1–2) (2009) 57–67.
[57] Y.H. Chew, Y.L. Shia, C.T. Lee, F.A.A. Majid, L.S. Chua, M.R. Sarmidi, et al., Modeling of glucose regulation and insulin-signaling pathways, Mol. Cell. Endocrinol. 303 (1–2) (2009) 13–24.
[58] C. Cobelli, A. Mari, Validation of mathematical models of complex endocrine-metabolic systems. A case study on a model of glucose regulation, Med. Biol. Eng. Comput. 21 (4) (1983) 390–399.

[59] A.R. Sedaghat, A. Sherman, M.J. Quon, A mathematical model of metabolic insulin signaling pathways, Am. J. Physiol. Metab. 283 (5) (2002) E1084–E1101.
[60] E. Nyman, C. Brännmark, R. Palmér, J. Brugård, F.H. Nyström, P. Strålfors, et al., A hierarchical whole-body modeling approach elucidates the link between in vitro insulin signaling and in vivo glucose homeostasis, J. Biol. Chem. 286 (29) (2011) 26028–26041.
[61] H. Heydarinejad, H. Delavari, D. Baleanu, Fuzzy type-2 fractional backstepping blood glucose control based on sliding mode observer, Int. J. Dyn. Control 7 (1) (2019) 341–354.
[62] T. Herrgårdh, H. Li, E. Nyman, G. Cedersund, An updated organ-based multi-level model for glucose homeostasis: organ distributions, timing, and impact of blood flow, Front. Physiol. 12 (2021).
[63] P. Palumbo, S. Ditlevsen, A. Bertuzzi, A. De Gaetano, Mathematical modeling of the glucose—insulin system: a review, Math. Biosci. 244 (2) (2013) 69–81.
[64] R.J. Marles, N.R. Farnsworth, Antidiabetic plants and their active constituents, Phytomedicine 2 (2) (1995) 137–189.
[65] P.D. Patil, et al., Past and current perspective on new therapeutic targets for Type-II diabetes, Drug Des. Devel. Ther. 11 (2017).
[66] N.D.T. Nguyen, L.T. Le, Targeted proteins for diabetes drug design, Adv. Nat. Sci. Nanosci. Nanotechnol. 3 (1) (2012), 013001.
[67] N. Tiwari, et al., Therapeutic targets for diabetes mellitus: an update, Clin. Pharmacol. Biopharm. 3 (1) (2014).
[68] L. He, alpha-Glucosidase inhibitors, Endocrinol. Metab. Clin. N. Am. 26 (3) (1997) 539–551.
[69] D.J. Drucker, M.A. Nauck, The incretin system: glucagon-like peptide-1 receptor agonists and dipeptidyl peptidase-4 inhibitors in type 2 diabetes, Lancet (London, England) 368 (9548) (2006) 1696–1705.
[70] M. Chen, Y. Liu, J. Jin, Q. He, The efficacy and safety of dipeptidyl peptidase-4 inhibitors for treatment of type 2 diabetes mellitus patients with severe renal impairment: a meta-analysis, Ren. Fail. 38 (4) (2016) 581–587.
[71] M.E. Okur, I.D. Karantas, P.I. Siafaka, Diabetes mellitus: a review on pathophysiology, current status of oral medication and future perspect, Acta Pharm. Sci. 55 (2017).
[72] K.S. Park, T.P. Ciaraldi, L. Abrams-Carter, S. Mudaliar, S.E. Nikoulina, R.R. Henry, PPAR-gamma gene expression is elevated in skeletal muscle of obese and type II diabetic subjects, Diabetes 46 (7) (1997) 1230–1234.
[73] R.C. Andrews, B.R. Walker, Glucocorticoids and insulin resistance: old hormones, new targets, Clin. Sci. (Lond.) 96 (5) (1999) 513–523.
[74] B. Davani, N. Portwood, G. Bryzgalova, et al., Aged transgenic mice with increased glucocorticoid sensitivity in pancreatic beta-cells develop diabetes, Diabetes 53 (Suppl 1) (2004).
[75] T. Saloniemi, H. Jokela, L. Strauss, P. Pakarinen, M. Poutanen, The diversity of sex steroid action: novel functions of hydroxysteroid (17β) dehydrogenases as revealed by genetically modified mouse models, J. Endocrinol. 212 (1) (2012) 27–40.
[76] K.Y. Trinh, R.M. O'Doherty, P. Anderson, A.J. Lange, C.B. Newgard, Perturbation of fuel homeostasis caused by overexpression of the glucose-6-phosphatase catalytic subunit in liver of normal rats, J. Biol. Chem. 273 (47) (1998) 31615–31620.
[77] M. Stumvoll, B.J. Goldstein, T.W. van Haeften, Type 2 diabetes: principles of pathogenesis and therapy, Lancet 365 (9467) (2005) 1333–1346.
[78] S. Ineedi, A.D. Kandasamy, A. Veeranjaneyulu, V. Kumar, G-protein coupled receptors for free fatty acids as novel targets for type 2 diabetes, Pharmacologyonline 2 (2009) 17–28.

[79] K. Shravanti, P.K. Kumar, M.B. Raju, I. Madhusudhanareddy, G. Atyam, A review on structure based drug design of protein tyrosine phosphatase 1B inhibitors for target for obesity and Type 2 diabetes mellitus, J. Pharm. Res. 3 (2010) 2939–2940.
[80] V. Gligorijević, N. Malod-Dognin, N. Pržulj, Integrative methods for analyzing big data in precision medicine, Proteomics 16 (5) (2016) 741–758.
[81] X. Zhao, L. Chen, Z.-H. Guo, T. Liu, Predicting drug side effects with compact integration of heterogeneous networks, Curr. Bioinforma. 14 (8) (2019) 709–720.
[82] P. Polishchuk, Interpretation of quantitative structure-activity relationship models: past, present, and future, J. Chem. Inf. Model. 57 (11) (2017) 2618–2639.
[83] S. Lee, K. Park, D. Kim, Building a drug-target network and its applications, Expert Opin. Drug Discovery 4 (11) (2009) 1177–1189.
[84] M.A. Yildirim, K.-I. Goh, M.E. Cusick, A.-L. Barabási, M. Vidal, Drug-target network, Nat. Biotechnol. 25 (10) (2007) 1119–1126.
[85] F. Cheng, C. Liu, J. Jiang, W. Lu, W. Li, G. Liu, et al., Prediction of drug-target interactions and drug repositioning via network-based inference, PLoS Comput. Biol. 8 (5) (2012), e1002503.
[86] Y. Luo, X. Zhao, J. Zhou, J. Yang, Y. Zhang, W. Kuang, et al., A network integration approach for drug-target interaction prediction and computational drug repositioning from heterogeneous information, Nat. Commun. 8 (1) (2017) 1–13.
[87] S. Kim, P.A. Thiessen, E.E. Bolton, J. Chen, G. Fu, A. Gindulyte, et al., PubChem substance and compound databases, Nucleic Acids Res. 44 (D1) (2016) D1202–D1213.
[88] D.S. Wishart, C. Knox, A.C. Guo, D. Cheng, S. Shrivastava, D. Tzur, et al., DrugBank: a knowledgebase for drugs, drug actions and drug targets, Nucleic Acids Res. 36 (Suppl_1) (2008) D901–D906.
[89] Protein Data Bank. 1971.
[90] E. Boutet, D. Lieberherr, M. Tognolli, M. Schneider, A. Bairoch, Uniprotkb/swiss-prot, in: Plant Bioinformatics, Springer, 2007, pp. 89–112.
[91] I. Lee, H. Nam, Identification of drug-target interaction by a random walk with restart method on an interactome network, BMC Bioinform. 19 (8) (2018) 9–18.
[92] X. Chen, Z.L. Ji, Y.Z. Chen, TTD: therapeutic target database, Nucleic Acids Res. 30 (1) (2002) 412–415.
[93] S. Günther, M. Kuhn, M. Dunkel, M. Campillos, C. Senger, E. Petsalaki, et al., SuperTarget and Matador: resources for exploring drug-target relationships, Nucleic Acids Res. 36 (Suppl_1) (2007) D919–D922.
[94] J.-Y. Shi, S.-M. Yiu, Y. Li, H.C.M. Leung, F.Y.L. Chin, Predicting drug-target interaction for new drugs using enhanced similarity measures and super-target clustering, Methods 83 (2015) 98–104.
[95] M. Kuhn, C. von Mering, M. Campillos, L.J. Jensen, P. Bork, STITCH: interaction networks of chemicals and proteins, Nucleic Acids Res. 36 (Suppl_1) (2007) D684–D688.
[96] M. Campillos, M. Kuhn, A.-C. Gavin, L.J. Jensen, P. Bork, Drug target identification using side-effect similarity, Science (80) 321 (5886) (2008) 263–266.
[97] L. Xie, J. Li, L. Xie, P.E. Bourne, Drug discovery using chemical systems biology: identification of the protein-ligand binding network to explain the side effects of CETP inhibitors, PLoS Comput. Biol. 5 (5) (2009), e1000387.
[98] P. Csermely, V. Agoston, S. Pongor, The efficiency of multi-target drugs: the network approach might help drug design, Trends Pharmacol. Sci. 26 (4) (2005) 178–182.
[99] F. Xie, J. Gu, Computational methods and applications for quantitative systems pharmacology, Quant. Biol. 7 (1) (2019) 3–16.
[100] J. Gu, Y. Gui, L. Chen, G. Yuan, H.-Z. Lu, X. Xu, Use of natural products as chemical library for drug discovery and network pharmacology, PLoS One 8 (4) (2013), e62839.

[101] H. Li, L. Zhao, B. Zhang, Y. Jiang, X. Wang, Y. Guo, et al., A network pharmacology approach to determine active compounds and action mechanisms of ge-gen-qin-lian decoction for treatment of type 2 diabetes, Evid. Based Complement Alternat. Med. 2014 (2014).
[102] G. Wang, L. Zeng, Q. Huang, Z. Lu, R. Sui, D. Liu, et al., Exploring the molecular mechanism of Liuwei Dihuang pills for treating diabetic nephropathy by combined network pharmacology and molecular docking, Evid. Based Complement. Alternat. Med. 2021 (2021).
[103] Q. Han, Q. Yu, J. Shi, C. Xiong, Z. Ling, P. He, Molecular characterization and hypoglycemic activity of a novel water-soluble polysaccharide from tea (Camellia sinensis) flower, Carbohydr. Polym. 86 (2) (2011) 797–805.
[104] H. Chen, M. Zhang, Z. Qu, B. Xie, Compositional analysis and preliminary toxicological evaluation of a tea polysaccharide conjugate, J. Agric. Food Chem. 55 (6) (2007) 2256–2260.
[105] S. Tian, Y. Li, D. Li, X. Xu, J. Wang, Q. Zhang, et al., Modeling compound—target interaction network of traditional chinese medicines for Type II diabetes mellitus: insight for polypharmacology and drug design, J. Chem. Inf. Model. 53 (7) (2013) 1787–1803.
[106] H.-L. Zhao, Y. Sui, C.-F. Qiao, K.Y. Yip, R.K.K. Leung, S.K.W. Tsui, et al., Sustained antidiabetic effects of a berberine-containing Chinese herbal medicine through regulation of hepatic gene expression, Diabetes 61 (4) (2012) 933–943.

CHAPTER 11

Computer-aided drug designing illuminate polypharmacology of natural products against multiple estrogen receptor

Shafi Ullah Khan[a,b], Ashraf Ullah Khan[b,c], Mohammad Amjad Kamal[d,e,f,g,h], and Thet Thet Htar[i]

[a]Product & Process Innovation Department, Qarshi Brands (Pvt) Ltd, Hattar Industrial Estate, Haripur, Pakistan
[b]Faculty of Pharmaceutical Sciences, Abasyn University Peshawar, Peshawar, Pakistan
[c]Pharmacological Sciences Research Lab, Department of Pharmacy, Faculty of Biological Sciences, Quaid-I-Azam University, Islamabad, Pakistan
[d]Institutes for Systems Genetics, Frontiers Science Center for Disease-related Molecular Network, West China Hospital, Sichuan University, China
[e]King Fahd Medical Research Center, King Abdulaziz University, Jeddah, Saudi Arabia
[f]Department of Pharmacy, Faculty of Allied Health Sciences, Daffodil International University, Dhaka, Bangladesh
[g]Enzymoics, Hebersham, NSW, Australia
[h]Novel Global Community Educational Foundation, Hebersham, NSW, Australia
[i]School of Pharmacy, Monash University Malaysia, Bandar Sunway, Selangor, Malaysia

1. Background

Drug development is an extended cycle that takes around up to 20 years and costs up to 3 billion US dollar for a medication to arrive at the market for clinical use [1]. It is a multistep interaction that starts with the distinguishing proof of reasonable target of the disease, target approval for drug undergoing discovery process, identification of hit to lead compounds, improving the lead compound, and its evaluation both preclinically and clinically [2,3]. Despite the great speculations and time brought about for the introduction of new chemical entity into the market, the rate of success in this regard to bring the chemical moiety into market is very low; however, the medicines wearing down rate is particularly high [4]. In most of the cases (up to 50%), the failure of drug to be employed for the ailment of the disease at a clinical trial phase has been accounted for because of absence of ideal pharmacokinetic properties on ingestion, conveyance, digestion, discharge, and poisonousness (ADME/Tox) [5,6]. The utilization of computers for the discovery and evaluation procedures in beginning of studies by driving organizations and exploration of discovery and development of drugs and advancement process with limiting

Computational Approaches in Drug Discovery, Development and Systems Pharmacology
https://doi.org/10.1016/B978-0-323-99137-7.00005-8

the expenses and setbacks in the last stage [5]. The utilization of reasonable medication plan as a vital piece of CADD (computational-aided drug design) gives valuable experiences into the comprehension of the limiting partiality and subatomic connection between ligand (drug) and receptor (target protein) [7]. Moreover, the lead distinguishing proof in drug development and research has been worked with the accessibility of supercomputing office, equal handling, and progressed projects, calculations, and apparatuses [6,8]. Moreover, late progressions in AI (artificial intelligence) and AI techniques have incredibly helped with investigating, learning, and clarifying the drug-related enormous information in the development and discovery of the new chemical moieties [8]. Various techniques utilized in the documentation of new inhibitors from compound information bases to incorporate pharmacophore demonstrating, quantitative structure activity relationship (QSAR), atomic mooring, measurable learning strategies, and the use of quantum mechanics [3,8]. CADD can be extensively subdivided into ligand- and structure-based medicine configuration draws near; both have been broadly utilized in the discovery as well as development of new chemical moiety process in the recognizable proof of reasonable lead particles [9]. While this construction put together medication configuration with respect to the three-layered construction of the objective receptor and its dynamic locales to comprehend the atomic cooperation between the receptor and ligand, the ligand put together medication configuration depends with respect to the information on ligands connecting with the given objective receptor [3]. Use of computational methods helped drug configuration has countless examples of overcoming adversity and keeps on assuming an imperative part in the medication disclosure process [9].

1.1 Breast cancer (BC) and evolution of its treatment

The breast cancer is the leading causes of cancer-related deaths worldwide, and in the United States approxiametly 42,700 deaths were reported in 2020 alone [10]. Despite the increase in the incidence rate, the new deaths due to the breast cancer has decreased significantly in the US and Europe [11]. This decrease in the mortality of the breast cancer has been attributed to the timely diagnosis, improvement in the systemic therapies, and continuous efforts to bring new effective drugs into the market [11]. The BC at the early stage that has invaded only the axillary lymph nodes has cure chances of 70%–80% [12]. However, the advance stage of the breast cancer is difficult to cure completely and only the quality of the life can be improved [12]. The breast cancer is classified into 5 types based on the immunohistochemistry analysis and predictive markers such as progesterone receptor, estrogen receptor (ER), proliferation marker Ki67, and epidermal growth factor receptor 2 [13]. These groups include luminal A-like (progesterone receptor positive (PR+)), estrogen receptor positive (ER+), human epidermal growth factor receptor 2 negative (HER-), luminal B-like HER2- (the expression of the ER and PR expression is less than luminal A-like, ER+), luminal B-like HER2 positive (the expression of the ER and PR is lower than the first one but ER+ and HER2+), nonluminal enriched HER2- (HER2+, PR-, ER-), and triple negative breast cancer which lack the expression of PR, ER, and HER2 [14,15]. Breast cancer with increased expression of HER2+, i.e., show increased expression of HER2, can be treated with the trastuzumab [15]. The cisplatin-based therapies are useful for the treatment of the triple-negative breast cancer. Increased expression of the Ki67 is associated with the increased cancer cell growth and can be used for cancer grading [16,17]. All these expression patterns of the receptor such as HER2 status, Ki67, and hormone receptor (HR) can be employed to pave the way for breast cancer treatment. The estrogen and progesterone play key role in breast growth and proliferation [17]. The estrogen and progesterone production occur in the ovaries in the premenopausal females, while after the menopause the estrogen synthesis is facilitated by the aromatase enzymes on the androgen's hormones [18]. The physiological effects including growth and tissue development of the estrogen are regulated by the ER. The estrogen has various subtypes, but ERα plays a crucial role in the progression and pathogenesis of breast cancer. More than 70% breast cancer express the ERα receptor and targeting this receptor precisely has been the mainstay in the treatment of breast cancer [19]. The breast cancer when express PR and ERα, this type of the breast cancer is regarded as hormone-positive HR+ breast tumor. The FDA approved for the treatment BCa various drugs such as ER modulators, i.e., tamoxifen, and selective ER degrader as adjuvant or neoadjuvant such as fulvestrant with radiation or surgery [18]. The effect of the HT on the clinical outcome of the breast cancer was evaluated using an aromatase inhibitor or ER antagonist [20]. It was assessed that the tamoxifen has been the gold standard for the premenopausal breast cancer for five years. While in the postmenopausal women have shown the superiority of AI over the tamoxifen and considered as a new standard treatment [21]. However, the combination therapies showed higher efficacy against the breast cancer such as HT combination with the mTOR inhibitors or combination of the mTOR and CDK4/6 inhibitors showed enhanced activity [21]. It is well established that tamoxifen therapies increase the survival in patients with breast cancer, relapses are reduced, and prevent the breast cancer in women with high risk. However, those women treated with tamoxifen showed resistance in about 40% cases [20].

1.2 Estrogens

The estrogen is a female sex hormone produced by the ovaries and in case of pregnancy produced by the placenta [22]. The estrogen has widespread effects on the female reproductive system including development, regulation, and maintenance of the secondary characteristics [22]. Furthermore, they also influence the cognitive function, bone formation, metabolism, cardiovascular activity, and neutrophils mobilization, etc. The estrogen synthesis is under the influence hypothalamic-pituitary-ovarian ovarian axis [23]. The hypothalamus release gonadotrophin-releasing hormone that induce the release of two hormones from the pituitary glands such as FSH and LH [23]. These two hormones regulate the activity and expression of the cytochrome *p*450 enzyme system and in turn facilitate the conversion of the androgens to estrogens conversion. While the FSH acts as a rate-limiting enzyme during the estrogen production. The naturally occurring estrogen are of four types such as estrone (E1), 17β-estradiol (E2), estriol (E3), and esterol (E4) [24]. The E1 and E2 production occurs in the ovaries, while placenta produces E3, and E4 production is facilitated by the fetal liver during the pregnancy [24]. The E2 is produced in the highest concentration and has high potency, i.e., its potency is 10 times higher than the E1 and 100 times potent than E3 [25]. The E2 after binding with the EBS induces the signaling cascade by stimulating the cytosolic ER and triggers its dimerization, nuclear shuttling, and for binding of the co-activator, it exposes its ER-AF2 site [26]. Within the nucleus, the ER DBD region interacts with the ERE for the transcription of DBD/DBD dimer. Following this, the ER forms complexes with the p160 family co-activator protein such as GRIP-1, AIB1, and SRC-1 [26]. It is noteworthy that all these ER activations and subsequent steps provide an important avenue for the targeting of the small molecular inhibitors and modulators [24].

1.3 Small-molecule inhibitors of estrogen

1.3.1 Focusing on EBS

Selective estrogen receptor modulators (SERMs)

The SERMs exert an antagonistic or agonistic effect on ER, which mainly depends upon the tissue in which it is expressed and the ERE promoter sequence [27]. The SERMs when acts as antagonist inactivate the ER by inducing the conformational changes [28]. Tamoxifen was developed during the synthesis of the potential nonsteroidal antiestrogen contraceptives and this SERM after approval by the FDA became the most important drug for the treatment of the ERa+ BC and opens the avenues for the development of additional SERMs [28]. Tamoxifen produces significant effects in both pre- and post-menopausal women; however, prolonged use was associated with the resistance emergence [29]. The resistance may be attributed to the alteration in HER2, ERa downstream signaling, or mutations in the PI3K/Akt/mTOR and NF-kB signaling. Furthermore, it also produces uterine tumors by inducing the growth of endometrial cells [29]. The success of the tamoxifen in the treatment of the BC, new chemicals compounds with different or similar cores were introduced such as toremifene, idoxifene, and droloxifene having the same core structure as triphenylethylene were synthesized [30]. After the approval of the tamoxifen for the BC treatment, the other agent that was approved for the BC treatment was toremifene [30]. It showed safety, tolerability, selectivity, and reduced the risk of the endometrial cancer development upon prolonged use. However, the first-generation SERMs showed cross-resistance, which necessitate the development of the second- and third-generation SERMs. These efforts lead to the development of raloxifene, which second-generation SERM showed good activity against the BCa cell lines [31]. However, it failed during the Phase II clinical trial because it showed no activity against the metastatic BC but was approved for the prevention of the BC in postmenopausal women having high risk. Further, it was reported that it reduced uterine tumorigenesis by 50% compared to tamoxifen [32]. However, it increased the risk of strokes, thromboembolism, and poor solubility. These limitations lead to the development of the third-generation SERMs such as arzoxifene [32]. It has a lower risk of endometrial cancer than the tamoxifen and a shorter time of treatment failure. Other SERMs of third generation were approved for osteoporosis such as bazedoxifene, lasofoxifene, and bazedoxifene [33]. The bazedoxifene is very active against the BCa and is approved for the osteoporosis as monotherapuetic agent in the US. Similarly, many small molecules have recently been named as fourth-generation SERM such as acobifene, which is the derivative of the benzopyran [33,34]. The easy availability of the ER-LBD structure and molecular docking programs have made it easy to assess the docking poses of the ligands binding within the target [34]. Several studies used docking to study the conformations and poses of the compounds to predict the activity in in vitro and in vivo experiments [34]. One study used computational analysis to assess the activity of the synthesized isatin derivatives with steomers [35]. The author utilized the Chem3D ultra for the designing of the ligands, for docking with the UCSF chimera prepared target, optimized with the Avogadro tool, and using AutoDock Vina for molecular docking. All the conjugates bind with their target protein with high binding energy than the tamoxifen; however, the experimental results do not always match with the computational results [35]. Furthermore, other studies also used in silico analysis for the poses assessment and the role of the side chain exploration in the antagonizing ERα mutant receptor with their proposed ligands. SBDD-based pharmacophore modeling and docking software facilitated the rapid screening and drug development. Numerous researchers are using CADD tools for novel drug development and perform the experimental validation to find the best inhibitors. Similarly, computational studies were performed for the drug designing against the ERα-EBS ligand binding domain [36]. In 2015, a similar study reported the use of PLANTS1.2 program for the repurposing of the COX-2 inhibitor, i.e., celecoxib for the ERα. Following docking, they utilized docking results to explore the protein-ligand interaction fingerprints [37]. Best docking conformations and poses with the best Tanimoto coefficient (Tc) with respect to the reference OHT fingerprints Tc were chosen after three runs and the method was validated by running the 1000 times [37]. Wilcoxin test showed that the results were almost equal to the standard threshold and can be repurposed against the ERα. However, the experimental data showed that the IC50 value of the celecoxib was high compared to the tamoxifen [30]. Wang et al. used the cyclopropyl derivatives and screened against the ERα to develop the selective SERMs using Discovery studio visualizer against both isoforms of ER, i.e., ERa and ERB [38]. The authors discover five compounds exhibited ERa activity but using FP assays nondetectable binding to ERB [39]. Pavlin et al. use computational assays to assess the influence of the Y357S mutation on the ERa along with the antagonistic impact on the specific mutation and to dig out the new inhibitors against the mutation. Using the Ligfilter, the NCI database was filtered based on the q0 rotatable bonds, Lipinski rule, and logP values calculated by the Schrodinger software QikPro to enhance the bioavailability of the ERa antagonist [39]. The GROMACS5.0.4 was used for MD to assess the behavior of ER mutants with Fulvestrant, AZD-9496, and Endoxifen. These models were subjected for docking with filtered set using Glide HTVS. The top 10% hits generated were docked by employing the Glide SP to choose the top 10% of the generated hits for further docking with Glide XP [40]. The ligands were chosen based on their GlideScore and consensus based on the concept that ligand interact properly with the one of the five-target generated previously. The ligands were screened with the Glide XP and chosen based on their score and whether they show acceptable bindings with two structures out of five mutant MD targets [38]. The experimental studies are required to confirm the in silico results because the in silico methods are unable to completely explain the interaction with the actual system. However, various simulation tools can be employed to assess the predictions [38]. In this regard, in 2012, Istyastono et al. investigated the eugenol and its analog using Monto Carlo and PLANTS1.2 simulation packages to assess the biological studies [41]. This studies utilized 4-(4-hydroxy-3-(prop-2-en-1-yl)phenyl)-2-(prop-2-en-1-yl)phenol exhibited higher binding affinities with the ER and served as a inhibitors of the ER receptors; however, these claims will be confirmed from the experimental studies. Similarly, the Muchtaridi et al. investigated the chalcEa and their analogs according to Lipinski's rule using AutoDock docking tool [41]. The same authors then utilized 3D pharmacophore modeling (using LigandScount4.1 Advanced validation by actives and decoys taken from DUD-E database) to perform the in silico analysis of all the derivatives of the chalcEA, and all the compounds showed higher binding energies [42]. The compounds with the dimethylaminoethoxy side chain exhibited highest binding energies, but the data lack the experimental support [43]. In the search for novel SERMs, Munir et al. used the computational tool, i.e., LigandScout for the preparation of structure of ERa using four pdb structure such as 1UOM, 2JFA, 4XI3, and 1R5K to develop the pharmacophore model by collecting the common parameters from all the structures [42]. Following this, the ZINC database was employed to reveal the ligands suitable fit the pharmacophore model employing the Lipinski rule-based filtering using LigscreeServer with the database of interest [44,45]. The authors selected three hits of out of ten, which exhibited ideal docking properties against both mutant and wild type of the protein target. The experimental validation should be performed to confirm the claims because computational tools lack the biological specificity in the biological system [43,45]. The SERMs tissue specificity for the agonistic and antagonistic profile and E2-independent coactivator binding sites pose a challenge for the CADD for the development and discovery of the novel inhibitors against the target proteins [44]. The MD simulation tools including the Simulation plus can be employed to assess the specificity of the ligand, but it still lacks the absolute the specificity in the biological system [46].

Selective estrogen receptor degraders (SERDs)

To deal with the partial agonism of the SERMs, full SERDs agonists were developed [47]. These compounds trigger the degradation of the ER by competitive antagonism with the EBS inducing the conformational changes in target ER for degradation [48]. The SERDs induce the destabilization in the ER by altering the H12 conformation in a way to enhance the hydrophobic surface exposure and prevent the dimerization of the ER [47].

1.4 Computer-aided drug design for estrogen receptor inhibitors

Conventionally empirical tools have been used for the discovery of the drugs against the ER and following this high-throughput screening along with the experimental validation plays a crucial role in the potential active hits identification [49]. Nowadays, the CADD tools have significantly contributed to the bioinformatics and chemoinformatics for more efficient processing and facilitating the drug development and discovery via molecular docking and FEP simulations tool [47]. The various other tools such as NMR, X-ray, and Cryo-EM have brought a significant revolution in the SBDD with higher reliability and practicality. It should be kept in mind that the interaction of the ligand with the target binding site is difficult to understand without suitable visualization tools [50,51]. In the recent time, the CADD techniques were significantly improved with respect to docking, molecular graphics, scoring functions, molecular dynamics simulation tools, and artificial intelligence (AI) tools or machine learning modeling [50]. Various tools of computer-aided drug designing significantly speed up the drug discovery process [50]. The lack of the experimental structure can be fulfilled by employing the homology modeling of the protein target using various modeling tools if viable templates of the target with sequence similarity are present or de-novo methods in a case when the templates are available [51]. The structural investigation of the IDP (intrinsically disordered proteins) is difficult to explore by employing the traditional methods of the structural solving tools [52].

For this purpose, the FRAGFOLD-IDP method can be used to dig out the precise and exact stretches within the protein that are intrinsically disordered, and using the IDP-LZerD algorithm models can be constructed [53]. The MD simulations can be used to simulate the possible stretches of the native protein structure for the commencement of the SBDD [54]. The X-ray structure availability of the target protein and ligand is very important for the assessment and identification of the binding pose for the SBDD

[55,56]. The various tools that are used for the binding site identification include the MOE SiteFinder tool, Q-SiteFinder, and PASS to investigate the ligand-target interactions and characteristics of the binding site of the target protein [57]. The various docking tools such as AutoDock Vina, ICM, and Glide have made it easier and possible to screen the database of the ligands effectively and predict the binding site and rank the ligand according to their binding energy [55,57].

1.5 Natural product-based computational analysis for breast cancer

1.5.1 Anticancer activity of medicinal plants

The phytochemicals isolated from various can be utilized for the cancer therapies as most of the plants extract showed marked activity against inflammation, oxidative stress, and tumors [58]. The various phytochemicals that showed promising activities include taxanes, derivatives from vinca plant, colchicine from the colchicum, triterpenoid acids, camtothecin, ellipticine, cephalotaxus, berberine, and combretastatins [56].

Echinacea

Echinacea belongs to the family of Asteraceae, and other most important species of this family include *E. angustifolia*, *E. purpurea*, and *E. pallida*, and *E. Purpurea* is commonly implicated in the treatment of the cancer and is called as coneflower [59]. It induces the number of natural killer cells, while the flavonoids content triggers the induction of the immune system [60]. The crude extract of the root and leaf showed significant activities against the BT-549 cell lines. *E. angustifolia* DC extract obtained with the ethyl acetate showed caffeic acid and echinacoside content using HPLC analysis when assessed against the MCF-7 and MDA-MB-2311 breast cancer cell line showed marked activity, while with paclitaxel the effect was synergistic [60].

Allium sativum

Allium sativum commonly named as garlic. The garlic contain the Allicin, which is sulfur-containing compound is associated with anticancer activities [61]. Similarly, other sulfur-containing compounds such as Ajoene decrease the tumor progression, while the selenium works as antioxidant [62]. The ripened extract of garlic facilitates the shielding of aggressive tumors. The Ajoene has been reported for inhibiting the growth of the human breast tumor cells. *A. sativum* revealed against the MCF-7 cancer cell line when formulated as silver nanoparticulate system [63].

Curcuma longa

Curcuma longa, also called as turmeric and contain curcumin as an ingredient, which is reported as potent anticancer agent and composed of the phenolic content [64]. The curcumin formulated as a nanoparticulate system has been reported for its antiinflammatory activities with low toxicity profile by inhibiting the NF-κB, AP-1, and STAT3 signaling and target the G2/M phase of cell division [64,65]. Additionally, the pulsed electric field activated *C. longa* exhibited significant inhibition of the MCF-7 breast cancer cell line and could be employed for the cancer with minimum toxicity. Similarly, the ethanolic extract of the *C. longa* showed marked activity against the MDA-MB-231 cancer cell lines [66].

Arctium lappa

Arctium lappa whose common name is Burdock. The seed of Burdock contains Arctigenin having strong anticancer activities by reducing growth and metastasis of the tumor cells [67]. Furthermore, Lappaol F was also isolated from the *A. lappa* L., which is reported for arresting the growth of the cancer cell and traget the G2 phase of the cell cycle [67]. The Lappaol F portrays anticancer activities and arrests the cell growth via CDK1 and Cyclin B1 signaling [68]. Similarly, several studies reported that the Lappaol F synergizes the activity of the doxorubicin against the MCF-7 and MDA-MB-231 cancer cells [69].

Synadenium cupulare

Synadenium cupulare leaf extract was employed for the synthesis and formulation of CdO/CdO3 nanocomposite utilizing the cadmium nitrate tetrahydrate [70]. Furthermore, the *S. cupulare* contains saponins, flavonoids, tannins, and glycosides which have been implicated in the antitumor activity of *Synadenium cupulare* [71].

Cimicifuga foetida

Cimicifuga foetida is also regarded as black cohosh generally [72]. Acetin derivative of this plant inhibits the growth of the MCF-7 cell line by targeting the Ras/MEK/JNK/ERK and mTOR/Akt signaling [72]. Furthermore, it also inhibits the TLR-4 receptor and its downstream signaling protein such as NF-kB and MyD88 in the TNBC. The cycloartane triterpenoid and KHF16 obtained from the *C. foetida* rhizomes target the G2/M phase of the cell cycle in the MDAMB-468 cells and MCF-7 cells [73].

Cymbopogon citratus

Cymbopogon citratus contains citral and is citrus containing plant [73]. The nanostructures lipid carrier-citral showed promising activity compared to the citral alone when treated the MDA-MB-231 cancer cells [74]. The essential oil of this plant exhibited anticancer activities against DMBA-induced breast cancer in female rats. Additionally, the polysaccharide portion of this plant exhibited significant anticancer activities against the breast cancer cell line by inducing apoptosis and decreasing the expression of the Bcl-2 gene [74].

Zingiber officinale

Zingiber officinale that is commonly known as ginger and has known anticancer effect [75]. The extract of the ginger showed marked anticancer activities against the TNBC. Furthermore, the *Z. officinale* inhibit the MCF-7 and other breast cancer cell line growth by inducing apoptosis marker and inhibit the antiapoptotic genes [76]. Furthermore, the NF-κB, Cyclin D1, and CDK-4 proteins were significantly altered. Fulbaria and Syedpuri the two Bangladeshi varieties showed marked inhibition of the growth and metastasis of the MCF-7 and MDA-MB-231 cancer cell lines [75].

Rhus coriaria

Rhus coriaria, contain phenolic acid, tannins, and flavonoids and is also called as Sumac. It portrays its anticancer activities by inhibiting the growth and metastasis via multi signaling pathway such as NF-κB, STAT3, and iNOS signaling [77]. The extract of these plants has been associated with the G1 phase arrest of the cell cycle. The extract of this plants showed promising activity against the breast cancer by inducing the autophagy and apoptosis via p38, JNK, and ERK1/2 [77]. It also regulates the tumor cell growth and progression by targeting the cyclin D1, p21, and c-Myc protein in the MCF-7 and MDA-MB-231 cells [78].

Ricinus communis L.

Ricinus communis L. fruit has been reported for the anticancer activity against the MDA-BA-231 and MCF-7 cells [79]. The fruit of the *R. communis* contain various compounds, which are medicinally very active such as p-coumaric acid, Epigallocatechin, Ricinine, and Ricinoleic acid [79]. It produces its anticancer activity by targeting the PPAR-gamma, NF-κB, and MAPKs signaling. The seed of the *R. communis* formulated with zinc nanoformulation showed significant inhibition of the breast cancer cells [80].

Drosera bormannii

It is also called as sundew plant, and it has been reported for potent anti-inflammatory and antitumor activities [81]. It portrays its anticancer activities by arresting the growth of the cancer cell line in the G2/M phase and facilitating the apoptosis process in the MCF-7 cells. It also regulates various genes such as p53, apoptotic, and antiapoptotic proteins [82]. The various compounds present in the *Drosera bormannii* include hexadecenoic acid, hexadecen-1-ol, tetradecanoic acid, and other fatty acids. These constituents may play a pivotal role in the anticancer activities of this plant [81].

Acacia hydasica

Acacia hydasica plant comprised of various active compounds such as catechin, methyl gallate, catechin-3-O-gallate, and 7-O-gallolyl catechin [83]. The various active constituent of this plant showed promising anticancer activities against the several cancer cell lines including the MCF-7 and MDA-MB-231 cells by targeting the apoptotic protein (caspase-3, caspapse-9, and bax), antiapoptotic proteins (Bcl-2), and NF-κB/MAPKs (JNK, ERK, p38) [84,85].

Saussurea lappa

The root of the *Saussurea lappa* plant contains sesquiterpene lactones such as dehydrocostuslactone and costunolide [85]. These two active ingredients are responsible for the anticancer activity against the breast cancer via multiple signaling pathways such as c-Myc/p53 and Pi3K/Akt. *Saussurea lappa* and its constituents suppress the growth and proliferation of the MDA-MB-231 cell growth and invasion by NF-κB and STAT3 signaling [85].

Centella asiatica

Centella asiatica possesses anticancer activities against the MCF-7 and MDA-MB-231 cancer cell lines [86]. The aqueous extract of this plant possesses anticancer activities by the inhibition of WAWE3 protein and inducing the Pi3K/Akt signaling in the MDA-MB-231 cells [86].

Eclipta alba

This plant contains a wedelolactone compound that inhibits the growth of various cancer cell lines such as MDA-MB-231, MCF-7, and T47D [87]. The chloroform extract of leaves showed disruption of the mitochondrial membrane and upregulate the apoptotic proteins, while inhibiting the anti-apoptotic proteins in various cancer cell lines [87].

1.6 Bioinformatics approaches

1.6.1 Frameworks pharmacology

The systems pharmacology basically deals with the drugs and proteins of the biological system and has significantly emerged in recent times [88]. The systems pharmacology also regarded as a network pharmacology approach can be utilized for the protein-protein interactions, the possible targets of the disease, and signaling cascades in a particular disease [89]. In recent years, based on the systems pharmacology various natural products were discovered and developed and potential mechanisms have been explored [90]. Likewise, network-based pharmacology has been used for the identification of a number of genes having a pivotal role in the disease development and progression. Recent study reported that wogonoside can be used to treat the angiogenesis in the TNBC using network biology [90]. A system pharmacology-based search was used to find the link between the Iranian chrysanthemum cultivators and well-established breast cancer drugs with their breast cancer associated protein target and to dig out the mechanism [91]. Among these compounds, the rutin showed potent activity against the MCF-7 breast cancer cell line. The systems pharmacology gives an insight into the network of the target compounds and signaling cascade having relation with the complex disease including breast cancer apart from the chosen and confirmed target [92]. Quantitative systems pharmacology connects the systemic biology with the pharmacodynamic as well as pharmacokinetic aspects and provides maximum information about the toxicity and efficacy of the drug employed for treating complex diseases such as breast cancer [92]. Recently, it has been proposed to combine the single-cell data in the special quantitative systems pharmacology to initiate the prediction of immunotherapy in TNBC [91].

1.6.2 Cheminformatics

The significant increase in epigenetics knowledge and data in the recent years has laid the foundation of the cheminformatics methods [93]. Hidden allosteric attachment sites and the interaction of proteins with other proteins are the hotpots for targeting epigenetics using computational tools [93]. Furthermore, the chemoinformations and modeling techniques have a substantial role in the development and discovery of the drugs [94]. Similarly, QSAR has also been employed as an important tool for the drug development and discovery process and can easily predict the anticancer agent efficacy using multitarget approach against various cancer cell lines in real-time [94]. Based on the cheminformatics, the selection of small molecules enhances the transported mediating targeting facilitates the drug effectiveness and increases the therapeutic index [94]. Along with web ontology language, the chemoinformatic tools can be utilized for assessing the pharmacogenetics and pharmacogenomics base for the breast cancer drug repositioning which leads to the exploration of new clinical indications and potential conflicting influence on the breast cancer drugs predictions [95]. Furthermore, the drug development and discover process can further be facilitated by the drug repurposing approaches and tries finds new uses for the existing drugs, which will significantly reduce the time and money in discovery of new moiety [95]. The most important aspect of the drug repurposing is to find the relationship between the drugs and diseases, and chemoinformatics tools can assist in this regard markedly [96]. Molecular modeling and other computational tools based on the chemoinformation have been significantly related with the discovery of new drugs from the natural sources, which includes the organization of information, their analysis and dissemination of that chemical information in the natural compounds database are the key uses of cheminformatics [97]. Furthermore, these tools also help in the selection of drugs from natural sources, molecular target identification and selection for natural compounds, natural product likeness quantification, and de novo design [96].

1.6.3 Latest trends in indigenous medicinal plant informatics and avenues to Battle Cancer

With the emergence of bioinformatics tools, omics, and information technology there is increased tendency to build data and knowledge bases of the natural products, herbal medicine and formulation and bio-active compounds from the plant's sources [96]. Several efforts have been made in this regard such as Phytochemistry and therapeutics, Indian Medicinal Plants, Indian Medicinal Plants Database, and Collective Molecular Activities of Useful Plants, and SymMap databases [98]. Moreover, the experts in the field of computational chemistry have developed novel in silico techniques for the assessment of the pharmacokinetic profile of the medicinal compounds and bioactive drugs [98]. These novel approaches are very applicable to the phytochemicals and plant bioactive molecules for the assessment of various properties using virtual screening, potential mechanism of action, and their discovery [99]. Many antitumor drugs were discovered and developed by the computational tools and network pharmacology based approaches to from the medicinal plants [100]. Based on this report, the computational tools can be successfully used to assess and discover anticancer medicine especially against the breast cancer from these plant sources including elucidation of the possible mechanism of action, pharmacokinetics analysis, and toxicokinetic profile of the drugs [101]. In fact, plant-derived products contain many phytochemicals, and these phytochemicals may be present in more than one plants, so the most important part of study would properly investigate the action of these compounds within the biological system rather than just knowing about the plant phytochemicals [101].

1.7 Drug designing tools

1.7.1 Structure-based drug design

The 3D structure availability of the protein's targets for different diseases and investigation of the limiting site cavity frames cornerstone of structure-based drug design and development (SBDDD) [102]. This methodology is explicit and adequately quick in distinguishing proof of lead atoms and their enhancement, which assists in understanding illness at a subatomic level. A portion of the normal techniques utilized in SBDDD incorporates structure-based virtual screening process (SBVS), docking, and simulation (MD) process [103]. These techniques utilize various methods, for example, evaluation of restricting energetics, communication of protein-ligands, and after restricting ligands within the protein triggering the conformational changes [104]. Being utilized by numerous pharma and computational experts, SBDDD as a computational procedure helped tremendously in the discovery and development process of various drugs and ensure the availability of drugs to the market [105]. The amprenavir discovery and development which is an inhibitor of the human immunodeficiency infection (HIV) protease utilizing modeling and MD analysis, raltitrexed against HIV which inhibits the thymidylate synthase enzyme utilizing SBDD, norfloxacin an inhibitor of the bacterial topoisomerase II and IV protein used against the gram-negative bacteria of the urinary tract employing the SBVS technique [106]. Similarly, the introduction of the carbonic anhydrase inhibitor dorzolamide for reducing the intraocular pressure treatment (glaucoma), using section-based drug screening for the cystoid macular edema, and INH (isoniazid) an anti-TB agent, which inhibit the enoyl-acyl-ACP reductase (InhA) was introduced through the pharmacophore and SBVS techniques [106]. The key steps involved with the SBDDD comprised of target protein structure identification and preparation, ligand-binding site (pocket) exploration, preparing the compounds library, docking analysis, simulation process optimization, and assessing the binding free energies [104].

Planning of the target structure preparation

Preparation of the target structure The rapid advancement in the structure elucidation and identification procedures such as NMR, X-ray analysis, and protein data bank availability have significantly increased [107]. Due to the experimental analysis limitation, most of the proteins structure have not been well characterized until now [108]. Computational tools such as threading, comparative homology modeling (HM), and ab initio have been very impressive in structural deciphering of proteins from their relative genome sequence [109]. HM is most acceptable and commonly used method for the determining the exact three-dimensional structure of protein from the amino acid sequence using an appropriate structural template. It involves multiple steps such as template identification, target model building, sequence alignment, refinement of the model, and validation of the model [108]. Protein threading is another approach for the prediction of the protein structure is often used whenever the target proteins have less sequence similarity with other proteins and target proteins is structurally similar with some protein in the PDB database [109]. The HM only consider the sequence similarity of the template and target protein, the protein threading also considers the structural information such as the secondary structure of the protein, pairwise interaction, solvent accessibility to improve the prediction more accurate [110]. The ab initio modeling is used when the target has no template in the existing biological databases. It takes into the account a generalized optimization problem to assess the dihedral angle of the studied protein structure which imparts stability to the structure [111].

Identification of the ligand-binding site The identification of the binding site within the protein is of utmost importance for performing the docking that is specific [112]. The binding site can be retrieved from the X-ray crystallographic analysis of the protein, which is bind with the co-crystallized ligand and site directed mutagenesis [112]. The exact binding site of the ligand have little or no information experimentally; however, various software can be used to specify the site of ligand binding such as CASTp, which help in the protein binding site prediction [113]. The heavier or bulky compounds are rejected during the process of lead identification within the binding site pocket [113].

Compound library preparation The compounds library is prepared from various databases such as ZINC, PubChem, ChEMBL, and MCULE where millions of compounds are present [112]. The molecular docking analysis is commenced with those compounds that fulfill the criteria of drug-Likeness such as Lipinski's rule of five, ADMET factors, and toxicokinetic parameters [114]. The Lipinski's rule devises five parameters such as molecular weight, partition co-efficient, number of H-bonds acceptors and donors [114]. While the ADMET analysis considers various parameters such as the BBB permeability, Cytochrome inhibition or activation, plasma protein binding, human intestinal absorption, and P-glycoprotein substrate. Besides the pharmacokinetic parameters, the toxicokinetic parameters such as drug safety, mutagenicity and synthetic accessibility are considered [112].

1.8 Molecular docking and scoring functions

Molecular docking is important computational tools to assess the receptor and ligand interaction at subcellular level, and the ligand is ranked according to their respective binding energy and affinity toward the protein using scoring functions [115]. The fruitful binding of the compound with the target protein depends upon two factors such as conformational localization of the ligand within the active pocket and affinity of the ligand which is assessed by the binding energy of each pose. Molecular docking can be classified into two types such as flexible protein docking and flexible ligand search docking [116]. The flexibility of ligand in case of the flexible ligand docking utilizes three algorithms such as stochastic method, systemic method, and simulation method; however, the flexible protein docking depends upon the molecular dynamics (MD) and MC (Monte Carlo) [116].

1.8.1 Molecular dynamic (MD) simulation

The MD analysis was first reported in the 1970s [117]. The MD process is a very powerful physical tool to assess the position of each atom with respect to the time within the molecule, and this interatomic interaction is based on Newton's law of motions [117]. The suitable force field is applied to assess the interaction between the atom of the molecules and find the overall energy status of the system [118]. This tool is extensively used because this system provides information about the motion and position of the system at every nanosecond, which is very difficult with other experimental techniques. Similarly, the condition of the simulation process can be modulated carefully, and condition of the system is well known [118]. This technique is widely used in the structure-based drug design and discovery because it provides information about the atomic level interaction binding energy, unbinding, and changes happening in the receptor conformation in detail which is very difficult with the other experimental procedures [119]. Additionally, it is also possible with the MD analysis to assess the dynamics of the ligand-receptor binding and unbinding and to quantify the kinetics, free energy, and thermodynamics process [105]. The various program that can be employed for the MD simulation includes YASARA, GROMACS, CHARMM, AMBER, and NAMD, etc. [119].

1.8.2 Ligand-based drug design

The ligand-based drug design is another approach for drug development and discovery and is extensively used when the target protein lacks a three-dimensional structure [120]. The information obtained from the active compounds targeting-specific receptors can be employed for the assessment of the physicochemical and structural parameters, which correspond to the biological activity since similarity in structure will leads to similar activities [121]. The widely used techniques in ligand-based screening are composed of QSAR, pharmacophore modeling, and AI [120].

Pharmacophore modeling

This modeling basically considers the spatial chemical feature within the ligand which is important for its interaction with the receptor [122]. The various chemical features that will be considered in this modeling include H-bond acceptor, H-bond donors, hydrophobic areas, aromatic ring systems, negatively charged ionizable groups, positively charged ionizable groups, and hydrophobic area [123]. Through this modeling approach, the ligand having different scaffolds but composed of similar functional groups can be assessed. The active conformation of the molecules can be added to this model within the target binding site. At the molecular alignment stage, while performing QSAR, this modeling can be used [123]. The various through which this modeling process can be performed include PHASE, LigandScout, Catalyst, and PharmMapper. This modeling process should have optimum specificity and sensitivity to reduce the false positive and negative results and can be validated by the external test set as independent factor [124]. If a receptor lacks 3D structure and lack library of known active compounds, then sequence derived 3D model is quite useful [124].

Quantitative structure-activity relationships (QSARs)

The QSAR process indicate the variation in the compound's bioactivity can be related to the changes in the molecular structure features [125]. The QSAR is extensively used in the process of drug invention process from hit to lead optimization and identification [126]. The statistical model is developed using correlation studies and finally, the biological activities of the new compounds is predicted [126]. The best QSAR modeling depends upon the increased number of data sets with pharmacological activities assessed from the experiments, the test set, and training ligands must be selected properly. There should be no correlation of the physicochemical features of the compounds which may leads to overfitting data, and finally, the applicability as well as predictivity of the final must be assessed using internal and external standards [125]. Depending upon the derived descriptor, the QSAR modeling is classified into six types which are as follows [127].

1. 1DSAR that focuses on the correlation between molecular parameters such as pKa and logP and their biological potentials.
2. 2D-QSAR in which the structural features such as 2D-pharmacophore are compared with biological activities.
3. 3D-QSAR that depends upon the noncovalent binding surrounding the ligands influence the biological activities.
4. 4D-QSAR is the extension of the 3D-QSAR, however, involves the configurations of ligand addition.
5. 5D-QSAR involves the addition into the 4D-QSAR using induced-fit models.
6. 6D-QSAR involves the addition of solvation models into the 5D-QSAR.

The examples of the 3d-QSAR tools comprised of PHASE, Catalyst, and comparative similarity index analysis. The QSAR modeling can be categorized into 2 types such as nonlinear and linear-based chemometric methods [127].

Artificial intelligence and drug discovery

The AI is machine leaning type that depends upon the computer's ability to utilize the data present [128]. Various computational tools used AI to predict the biological and toxicological behavior of the chemical moiety [129]. Additionally, it has been employed to assess protein folding, interaction of protein with other proteins, QSAR, virtual screening, and investigating the ADMET features. Two powerful tools such as machine learning (ML) and deep learning (DL) to design the drug rationally [129]. ML have been used widely in drug development such as support vector machine (SVM), Naïve Bayesian (NB), and Random Forest. While example of the DL includes deep neural network (DNN), convolutional neural network (CNN), autoencoder, and recurrent neural network (RNN). The conventional QSAR analysis can effectively predict various features such as solubility and logP [130]. However, the QSAR may not predict the side effects and efficacy of compounds because this method uses a small set and has limited space occupancy. The huge data using the HTS (high-throughput screenings) tools are very challenging for machine learning and QSAR analysis [129]. The AI fills the gap of dealing with such a bid data of multidimensional nature and high volume to fruitfully assess the drug efficacy and ADRs in human subjects [131]. The most encouraging technique to deal with the huge data in the present time is using deep learning which was first implemented in the drug development process in 2012 by Merck using QSAR [131]. The results were promising in the sense that they exactly predicted the ADMET features in contrast to the traditional method of machine learning. However, despite its usefulness, AI is a challenging process because it is a data mining tool that depends upon the amount and quality of the data available [130].

1.8.3 Computational tool use CADD

The CADD tools are based on mathematical calculation to quantify and assess the properties of the potential drug candidate for clinical practice [132]. This process utilizes a number of software available commercially or publicly which are discussed below [132].

1. The widely employed simulation codes are AMBER, CHARMM, GROAMCS, OpenMM, and NAMD. The above software can be run on various computer such as running on multicore processing unit and graphics processing units (widely used for video games) [133].
2. The 3D structure protein, RNA, and other molecules may be retrieved from the Protein Data Bank, after confirming its solvation with NMR or X-ray crystallography. Furthermore, the 3D structure can also be designed by HM method utilizing MODELER or an online tool such as SWISS-MODEL [133].

3. For the commencement of the MD analysis, database screening, HM, and empirical force field are necessary for the molecule of interest [134]. These force fields are used by the software to calculate the force and associated energy, e.g., ligand-protein complex. Force fields from the AMBER and CHARMM families are employed for the description of the external as well as internal energetic features of a system during simulation [134]. When within the existing force field parameters are missing, e.g., for small drug-like molecules CGenFF or Antechabmer program can be employed for the automated parameter generation for the completion of the force field. Importantly, when utilizing the force field for different parts of the same system such as ligand and protein their compatibility is of utmost importance, e.g., Antechamber should be used with AMBER and CHARMM with CgenFF [135]. Moreover, during the calculation of parameters, it is important to check the parameters with respect to their preciseness when dealing with the energy as a conformational function [135].
4. When there is no information regarding the target binding site is available, the possible binding site can be recognized by computational methods. The computational program recognizes the possible site of binding by assessing the geometrical match and binding energy for a diverse number of compounds to the proposed sites on the protein. The programs for binding site identifications include ConCavity and FINSITE [136].
5. The VS tool is employed to screen a large number of compound database using in silico approach and determine the potential binding energy for a query target. The various software used for VS includes Pyrex, AutoDock, AutoDock Vina, and Gold. While the Pharmer program uses a 3D pharmacophore database for screening against the protein target [137].
6. The commercially available computational tools include OpenEye, Discovery Studio, MOE, and Schrodinger. These programs can be excessed at discount for academic users and include most of the features used to LBDD and SBDD [137].

1.8.4 MD simulations

The MD simulation is used to provide an insight into the atomic-level interaction between ligand and protein, to generate conformational sets for ligand and target to take flexibility into the for LBDD and SBDD and to find the binding free energy following combination with other tools [138]. The following steps are important for running a successful MD simulation. A suitable web-based approach to commence a number of steps is below in the CHARMM-GUI at www.charmm-gui.org [139].

1. Retrieve the 3D structure from the PDB site or generate a structure using HM [139].
2. Perform the refining of the structure by manuring the orientations of the side chain, add H-atoms, and for titratable residue find the proper protonation state using various software. Retain or removed ions, and crystal waters cofactors depend upon the study protocols [139].
3. Select a force field such as CHRMM36 for the description of the system and code for running MD. According to the program, prepare the input files. In case, if the force field parameters are missing, then use CGenFF program to develop parameters or chose the force field by following appropriate parameter protocols [138].
4. For specific solvent MD, use periodic boundary conditions for the solvation system in water box, which can be done by employing the CHARMM-GUI. Perform the minimization and equilibrium of the system stepwise to facilitate the relaxation of the bad atomic contacts and obtain the geometries in the relaxed form [139].
5. Mostly, the harmonic restriction is first applied to the system's nonwater components and subsequently reduced through the MD equilibrium and minimization process. This process leads to the decreased alteration in the structure of the protein due to close atomic interaction during initial modeling. The NVT canonical MD ensemble is most utilized first for equilibration and then it is followed by the NPT MD ensemble to facilitate the PBC box size according to the pressure and temperature at 1 atmospheric and 298 K, respectively [139].
6. Perform the simulation using an NPT ensemble for the phenomenon under consideration for the time scale. Usually, the time scale phenomenon involves the nanosecond, and microsecond time scale; however, some phenomena occur very rapidly. The event of interest is observed such as alteration in the protein binding site following interaction with the ligand, and it also taken into consideration that the changes in the phenomenon occur markedly with the passage of time or remain within an acceptable range [139].
7. The MD process quality is observed using RMSD trajectories during the whole simulation process. The RMSD is typically increased followed by the fluctuating stable values. However, the simulation is run for additional time, then the simulation process becomes stable and the RMSD value becomes stable [140].

8. During the ligand-protein complex analysis, various other properties can be assessed such as the H-bonding profile and interaction energies along with the trajectories analysis. Moreover, to extract the different conformation from the trajectories, structural clustering algorithms can be employed [140].

1.8.5 Site identification by ligand competitive saturation (SILCS)

The SLICS is another novel tool of ligand design. It utilizes all-atom MD simulation (explicit solvent) including propane, methanol etc. to recognize the binding site and mode on the target by the 3D functional groups [141]. These patterns can be used for both qualitatively such as ligand design and quantitatively to estimate the binding affinities of the different ligands [142]. The SLICS for the simulation process uses an updated version of the GCMC/MD (oscillating μ_{ex} Grand Canonical Monte Carlo/MD). The updated SLICS can target the occluded or deep binding sites including GPCRs and nuclear receptors [142].

1. The system preparation is use similar protocols as described above for the simulation. However, to this system, we can add solute molecules such as propane, formamide, methanol, and benzene along with water molecules [143].
2. Restrain weakly the Cα carbon atoms backbone only with a force constant of 0.12 kcal/mol/Å for all the residues of the target protein or residue of the core region only within the protein in case of required flexibility of selected regions. The utilization of the Cα restraints inhibits the translation and rotation of the target protein in a box and avoids the potential denaturation of the target from the small solute molecule which surrounds the protein [143].
3. With the steepest descent algorithms, the system is minimized up to 5000 steps with the help of PBC with 250 ps equilibration, and the temperature regulation is facilitated by the rescaling velocity [144].
4. During GCMC, the exchange of water and solute molecules takes place between their simulation system and gas-phase reservoirs. The water exchange and the excess chemical potential provided to drive the solute periodically by oscillation for water or solute every 3 cycles depending upon the concentration of the target [145]. The calculations are run for 100 or above cycles and the average chemical potential is near to the free energy (experimental hydration) for both water and solute. The GCMC can move in three different moves such as deletion, insertion, rotation, and translation with acceptance probabilities facilitated by the criteria of Metropolis [145].

5. At the end of the GCMC cycle, the end configuration is utilized as a configuration of initiation for 0.5–1 ns simulation. During this MD process, the target protein shows structural conformational changes and obtains additional water and solutes samples around the protein [146]. Prior to the MD production, 100 ps equilibration and SD minimization of 500 steps are performed. From the MD production, the last conformation achieved is utilized for the next GCMC cycle starting conformation [144].
6. The "FragMaps" is basically the 3-Dimensional probability distribution of solute selected atoms and is constructed from the GC-MC/MD analysis [147]. On a Boltzmann transformation, these are modified to GFE FragMaps, which assess the quantitate affinities of the ligand along with the individual atoms' contributions. The BFE FragMaps facilitate the ligand-based docking using utilizing the approach of the MC-SLICS or pharmacophore models calculation can be performed using SLICS-Pharm [147].

1.8.6 Database preparation

The VS using commercially available free databases of compounds is very important source for target proteins using low-molecular weight compounds. While the ZINC provides an in-house database preparation for performing a different task [148].

1. From the chemical vendors such as Chemdiv, Chembridgem Specs, Maybridge, etc., download the database. These databases provide compounds in the SDF 2D format and can converted accordingly [149].
2. The 2D SDF format is converted to the 3D format, i.e., MOL2 by various software including RDKit, Open Babel, etc. The structure preliminary geometry in the 2D format is optimized during the conversion to the 3D format so that bad contacts is avoided. The H-atoms that are missing are added, and a proper state of protonation that is pH 7.2 is achieved [149]. Various tautomer in case of further screening can be produced for rigid type of ligand docking. Similarly, multiple rotamers around 100 to 200 can also be produced for consideration of the accessible conformation for each molecule [150].
3. Force field base minimization is utilized to for 3D structure additional optimization to achieve the most accurate structure chemically and if required to assign atomic charges during the consequent screening process. For the said purpose, GAFF, MMFF94, and CGenFF force filed for organic molecules can used [150].

4. Once the database is prepared from the freely available vendors, to easyly manage the data in-house consistent identifiers are used for compounds tagging [151]. The physical and vendor information for every compound under consideration is added, which will facilitate the subsequent analysis easy. In case, if the data is very large, for more efficient use it can be divided into various pieces. Finally, the data is saved in a format which is for the software to handle it easily such as MDF format for MOE and MOL2 format for Dock [151].

1.8.7 Docking-based VS

The docking process involves the modeling of the ligand in the target putative binding site in a very optimized way, which can be assessed by the combination of scoring function and conformational sampling [152]. For docking analysis, various softwares are available and they differ from each other based on their ligand-target interaction scoring and the conformational method of ligand binding within the active pocket of the target. Below is the protocol described for the DOCK software to perform typical VS docking [152].

1. The most important step is the preparation of the target structure for the DOCK in the required format. After the preparation of the target protein, the active pocket with which the ligand bind should be defined using either binding site prediction software or utilizing the experimental information [153]. The docking process is based on the target single conformation and the MD program can be employed to generate multiple conformations from the individual docking process. In this condition, all the compounds are docked against the said target and the compounds are ranked based on the most favorable docking score [152].
2. Following this, select a scheme of scoring and sampling method for molecular docking [153]. The DOCK program basically uses the conformation sampling method and incremental ligand construction, which triggers the division of the ligands into individual fragments and collect these ligand fragments within the binding site in several different poses. Physical force field base scoring is used to score the binding poses and is comprised of electrostatic terms and van der Walls force [153].
3. The entire ligand database is docked against the single target or multiple information as described above for MD simulation [153]. The compounds are ranked and evaluated further based on their binding score. To assess the efficiency and reliability of the docking process, multiple step VS should be used [3].

4. Multiple steps VS using DOCK, the first phase involves fast and coarse optimization process for every compound of the database for one target or multiple targets [3]. In the first phase of docking, about 50,000 compounds are chosen based on their van der Walls energies. In this process facilitate the selection of the compounds with maximum steric complementarity against the target rather than the selected based on the favorable electrostatic binding interaction that is matchable with the binding site shape [3].
5. Second round of the VS is performed on the 50,000 compounds screened during the first round [154]. During the second round, the optimization is very rigorous which requires additional steps of minimization and to assess the target flexibility into consideration multiple protein conformations are employed. Out of 50,000 compounds, top 1000 hits based on the molecular weight normalized total energies such as van der Walls and electrostatic terms are chosen for further analysis [154].
6. During the final round, about 100 compounds are selected having diverse biological properties and with acceptable ADME parameters [155]. The diversity is crucial because it will facilitate the selection of biological potent compounds and provides lead compounds diversity which will the chances of compounds having high clinical trials success probability [155]. The selected 100 compounds is clustered to maximize the diversity of selected compounds based on the structure and physicochemical parameters. Lipinski's rule of 5 and bioavailability descriptors can be employed to filter the compounds with the best ADME properties [154].

1.8.8 SILCS-pharm

In contrast to the VS docking, there is an alternate type of docking such as target-based pharmacophore VS. This approach very rapidly filters the database against the target for potential binders [156]. The pharmacophore modeling is basically dependent on the special features of the chemical compounds that are required for ligand-target interaction. It signifies the simplification of the comprehensive information utilized by the docking protocols, so its requirement for the computational analysis is lowered [155,156]. Pharmacophore generation can be performed by several methods; however, we will discuss the SLICS method of pharmacophore generation as discussed in the above section [157].

1. The desired target pocket should be defined similar to the VS docking [156].

2. GFE FragMaps from the SLICS was employed for the pharmacophore model generation as input into the SLICS-Pharm code [157]. The pharmacophore feature sizes are defined using the GFE cutoff for FragMaps, and the visualization of the FragMaps can be done the VMD [157]. The contour value is adjusted to get well separated, local FragMaps regions as defined by the energy. The GFE value should be optimized in case of lower contour value few or no pharmacophore for VS and in case of a high contour value will leads to many bulky features [157].
3. During pharmacophore generation using the SLICS-Pharm program FragMap voxels as per the definition of the GFE cutoffs clustering into the SLICS features intermediate and is converted to the pharmacophore standard features [158]. The pharmacophore models or hypotheses generated finally are ranked by the summation of all GFE features. The higher GFE scores reflect an effective model for use in the VS as the strength of the functional group binding generated by the SLICS are defined by the GFE [158].
4. After all the above steps, the pharmacophore VS programs such as MOE or Pharmer is then utilized for the filtration of compounds in a database chosen SLICS-Pharm. The RMSD analysis indicates the agreement between the parameters of the pharmacophore model which is related to the query compounds functional group and can be employed for the ranking of the final ligand list [159].
5. As described above, low energy multiple conformations for every ligand in the data set before the pharmacophore VS should be pre-generated as the posing algorithm do not include ligand flexibility [159].
6. When the ligand selection is finalized depending upon the RMSD, an alternative method can be employed for the compounds ranking in a method regraded as consensus scoring. For example, SLICS ligand free energy scoring can be employed for re-ranking the list to provide the free energy-based ranking [160]. The list of the compound is finalized for experimentation and can be obtained from the scoring of LGFE and RMSD scores for hit potential maximization [160].

1.9 Similarity search

When the lead compounds are recognized from the experiments, the LBDD analysis can be used to initiate the SAR development or to find additional hit compounds [161]. In these methods, the most important one is a similarity search that is rapid and straightforward. In this method, the physicochemical or structural similarity is considered. The same method can be used to validate the lead, which is the compound having multiple analogs with diverse biological activities for SAR development and is adequate for additional studies [161].

1. Prepare the proposed compound in a proper format that is suitable for similarity search for recognition [162].
2. The fingerprint types are selected for recognizing the compound from the database. The fingerprint for a compound to assess the various properties such as physical, structural, and chemical features [162]. The structural fingerprints such as the presence of specific bonds, atoms, or rings in a compound, which is encoded by BIT MACCS and facilitate the compound's recognition with a similar structure to that of lead [163]. This will improve the binding affinities and pave the way for SAR development. The MPMFP encodes the physicochemical fingerprint of the compounds including polarity, MW, and solvation energy, and assists in the recognition of compounds with similar physicochemical properties and different structures [163]. This method helps in the identification of the hits with different structural scaffolds in contrast to the lead compound and having novel biological activities, while this process is called as lead hopping [164].
3. The similarity comparison method was chosen, and the search is performed against the in silico database [165]. Various similarity tools are available to quantify the degree of similarity between two molecules such as the Tanimoto coefficient. This can be utilized for the huge database screening in a short period of time. The compounds having similarity with the query molecule shows higher coefficient [164].

1.9.1 Lead optimization using SAR

When the number of hits with activity data exist against a specific target, it is easy to develop the SAR models, and new compounds with better activity can be predicted [166]. The LBDD SAR model employs the regression analysis for the lead series descriptors establishment relative to their activities. Based on this method, the prediction of the modified compounds can be done quantitatively [166]. The descriptors may be chemical or physical features of the ligand and even geometric parameters for the special functional groups, i.e., the pharmacophore group within the compounds can be considered [165]. The information regarding these properties with their relative activity can be employed to design new, and synthetic compounds by the medicinal chemist for quantitative evaluation. During the SAR development utilizing pharmacophore features, the conformations that are responsible for the activities should be employed. The below protocols will illustrate the SAR development using in-house conformational pharmacophore samples [165].

1. For all the known ligands, Langevin dynamic-based MD analysis is performed [167]. By employing the explicit solvent or treatment with the implicit solvent model including generalized Born continuum solvent model for the inclusion of the aqueous solvation effects of the simulated ligands [167]. The MD simulation should be run for 10 ns, and sampling of ligand conformations is assessed for the convergence. In case of inadequate sampling, the MD can be enhanced or performed utilizing enhanced sampling methods including Hamiltonian Replica Exchange methods and temperature, while the snapshots are saved for further analysis at 0.2 ps [167].
2. The pharmacophore group which are common in the hit compounds and indicates well-conserved functional groups including aromatic rings and H-bond acceptor and donors are recognized [168]. The angles and distances between the pharmacophore are assessed during the whole trajectories and the probability distribution is obtained on this basis [167].
3. Analysis can be performed on both 1D and 2D distribution. The 1D probability distribution involves the functional groups distance or the 3 functional groups mutual angles. The 2D probability distribution indicates all possible angle pairs or possible distance [168]. For every hit, the 1D and 2D distribution is noted. The most efficient compound is formed as a reference criterion. The distribution of the similarity is quantified using overlap coefficient between all other compounds which will be compared against the reference compounds [168].
4. The overlap coefficient (OC) is than set as an independent variable for the regression analysis for experiment validation [169]. The 1D and 2D pharmacophores probability distribution are used to recognize the yield showing an encouraging correlation with the experiments data by employing OCs different combinations [169]. Multiple SAR model can be generated for a significantly large database. The compounds which show activities are arranged into test and training dataset, while the SAR is developed for the training set and the test compound set is used as reference for filtration [169].
5. The expansion of the regression model can be done by considering various physicochemical features including MW, and polar solvent accessibility [170].

6. The ideal CSP-SAR model can be utilized to assess the query compounds predicted potencies and the most active compound is proceeded for the experimentations. Usually, for different activities such as both undesirable and desirable characteristics multiple models are there to design compounds [170].

1.9.2 Single-step free energy perturbation (SSFEP)

The free energy perturbation demand computationally required a highly accurate method because of its higher level and employed for the binding free energy changes quantification associated with the compound modification [171]. Single step free energy perturbation can be employed to save the time required for computational analysis. This approach utilizes a precomputed MD analysis of the ligand-target complex, and the free energy difference can be assessing rapidly due to the small and single non-H atom alteration. Compared to the many MD simulations that require the introduction of the chemical modification into the FEP standard procedure [172]. SSEFP provides rapid predictions in the binding energies changes associated with structural modifications and has important implications in the lead optimization. This method can be employed with the following protocols using various simulation programs [171].

1. Perform 10 ns simulation for the ligand-protein complex and ligand alone in the solution set for the MD [172].
2. The binding energy evaluation of the ligand with the environment for initiation, modified and unmodified condition of the simulation in both environments, i.e., ligand-protein complex and ligand alone [173].
3. The energy difference is calculated based on the FEP formula or Bennett acceptance ratio in the presence of target and in the aqueous environment [173]. The protein and aqueous solution differences in the free energy differences gives the overall free energy difference of the system [173].

2. Case studies of polypharmacology of natural product against multiple estrogen receptor

2.1 Retrospective validation of virtual screening approach

Virtual screening provides an approach for prioritizing drugs for experimental validation; however, the virtual screening algorithm chosen is dependent on the data collection and evaluation strategy. There are two types of virtual screening approaches: structure-based and ligand-based methods. Validation of virtual screening can be done retrospectively, prospectively, or both. In retrospective validation, previously published data is used to create a new model and evaluate its usefulness in screening novel drugs against a target protein or receptor. In the case of prospective validation, the top hit compounds are validated in the laboratory via experiments. In this paper, we describe a retrospective virtual screening approach for determining the polypharmacology of natural compounds against ERs in breast cancer [174]. In retrospective validation, there are many steps involved to virtual screen the large data set of compounds.

- Retrieval of ER ligands data sets (active and decoy)
- Assessment of new query models via different statistical matrices
- Virtual screening of compound using validate query model
- Ligand-based virtual screening
- Structure-based virtual screening
- Visualization of binding interaction
- Selection of best hit compounds

2.1.1 Retrieval of estrogen receptor ligands data sets (active and decoy)

ERs are divided into two categories: ER and G protein-coupled receptor GPR30 (GPER). The information for ER ligands was obtained from the Directory of Useful Decoys Enhanced: DUD-E [175]. DUD-E is a valuable directory that provides challenging decoys to aid in the benchmarking of molecular docking. DUD:E has a total of 22,886 active molecules with affinities for 102 targets, with an average of 224 ligands per target. DUD: E additionally includes roughly 50 decoys for each active, each with similar physicochemical features but a different 2-D topology. In the case of GPER-1, previously published literature yielded fifteen (15) potentially active GPER-1 ligands. For every selected active GPER-1, DecoyFinder v 2.0 was used to generate chemically different decoy GPER-1. A drug-like subset of ZINC15 was utilized as a search database to avoid biases and to resemble actual decoy GPER-1. For the development of decoys GPER-1 ligands, strict criteria were used based on five physical descriptors from the Directory of Useful Decoys (DUD) database [174,175]. Tanimoto thresholds for active ligand vs decoy and decoy versus decoy were set to 0.90, whereas acceptors and donors of hydrogen bonds were set to ± 0. The molecular weight and rotational bond were set to ± 40 Da and ± 0, respectively [176].

2.1.2 Assessment of new query models via different statistical matrices

After the development of prerequisite ER ligand data sets, retrospective validation of both LBVS and SBVS was performed using the receiver operating characteristic (ROC) plot and the early enrichment factor (EF) at 0.5%, 1%, and 2%, as described in earlier works [174,177]. The false-positive rate (FPR) of 1% (EF1 percent) is used to calculate the enrichment in true positives (TP): EF percent=TP/FPR percent. Using the Rocker tool, early enrichment rates of 0.5%, 1%, and 2% were calculated for each virtual screening parameter [177].

2.1.3 Ligand-based virtual screening of natural compound using validate query model

Ligand-based virtual screening (LBVS) does not need target protein or receptor information. It requires a known endogenous or synthetic ligand for screening new compounds against a target protein. In this case, a shape-based virtual screening and electrostatic potential similarity calculation were used to perform LBVS.

Shape-based virtual screening

The rapid overlay of 3D chemical structures (ROCS v3.2.2) tool from OpenEye Scientific Software is used to perform shape-based virtual screening [178]. Estradiol (E2), an endogenous ER agonist, and G-1, (1-((3*aR*, 4*S*,9*bS*)-4-(6-bromobenzo[*d*][1,3]dioxol-5-yl)-3*a*,4,5,9*b*-tetrahydro-3*H*-cyclopenta[*c*]quinolin-8-yl)ethan-1-one), a GPER-1 selective agonist, were used in the generation of ROCS query model. Prerequisite different conformations of both E2 and G-1 were calculated using OMEGA tool by employing default settings of no more than 200 conformers per molecule, and the lowest energy conformer of E 2and G-1 was chosen to generate the final ROCS overlay model.

Natural product databases NPASS Database—BIDD was utilized to test both query models generated with ROCS as a large data set of natural products [179]. TanimotoCombo was employed as a scoring feature in ROCS since it quantifies both ShapeTanimoto and ColorTanimoto (molecular shape overlay) (chemical functionality overlaps). In next step, electrostatic potential similarity screening was also performed on hit compounds with a TanimotoCombo score greater than 0.5.

Electrostatic potential similarity

ET_Comb score of EON v 2.2.0.26, which is a combination of ShapeTanimoto (ST) and PB Electrostatic Tanimoto (ET pb) score, was utilized to further narrow down the hit compounds after they were aligned using ROCS [180]. Compounds with an ET_Comb score greater than 1 were selected for further structure-based virtual screening (SBVS).

2.1.4 Structure-based virtual screening

SBVS requires a target protein structure that will be employed in the virtual screening procedure. Molecular docking studies need a co-crystalize or homology model protein structure to perform SBVS. In this case, X-ray crystallographic structure of ER and our previously published GPER1 homology model were used in SBVS [174,181].

Binding site identification of ER and GPER-1 protein

After the selection of targeted protein or receptor structure, binding site identification is very crucial for successful SBVS. In this case, the X-rays crystallographic structure of ER in complex with 4 hydroxy tamoxifen was used to identify the binding sites in the ER, whereas the Atlas of Surface Topography of Proteins (CASTp) server was used to predict the putative binding sites in the homology model GPER-1 receptor [180,182].

Docking-based virtual screening

The molecular docking-based virtual screening technique can be utilized to further narrow down the top hits obtained by ROCS and EON screening to gain insight into the binding affinity with ERs. Preparation of target protein, ligand data set, and binding site analysis need to optimized before molecular docking and MD simulation.

Preparation of ER and GPER1 protein structures

In order to perform molecular docker, target proteins must be prepared. The pdb2receptor tool in OEDocking was used to create ER and GPER-1 structures, which were then optimized at a pH of 7.0. The binding site was also specified within 10 Å of the indicated active site prior to docking computation.

Validation of docking protocol Prior to molecular docking of a big data set against a target protein, the technique must be validated with a co-crystal ligand or a previously described ligand. Estradiol was redocked in the ER receptor before docking of a huge data set of compounds in the ER, and previously known GPER-1 ligands, were also docked before docking of natural product database chemicals in the case of GPER-1 docking. Estradiol was redocked in the ER receptor before docking of a huge data set of compounds in the ER, and previously known GPER-1 ligands, were also docked before docking of natural product database chemicals in the case of GPER-1 docking.

Preparation of ligand data set for docking-based virtual screening Prior to molecular docking of the ligand within the target protein, the ligand must be properly tuned. In this scenario, OMEGA2.5.1 was used to construct and optimize multiconformers for all ROCS and EON hits [180]. In the generation of conformers, the default settings of OMEGA were used (maximum 200 conformers per molecule).

Molecular docking calculation of natural products data set in ER and GPER1 Molecular docking of all virtual hits from the ROCS and EONS screenings was performed using the FRED v3.2.0 programme in OpenEye Scientific Software. After protocol refinement [183], ROCS and EON hits were docked using the optimized docking process. A maximum of 10 poses were generated for each compound, with the best-hits chosen based on the lowest Chemgauss4 score. The binding orientation of docked poses was visualized using Discovery Studio Visualizer and Chimera v1.1 [183].

2.2 Results

2.2.1 Retrospective validation of ligand- and structure-based virtual screening approach

We used a sequential ligand- and SBVS of a large database to find new polypharmacology modulators for ER and GPER-1. Our virtual screening approach was evaluated using retrospective statistical indicators. Data from directory of usable decoys, enhanced (DUD-E) (http://dude.docking.org/), DUD-E was used for retrospective validation because we needed active and decoy datasets. The active and decoy data sets for ER were collected from the DUD:E webpage; however, there is no GPER-1-specific active and decoy data set accessible at this time. DUD-E (http://dude.docking.org/) is an up-to-date directory of deployable decoys that includes actives and decoys for 102 different targets [19]. We generated 509 decoys based on the fifteen active GPER-1 ligands using DecoyFinder V 2.0. These decoys have the same physical qualities as actives, but they are chemically distinct in order to act as false positives [174,184].

E2 and G1's query models were built using their respective three-dimensional structures. Several conformers of E2 and G1 were generated using OMEGA 2.5 to mimic the cocrystallographic ligand. The optimal conformer of E2 and G1 was chosen based on the ShapeTanimoto, ColorTanimoto, and TanimotoCombo properties (Fig. 1). The selected conformer would be enough to distinguish the difference between active ER

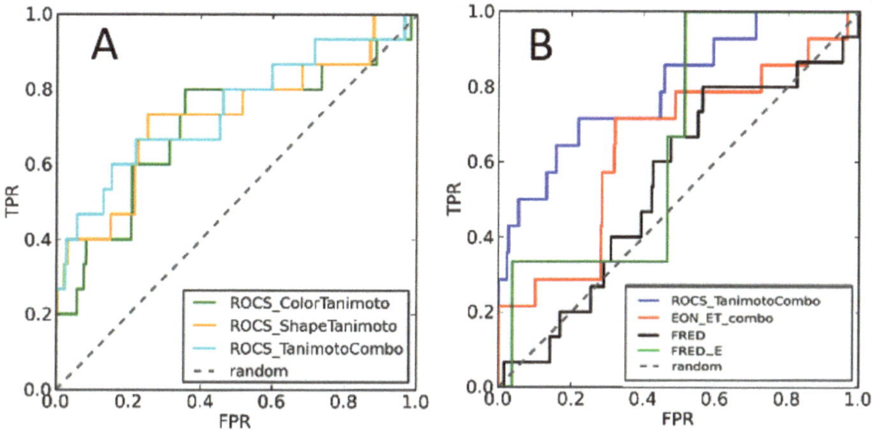

Fig. 1 ROC curves. (A) The TanimotoCombo, ColorTanimoto, and ShapeTanimoto of G-1 were used in the ROC-AUC virtual screening. (B) ROC-AUC plot comparison: TanimatoCombo score (blue), electrostatic potential (red), SBVS technique using the entire GPER-1 data set (black), and SBVS approach utilizing just selective GPER-1 ligands (red) (green).

and GPER-1 ligands and decoys. Different statistical matrices, such as the area under the curve (AUC) and the early EF can be used to evaluate the query model's usefulness in distinguishing between active and decoy ligands. In the present case, at 0.5%, 1%, and 2% rates, the overall performance of virtual screening of query model was evaluated using the AUC and the early EF.

Fig. 1 shows the ROC plots of conformer 1 for each LBVS parameter, with the fraction of active ER and GPER-1 ligand (true positives, TP) on the y-axis and the fraction of decoys (false-positives rate, FPR) on the *x*-axis. With an AUC of 0.797, the E2 and G1 conformer 1 had the best overall performance, suggesting that 79.7% of the ligands in the data set were ranked higher than the decoys. In terms of EF percentiles, we used EF 1% or below to evaluate our data. TanimotoCombo's EF 1% of conformer 1 was found to be 28.1. Matrix analysis for virtual screening based on EON ET, on the other hand, revealed a lower AUC of 0.649 and an EF1% of 21.4.

In the instance of SBVS, the AUC decreased to 0.546 with an EF 1 percent of 6.7, probably due to GPER-1's bigger active site, which allows it to interact with a wider range of molecular configurations. However, docking of only selected GPER-1 ligands (G1, G15, and G36) and their decoys increased SBVS statistical matrix AUC from 0.546 to 0.660, along with an increase in EF to 7.6 at a false-positive rate of 1% (Fig. 1).

Overall, the retrospective validation results backed up our method of sequentially screening database compounds with LBVS and then SBVS. The method is reliable for distinguishing between active and decoy E2 and GPER-1 ligands.

2.2.2 Ligand-based virtual screening (LBVS)

Shape-based virtual screening

Shape-based screening (SBS) has established itself as an important virtual screening technology. The method relies on the idea of the shape and electrostatic potential similarity to find novel molecules with comparable binding modes to the active site. The SBS is an effective technique for discovering and optimizing new inhibitors with excellent potency and selectivity [183,185]. Furthermore, SBS does not require a target 3D structure or a well-developed SAR model, which are both required to generate a credible pharmacophore model; instead, all that is required is a known active molecule as input.

ROCS was used to do the shape-based virtual screening. ROCS is a shape-based approach for analyzing molecular similarity quickly. E2 and G-1 (estrogen and GPER-1 selective and potent agonist) was chosen as the query component for the construction of the shape-based screening model after a thorough review of the literature for ER and GPER-1 ligands [186]. Fig. 2 shows the pharmacophoric characteristics of E2 and G-1. It has been assumed that screening hits with a molecular structure similar to E2 and G-1 would have high ER and GPER-1 regulation activity [174,185].

In case of E2 as a ROCS query model, eight diverse pharmacophore features were assigned. Among these two are hydrogen bond acceptor, two are hydrogen bond donor, while four were based on rings in E2. Moreover, in case of G1 as a query model, ten distinct pharmacophore characteristics were assigned. Among these ten features, five ring features were based on tetrahydro-3H-cyclopenta[*c*]quinoline and benzo[d][1,3]dioxole core. The three hydrogen bond acceptor features of the query model were given by the two oxygen atoms in the benzo[d][1,3]dioxole core and one oxygen atom in the acetophenone group. In addition, the amine and bromine (Br) each had a hydrogen-bond donor as well as a hydrophobic characteristic.

The resulting ROCS query model was then used to perform virtual screening on the NPASS natural product database. TanimotoCombo score (ROCS TC), which includes both ShapeTanimoto (ROCS ST) and Color-Tanimoto (ROCS CT), was used to assess the structural complementarity

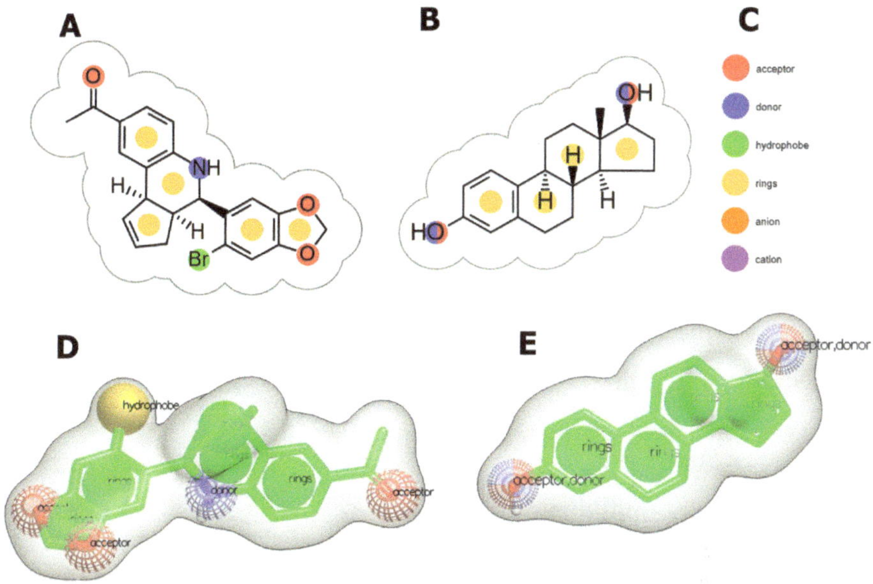

Fig. 2 Ligand-based pharmacophore feature of E2 (ER agonist) and G-1 (GPER agonist) as a query model. (A) and (B) illustrate the color-based pharmacophore feature of G-1 and E2, while (D) and (E) shows the shape-based pharmacophore feature of G-1 and E2. (C) describes the respective colors of each feature in color-based pharmacophore model.

between the template and the screened compounds. The top 5000 hits were kept for further in silico screening after shape-based virtual screening with ROCS TC. As shown in Fig. 3, the top hit compound had the greatest ROCS TC score of 1.861, while the bottom hit compound had the lowest ROCS TC score of 1.204.

Analyses of ROCS result by aligning the natural products compounds, and E2 query model calculates similarities such as volumes and chemical characteristics. A Default TanimotoCombo (TC) score ranging from 0 to 2 is used to analyze and illustrates the similarity. A TanimotoCombo score close to 2 indicates that molecules have an excellent shape and chemical feature match, whereas a number close to 0 indicates that molecules have poor shape and chemical feature dissimilarities. In case of E2 ROCS analysis, TC was found to be in the range of 0.4–1.80 as shown in Fig. 3. While in case of G-1 ROCS analysis, TC was found to be in the range of 0.2–0.9.

Electrostatic potential similarity

During EON screening, a single lowest-energy conformer of G-1 was chosen as a query model and was utilized for all electrostatic potential

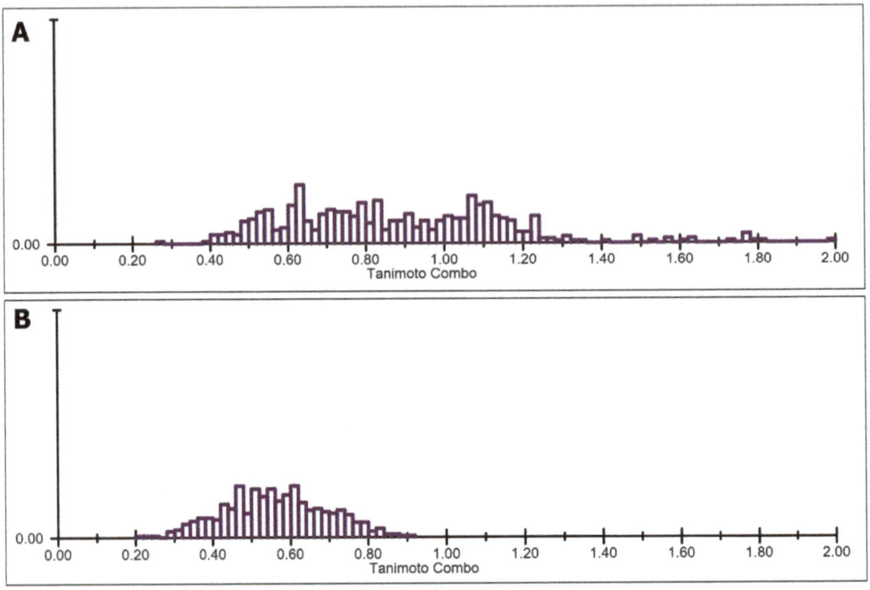

Fig. 3 (A) A histogram illustration of ROCS TanimotoCombo (ROCS TC) score distribution for the top 500 hits based on E2. (B) A histogram illustration of ROCS TanimotoCombo (ROCS TC) score distribution for the top 500 hits based on G-1.

comparisons with ROCS hits compounds. The EON Combo score, which is a combination of ShapeTanimoto (ST) and PB Electrostatic Tanimoto (ET pb), was used to rank the ligands. The EON map of G-1 and E2 is shown in Fig. 4.

2.2.3 Structure base virtual screening using receptor structure

Identification of receptor-binding sites

Binding site of ER was identified using the cocrystalized ligand 4-hydroxytamoxifen (4-OHT) as shown in Fig. 5.

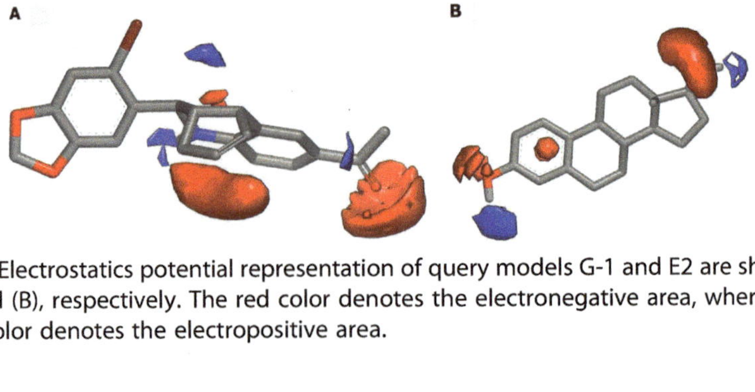

Fig. 4 Electrostatics potential representation of query models G-1 and E2 are shown in (A) and (B), respectively. The red color denotes the electronegative area, whereas the blue color denotes the electropositive area.

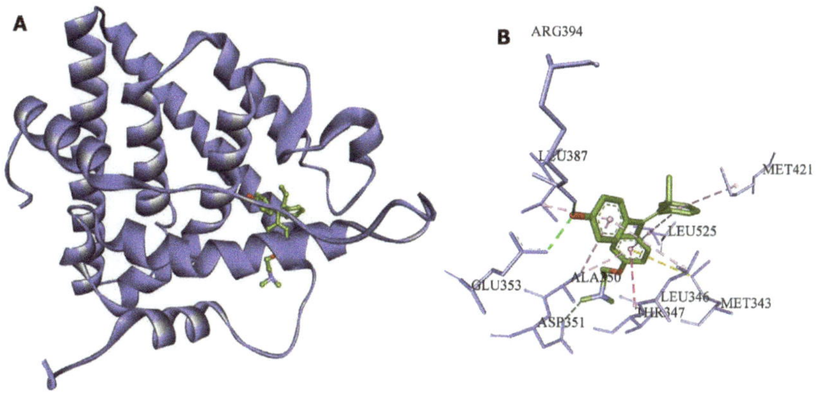

Fig. 5 4-Hydroxytmoxefin-binding interactions with ER. Hydrogen bonds, hydrophobic bonds, and electrostatic bonds are shown in green, pink, and yellow dotted lines, respectively. The interacting residues of ER are depicted in magenta-colored sticks.

In case of GPER1-binding site, our previously reported homology model was used for identification of active pocket. For active pocket identification, CASTp (computed Atlas of Surface Topography of Proteins) server was used to predict the active pocket. CASTp analysis predict 40 different catalytic sites in the GPER-1. Based on solvent accessible (SA) area the preeminent active site was fund with SAS of 1477.1 and a volume of 1396.0. All other predicted binding sites had relatively lower SA lower than 140. The best predicted binding has 73 amino acid residues. Likewise, the topological regions of these chosen amino acid residues were identified for future docking investigations. Table 1 enlists the detailed analysis of amino acid residues involved in making active site of GPER-1.

2.2.4 Docking-based virtual screening

After prerequisite preparation and selectin of binding site, molecular docking of all ROCS and EON hits compounds were executed using FRED docking software. The FRED programme has a strong track record of applicability in structure-based drug development. Huabin Hu et al. have determined FRED (Chemgauss4 score) as the best docking score function among three alternative docking score functions [186]. A total of 200 conformers per ligand were created and used as input. Because ER and GPER-1 are two distinct class of ERs involved in breast cancer. So, these were selected to identify new ER modulator having affinity with ER and GPER-1. Redocking of 4OHT within the active site has revealed different binding interaction with amino acid residue of ER as shown in Table 2.

Table 1 CASTp projected the solvent accessible (SA) area, volume, and interacting amino acid residue in the active site.

Active site	Area (SA)	Volume (SA)	Interacting amino acid residues within the active pocket of GPER-1
1	1477.1	1396.0	Leu49, Ser50, His52, Gln53, Gln54, Ile57, Gly58, Leu61, Ser62, Tyr65, Phe68, Leu108, Val109, Asp111, Ser112, Ile114, Glu115, Val116, Asn118, Leu119, His120, Arg122, Tyr123, Cys130, Met133, Ser134, Leu137, Gln138, Asn140, Met141, Ser144, Val145, Pro192, Val196, His200, Asp202, Ala204, Cys205, Phe206,Cys207, Phe208, Asp210, Arg212, Glu213, Val214, Gln215, Trp216, Glu218, Val219, Gly222, Phe223, Ile224, Phe268, Phe269, Trp272, Leu273, Glu275, Asn276, Phe278, Ile279, Ser280, His282, Leu283, Arg286, Phe298, His300, Ala301, His302, Leu304, Thr305, Asn310, Leu311, Phe314, Asn316, Ser317

Table 2 Detailed binding interaction of 4-hydroxytamoxefin with amino acid residue of ER.

Category of bond	Types of bond	Amino acid residue of ER involved in binding interaction	Moiety of 4OHT involved in binding interaction
Hydrogen bond	Conventional Hydrogen Bond	A:ARG394:NH2	A:OHT600:O4
Hydrogen bond	Conventional Hydrogen Bond	A:GLU353:OE2	A:OHT600:O4
Hydrogen bond	Carbon Hydrogen Bond	A:ASP351:OD1	A:OHT600:C25
Other	Pi-Sulfur	A:MET343:SD	A:OHT600
Hydrophobic	Amide-Pi Stacked	A:LEU346:C,O; THR347:N	A:OHT600
Hydrophobic	Pi-Alkyl	A:MET421	A:OHT600
Hydrophobic	Pi-Alkyl	A:LEU525	A:OHT600
Hydrophobic	Pi-Alkyl	A:LEU346	A:OHT600
Hydrophobic	Pi-Alkyl	A:ALA350	A:OHT600
Hydrophobic	Pi-Alkyl	A:LEU387	A:OHT600
Hydrophobic	Pi-Alkyl	A:ALA350	A:OHT600
Hydrophobic	Pi-Alkyl	A:LEU525	A:OHT600

Table 3 Detailed binding interaction of G-1 with amino acid residue of GPER-1.

Category of bonding	Types of bond	Amino acid residue of GPER involved in binding interaction	Moiety of G-1 involved in binding interaction
Hydrogen bond	Conventional Hydrogen Bond	A:ASN276:HD22	G-1:O23
Hydrogen bond	Conventional Hydrogen Bond	A:GLU218:OE1	G-1:H44
Hydrogen bond	Carbon Hydrogen Bond	A:ASP210:OD2	G-1:H37
Electrostatic	Pi-Anion	A:GLU218:OE2	G-1
Hydrogen bond	Pi-Donor Hydrogen Bond	A:GLN138:HE22	G-1
Hydrophobic	Alkyl	A:ILE279	G-1
Hydrophobic	Alkyl	A:LEU137	G-1:Br26
Hydrophobic	Alkyl	A:MET141	G-1:Br26
Hydrophobic	Pi-Alkyl	A:MET141	G-1
Hydrophobic	Pi-Alkyl	A:ILE279	G-1

In case of GPER-1, docking, G-1 was docked using the same methodology as stated in above method portion. Docking of G-1 within the active site of GPER-1 has revealed different binding interaction with amino acid residue of GPER as shown in Table 3 and Fig. 6.

Virtual screening of NPASS data set compounds against ER and GPER-1 revealed many compounds with significant binding affinity and interactions. Details of top 5 compounds common against both ER (ER and GPER-1) are shown in Table 4 and Figs. 7 and 8.

Top 5 five hits common in both ER and GPER revealed using the ligand and structure-based virtual screening approach. These potential polypharmacology hit compounds were obtained after narrow downing the large database of NPASS which contained more than 35,000 natural product compounds from various sources. The ligand-based VS approaches using ROCS and EONS narrowed down this large database into 5000 compounds which were further narrow down to 500 using structure-based VS approach against ER and GPER. Among these 500 top hits, the common hit that have affinity with ER and GPER were curated and selected as potential

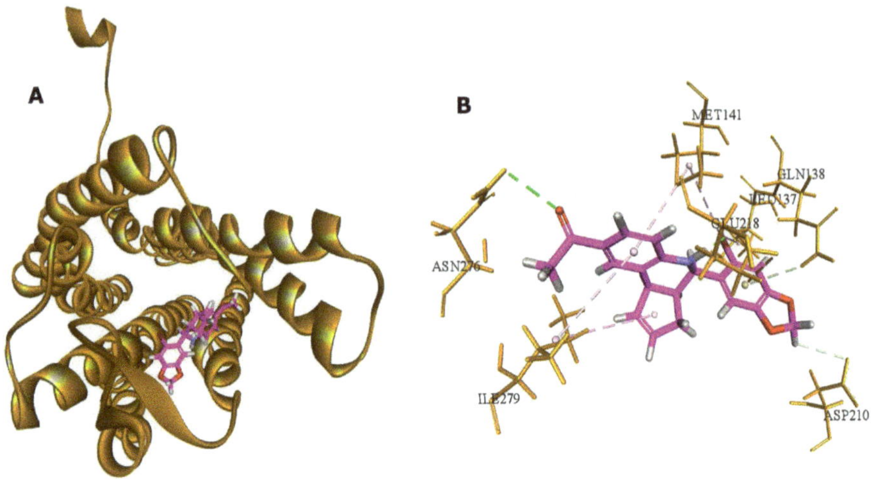

Fig. 6 G-1-binding interactions with GPER. Hydrogen bonds, hydrophobic bonds, and electrostatic bonds are shown in green, pink, and yellow dotted lines, respectively. The interacting residues of ER are depicted in magenta color sticks.

Table 4 ChemGuass4 Score of top 5 common hit compounds as polypharmacology agent against ER and GPER.

Natural product compound ID	Chemical structure	CHEMGUASS4 score	
		ER	**GPER**
NPC11216	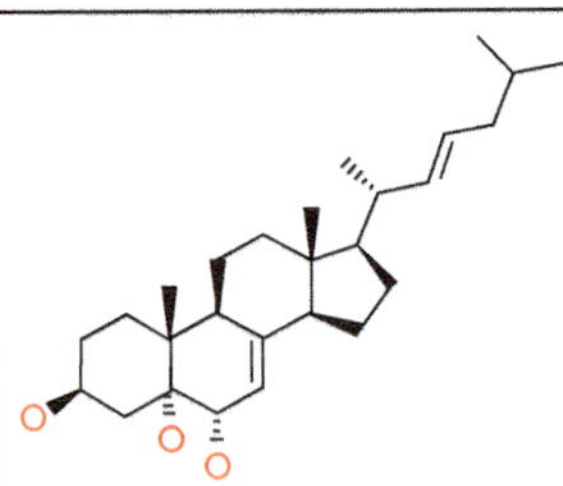	−10.41	−12.79
NPC203113	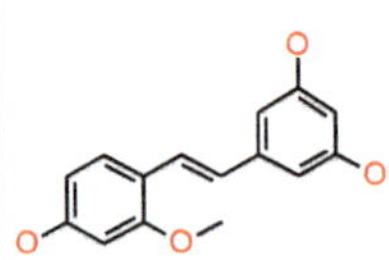	−12.17	−11.02
NPC214138	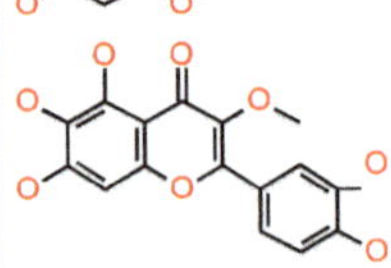	−12.90	−11.00
NPC474200	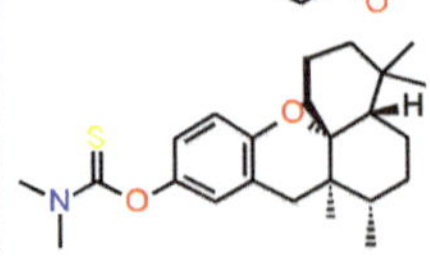	−14.46	−10.58
NPC478162	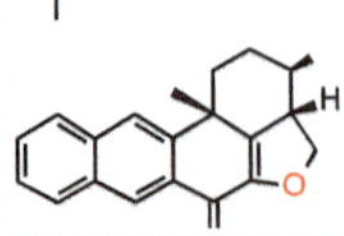	−11.37	−10.24

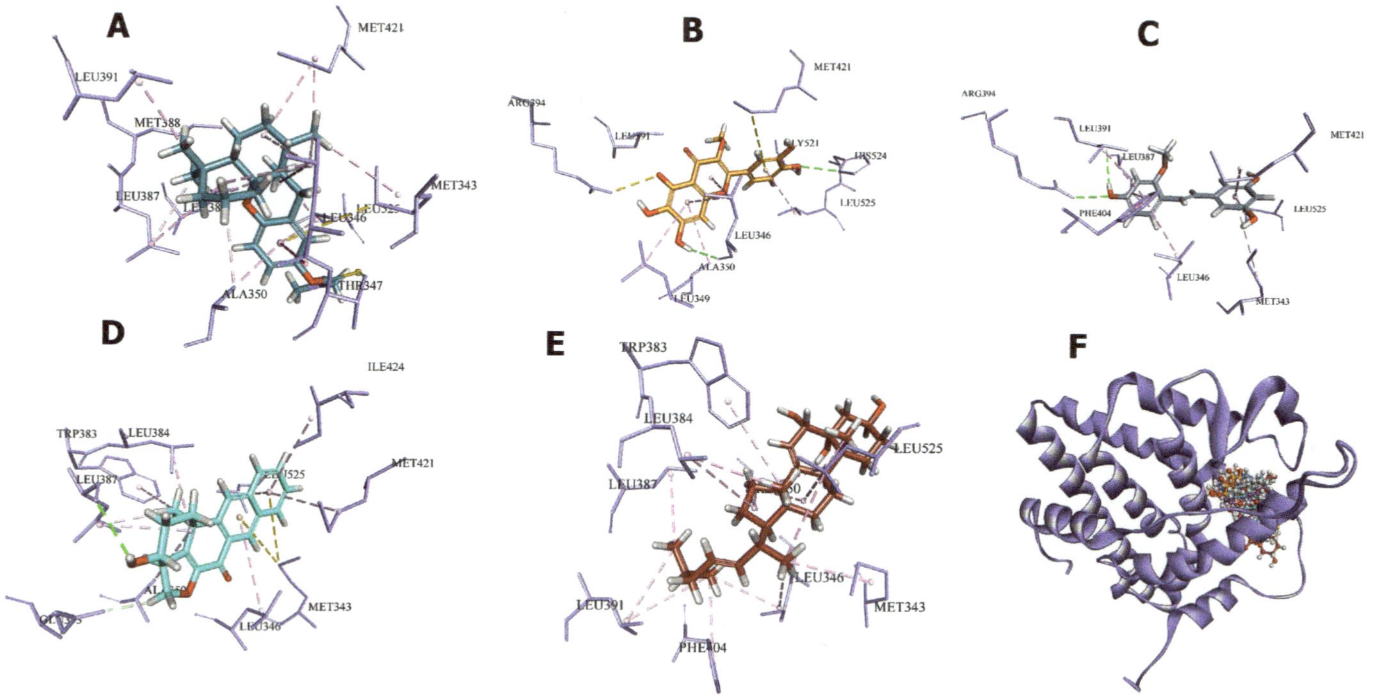

Fig. 7 Binding interaction of amino acid residue of ER and top 5 common hit compounds as polypharmacology agent against ER and GPER.

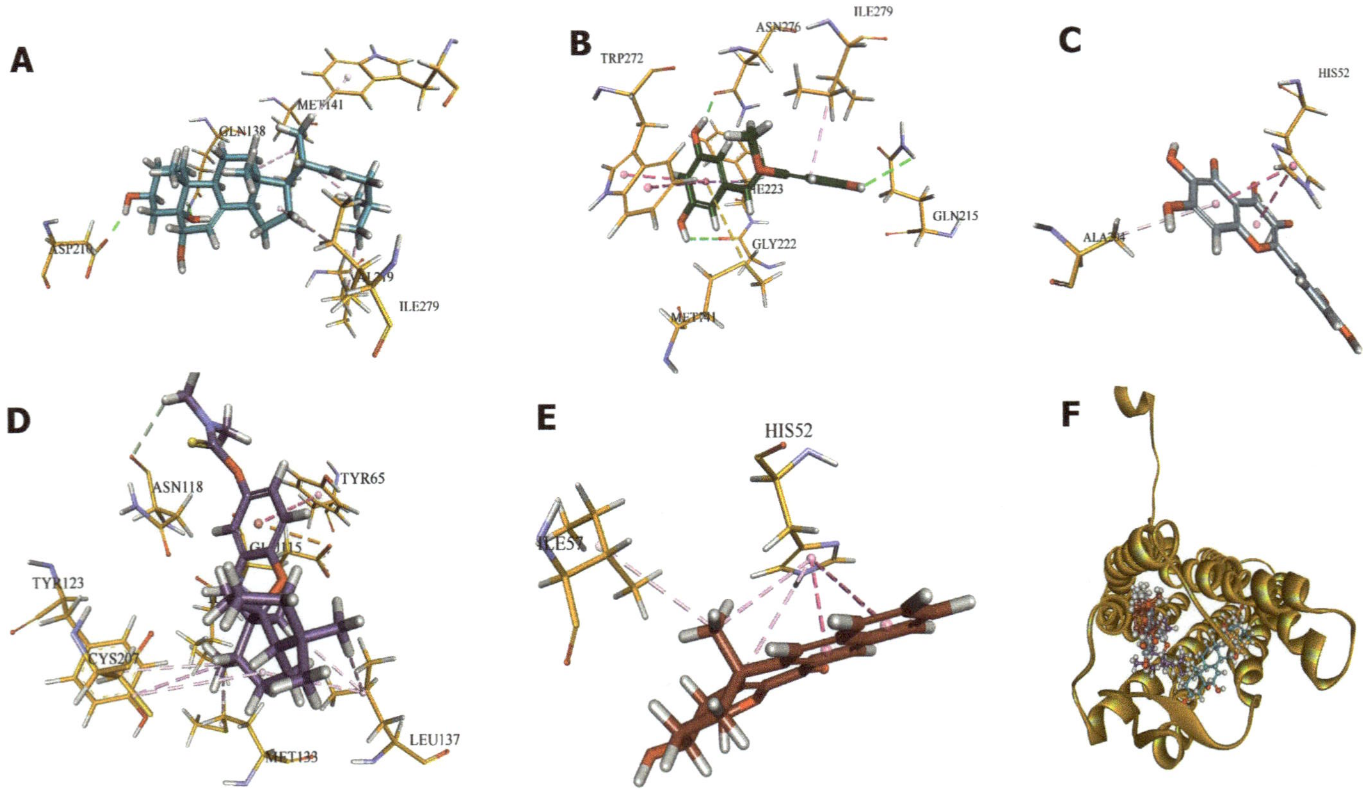

Fig. 8 Binding interaction of amino acid residue of GPER and top 5 common hit compounds as polypharmacology agent against ER and GPER.

polypharmacology compounds. Compound code in the database, chemical structures, and FRED Chemgauss4 score scores of top five best-identified scaffolds are shown in Table 4 and illustration of their binding with respective target are shown in Figs. 7 and 8.

References

[1] Y.-S. Sun, et al., Risk factors and preventions of breast cancer, Int. J. Biol. Sci. 13 (11) (2017) 1387.
[2] O.J. Scully, et al., Breast cancer metastasis, Cancer Genomics Proteomics 9 (5) (2012) 311–320.
[3] C. Jin, et al., Effect of substitution on the aniline moiety of the GPR88 agonist 2-PCCA: synthesis, structure-activity relationships, and molecular modeling studies, ACS Chem. Nerosci. 7 (10) (2016) 1418–1432.
[4] X. Lin, et al., A review on applications of computational methods in drug screening and design, Molecules 25 (2020) 1375, https://doi.org/10.3390/molecules25061375.
[5] A. Ganeshpurkar, et al., Protein-protein interactions and aggregation inhibitors in Alzheimer's disease, Curr. Top. Med. Chem. 19 (7) (2019) 501–533.
[6] K. Zeilinger, et al., Cell sources for in vitro human liver cell culture models, Exp. Biol. Med. 241 (15) (2016) 1684–1698.
[7] A. Rezaei Kolahchi, et al., Microfluidic-based multi-organ platforms for drug discovery, Micromachines 7 (9) (2016) 162.
[8] L.H. Santos, et al., Computational drug design strategies applied to the modelling of human immunodeficiency virus-1 reverse transcriptase inhibitors, Mem. Inst. Oswaldo Cruz 110 (7) (2015) 847–864.
[9] D.D. Wang, et al., Computationally predicting binding affinity in protein–ligand complexes: free energy-based simulations and machine learning-based scoring functions, Brief. Bioinform. 22 (3) (2021) bbaa107.
[10] S.M. McKinney, et al., International evaluation of an AI system for breast cancer screening, Nature 577 (7788) (2020) 89–94.
[11] N.F. Boyd, et al., Breast tissue composition and susceptibility to breast cancer, J. Natl. Cancer Inst. 102 (16) (2010) 1224–1237.
[12] K. Zeng, et al., The pro-metastasis effect of circANKS1B in breast cancer, Mol. Cancer 17 (1) (2018) 1–19.
[13] P.J. Stephens, et al., The landscape of cancer genes and mutational processes in breast cancer, Nature 486 (7403) (2012) 400–404.
[14] L. Fan, et al., Breast cancer in China, Lancet Oncol. 15 (7) (2014) e279–e289.
[15] M.J. Higgins, J. Baselga, Targeted therapies for breast cancer, J. Clin. Invest. 121 (10) (2011) 3797–3803.
[16] A.G. Waks, E.P. Winer, Breast cancer treatment: a review, JAMA 321 (3) (2019) 288–300.
[17] S. Libson, M. Lippman, A review of clinical aspects of breast cancer, Int. Rev. Psychiatry 26 (1) (2014) 4–15.
[18] A. Prat, C.M. Perou, Deconstructing the molecular portraits of breast cancer, Mol. Oncol. 5 (1) (2011) 5–23.
[19] C. Downs-Holmes, P. Silverman, Breast cancer: overview & updates, Nurse Pract. 36 (12) (2011) 20–26.
[20] J.J. Sariego, Breast cancer in the young patient, Am. Surg. 76 (12) (2010) 1397–1400.
[21] W.D. Foulkes, I.E. Smith, et al., Triple-negative breast cancer, N. Engl. J. Med. 363 (20) (2010) 1938–1948.

[22] A.G. Waks, et al., Breast cancer treatment, JAMA 321 (3) (2019) 316.
[23] D. Zardavas, et al., Clinical management of breast cancer heterogeneity, Nat. Rev. Clin. Oncol. 12 (7) (2015) 381–394.
[24] X. Dai, et al., Breast cancer cell line classification and its relevance with breast tumor subtyping, J. Cancer 8 (16) (2017) 3131.
[25] L. Wang, Early diagnosis of breast cancer, Sensors 17 (7) (2017) 1572.
[26] E.S. McDonald, et al., Clinical diagnosis and management of breast cancer, J. Nucl. Med. 57 (Suppl. 1) (2016) 9S–16S.
[27] R. Xiong, et al., Novel selective estrogen receptor downregulators (SERDs) developed against treatment-resistant breast cancer, J. Med. Chem. 60 (4) (2017) 1325–1342.
[28] H.K. Patel, et al., Selective estrogen receptor modulators (SERMs) and selective estrogen receptor degraders (SERDs) in cancer treatment, Pharmacol. Ther. 186 (2018) 1–24.
[29] S. He, et al., 27-Hydroxycholesterol, an endogenous selective estrogen receptor modulator, Maturitas 104 (2017) 29–35.
[30] F. Li, et al., The selective estrogen receptor modulators in breast cancer prevention, Cancer Chemother. Pharmacol. 77 (5) (2016) 895–903.
[31] J.H. Pickar, et al., Selective estrogen receptor modulators and the combination therapy conjugated estrogens/bazedoxifene: a review of effects on the breast, Post Reprod. Health 21 (3) (2015) 112–121.
[32] K. An, Selective estrogen receptor modulators, Asian Spine J. 10 (4) (2016) 787.
[33] G.S. Tria, et al., Discovery of LSZ102, a potent, orally bioavailable selective estrogen receptor degrader (SERD) for the treatment of estrogen receptor positive breast cancer, J. Med. Chem. 61 (7) (2018) 2837–2864.
[34] A.J. Ellis, et al., Selective estrogen receptor modulators in clinical practice: a safety overview, Expert Opin. Drug Saf. 14 (6) (2015) 921–934.
[35] S.E. Wardell, et al., Evaluation of the pharmacological activities of RAD1901, a selective estrogen receptor degrader, Endocr. Relat. Cancer 22 (5) (2015) 713–724.
[36] S.E. Wardell, et al., Efficacy of SERD/SERM Hybrid-CDK4/6 inhibitor combinations in models of endocrine therapy–resistant breast cancer, Clin. Cancer Res. 21 (22) (2015) 5121–5130.
[37] C. Holmberg, et al., NRG oncology/national surgical adjuvant breast and bowel project decision-making project-1 results: decision making in breast cancer risk reduction, Cancer Prev. Res. 10 (11) (2017) 625–634.
[38] P. Fan, New insights into acquired endocrine resistance of breast cancer, Cancer Drug Resist. 2 (2019) 198.
[39] B. Ljepoja, et al., MiRNA-27a sensitizes breast cancer cells to treatment with selective estrogen receptor modulators, Breast 43 (2019) 31–38.
[40] J. Leignadier, et al., Improving the efficacy of hormone therapy in breast cancer: the role of cholesterol metabolism in SERM-mediated autophagy, cell differentiation and death, Biochem. Pharmacol. 144 (2017) 18–28.
[41] V.G. Vogel, Ongoing data from the breast cancer prevention trials: opportunity for breast cancer risk reduction, BMC Med. 13 (1) (2015) 1–4.
[42] Y.-J. Yang, et al., Clinical significance of fatty liver disease induced by tamoxifen and toremifene in breast cancer patients, Breast 28 (2016) 67–72.
[43] M.A. Thorat, et al., Breast cancer prevention in high-risk women, Best Pract. Res. Clin. Obstet. Gynaecol. 65 (2020) 18–31.
[44] N. Thongon, et al., Selective estrogen receptor modulator (SERM)-like activities of diarylheptanoid, a phytoestrogen from curcuma comosa, in breast cancer cells, pre-osteoblast cells, and rat uterine tissues, J. Agric. Food Chem. 65 (17) (2017) 3490–3496.
[45] T. Traboulsi, et al., Antiestrogens: structure-activity relationships and use in breast cancer treatment, J. Mol. Endocrinol. 58 (1) (2016) R15.

[46] C.M. Vachon, et al., A polygenic risk score for breast cancer in women receiving tamoxifen or raloxifene on NSABP P-1 and P-2, Breast Cancer Res. Treat. 149 (2) (2015) 517–523.
[47] B. Sharma, et al., Diastereoselective approach to rationally design tetrahydro-β-carboline–isatin conjugates as potential SERMs against breast cancer, RSC Adv. 9 (17) (2019) 9809–9819.
[48] V.G. Vogel, Breast cancer risk reduction: notable achievements and remaining challenges, Breast J. 26 (1) (2020) 86–91.
[49] G. Luo, et al., Design, synthesis, biological evaluation and molecular docking studies of novel 3-aryl-4-anilino-2H-chromen-2-one derivatives targeting ERα as anti-breast cancer agents, Bioorg. Med. Chem. Lett. 27 (12) (2017) 2668–2673.
[50] B. Sharma, et al., Design, synthesis, antiproliferative evaluation, and molecular docking studies of N-(3-hydroxyindole)-appended β-carbolines/tetrahydro-β-carbolines targeting triple-negative and non-triple-negative breast cancer, ACS Omega 5 (45) (2020) 28907–28917.
[51] Y. Suryani, et al., Insilico docking studies of daidzeion compounds as selective estrogen receptor modulator (SERMS) breast cancer, in: MATEC Web Conferences, EDP Sciences, 2018.
[52] S. Lakshmi, et al., Comparative differential cytotoxicity of clinically used SERMs in human cancer lines of different origin and its predictive molecular docking studies of key target genes involved in cancer progression and treatment responses, Curr. Res. Pharm. Drug Discov. (2021) 100080.
[53] G. Kaur, et al., Design, synthesis, and anti-breast cancer evaluation of new triarylethylene analogs bearing short alkyl-and polar amino-/amido-ethyl chains, Bioorg. Med. Chem. Lett. 26 (8) (2016) 1963–1969.
[54] F.Z. Karadayi, et al., Design, synthesis, anticancer activity, molecular docking and ADME studies of novel methylsulfonyl indole-benzimidazoles in comparison with ethylsulfonyl counterparts, New J. Chem. 45 (20) (2021) 9010–9019.
[55] M. Muchtaridi, et al., Molecular docking and 3D-pharmacophore modeling to study the interactions of Chalcone derivatives with estrogen receptor alpha, Pharmaceuticals 10 (4) (2017) 81.
[56] A. Khan, et al., Antinociceptive properties of 25-methoxy hispidol A, a triterpinoid isolated from Poncirus trifoliata (Rutaceae) through inhibition of NF-κB signalling in mice, Phytother. Res. 33 (2) (2019) 327–341.
[57] H. Yuseran, et al., Molecular docking of genistein on estrogen receptors, promoter region of BCLX, caspase-3, Ki-67, cyclin D1, and telomere activity, J. Taibah Univ. Medical Sci. 14 (1) (2019) 79–87.
[58] R. Afridi, et al., Anti-hyperalgesic properties of a flavanone derivative Poncirin in acute and chronic inflammatory pain models in mice, BMC Pharmacol. Toxicol. 20 (1) (2019) 1–16.
[59] N.E. Thomford, et al., Natural products for drug discovery in the 21st century: innovations for novel drug discovery, Int. J. Mol. Sci. 19 (6) (2018) 1578.
[60] N. Herfindo, et al., Synthesis, antiproliferative activity and molecular docking studies of 1, 3, 5-triaryl pyrazole compound as estrogen α receptor inhibitor targeting MCF-7 cells line, Molekul 15 (1) (2020) 18–25.
[61] J. Quackenbush, et al., Computational analysis of microarray data, Nat. Rev. Genet. 2 (6) (2001) 418–427.
[62] J. Fang, et al., In silico polypharmacology of natural products, Brief. Bioinform. 19 (6) (2018) 1153–1171.
[63] J. Fang, et al., Quantitative and systems pharmacology. 1. In silico prediction of drug–target interactions of natural products enables new targeted cancer therapy, J. Chem. Inf. Model. 57 (11) (2017) 2657–2671.

[64] H. Ali, et al., Attenuation of LPS-induced acute lung injury by continentalic acid in rodents through inhibition of inflammatory mediators correlates with increased Nrf2 protein expression, BMC Pharmacol. Toxicol. 21 (1) (2020) 1–14.
[65] E. Sana, et al., Topical delivery of curcumin-loaded transfersomes gel ameliorated rheumatoid arthritis by inhibiting NF-κβ pathway, Nanomedicine 16 (10) (2021) 819–837.
[66] E.A. Crane, et al., Capturing biological activity in natural product fragments by chemical synthesis, Angew. Chem. 55 (12) (2016) 3882–3902.
[67] M. Ervina, et al., In silico estrogen receptor alpha antagonist studies and toxicity prediction of Melia azedarach leaves bioactive ethyl acetate fraction, J. Adv. Pharm. Technol. Res. 12 (3) (2021) 236–241.
[68] A. Yang, et al., MYC inhibition depletes cancer stem-like cells in triple-negative breast cancer, Cancer Res. 77 (23) (2017) 6641–6650.
[69] E. Persi, et al., Systems analysis of intracellular pH vulnerabilities for cancer therapy, Nat. Commun. 9 (1) (2018) 1–11.
[70] M. Suleman, et al., Mutational landscape of pirin and elucidation of the impact of most detrimental missense variants that accelerate the breast cancer pathways: a computational modelling study, Front. Mol. Biosci. 8 (2021).
[71] R.M. Meyers, et al., Computational correction of copy number effect improves specificity of CRISPR–Cas9 essentiality screens in cancer cells, Nat. Genet. 49 (12) (2017) 1779–1784.
[72] X. Zhang, et al., Breast cancer neoantigens can induce CD8+ T-cell responses and antitumor immunity, Cancer Immunol. Res. 5 (7) (2017) 516–523.
[73] W.W. Du, et al., A circular RNA circ-DNMT1 enhances breast cancer progression by activating autophagy, Oncogene 37 (44) (2018) 5829–5842.
[74] J. Ma, et al., The therapeutic significance of mutational signatures from DNA repair deficiency in cancer, Nat. Commun. 9 (1) (2018) 1–12.
[75] L.J. Smith, et al., Diels–Alder click-cross-linked hydrogels with increased reactivity enable 3D cell encapsulation, Biomacromolecules 19 (3) (2018) 926–935.
[76] A.A. Elfiky, Natural products may interfere with SARS-CoV-2 attachment to the host cell, J. Biomol. Struct. Dyn. 39 (9) (2021) 3194–3203.
[77] H. Alshetaiwi, et al., Defining the emergence of myeloid-derived suppressor cells in breast cancer using single-cell transcriptomics, Sci. Immunol. 5 (44) (2020).
[78] A. Ali, et al., Steroidal alkaloids efficient aromatase inhibitors with potential for the treatment of postmenopausal breast cancer, Chem. Biol. Drug Des. 95 (2) (2020) 233–239.
[79] F. Xing, et al., Activation of the c-Met pathway mobilizes an inflammatory network in the brain microenvironment to promote brain metastasis of breast cancer, Cancer Res. 76 (17) (2016) 4970–4980.
[80] A.E. Modell, et al., Systematic targeting of protein–protein interactions, Trends Pharmacol. Sci. 37 (8) (2016) 702–713.
[81] A. Rayan, et al., Nature is the best source of anticancer drugs: indexing natural products for their anticancer bioactivity, PLoS One 12 (11) (2017), e0187925.
[82] A.G. Atanasov, et al., Natural products in drug discovery: advances and opportunities, Nat. Rev. Drug Discov. 20 (3) (2021) 200–216.
[83] A. Ashworth, et al., Synthetic lethal therapies for cancer: what's next after PARP inhibitors? Nat. Rev. Clin. Oncol. 15 (9) (2018) 564–576.
[84] B. Zhang, et al., Matrine is identified as a novel macropinocytosis inducer by a network target approach, Front. Pharmacol. 9 (2018) 10.
[85] J.N. Nwodo, et al., Exploring cancer therapeutics with natural products from African medicinal plants, part II: alkaloids, terpenoids and flavonoids, Anticancer Agents Med Chem. 16 (1) (2016) 108–127.

[86] C.P. Bracken, et al., A network-biology perspective of microRNA function and dysfunction in cancer, Nat. Rev. Genet. 17 (12) (2016) 719–732.
[87] R.S. Lee, et al., A curated mammography data set for use in computer-aided detection and diagnosis research, Sci. Data 4 (1) (2017) 1–9.
[88] F. Cheng, et al., Systems biology-based investigation of cellular antiviral drug targets identified by gene-trap insertional mutagenesis, PLoS Comput. Biol. 12 (9) (2016), e1005074.
[89] Z. Zhou, et al., Applications of network pharmacology in traditional Chinese medicine research, BMC Complement. Altern. Med. (2020).
[90] Y.-H. Bi, et al., Antitumor mechanisms of curcumae rhizoma based on network pharmacology, Evid. Based Complement. Alternat. Med. (2018).
[91] J. Zhang, et al., Uncovering the pharmacological mechanism of Chaibei Zhixian decoction on epilepsy by network pharmacology analysis, Evid. Based Complement. Alternat. Med. (2019).
[92] K. Yang, et al., Exploring the pharmacological mechanism of Danzhi Xiaoyao powder on ER-positive breast cancer by a network pharmacology approach, Evid. Based Complement. Alternat. Med. (2018).
[93] O.A. Raevsky, et al., Applications of multi-target computer-aided methodologies in molecular design of CNS drugs, Curr. Med. Chem. 25 (39) (2018) 5293–5314.
[94] X. Yang, et al., Study on the multitarget mechanism and key active ingredients of herba siegesbeckiae and volatile oil against rheumatoid arthritis based on network pharmacology, Evid. Based Complement. Alternat. Med. (2019).
[95] X. Lin, et al., A review on applications of computational methods in drug screening and design, Molecules 25 (6) (2020) 1375.
[96] Y.-L. Wang, et al., Prediction of quality markers of traditional Chinese medicines based on network pharmacology, Chin. Herb. Med. 11 (4) (2019) 349–356.
[97] V. Bezhentsev, et al., Identification of potential drug targets for treatment of refractory epilepsy using network pharmacology, J. Bioinform. Comput. Biol. 16 (01) (2018) 1840002.
[98] Z. Wu, et al., SDTNBI: an integrated network and chemoinformatics tool for systematic prediction of drug–target interactions and drug repositioning, Brief. Bioinform. 18 (2) (2017) 333–347.
[99] S. Ekins, The next era: deep learning in pharmaceutical research, Pharm. Res. 33 (11) (2016) 2594–2603.
[100] Y.B. Laskar, et al., Hibiscus sabdariffa anthocyanins are potential modulators of estrogen receptor alpha activity with favourable toxicology: a computational analysis using molecular docking, ADME/Tox prediction, 2D/3D QSAR and molecular dynamics simulation, J. Biomol. Struct. Dyn. (2021) 1–23.
[101] S. Alam, et al., 3D-QSAR studies on maslinic acid analogs for anticancer activity against breast cancer cell line MCF-7, Sci. Rep. 7 (1) (2017) 1–13.
[102] L. Abdel-Ilah, et al., Applications of QSAR study in drug design, Int. J. Eng. Res. Technol. 6 (06) (2017).
[103] L. Simon, et al., In silico drug-designing studies on flavanoids as anticolon cancer agents: pharmacophore mapping, molecular docking, and Monte Carlo method-based QSAR modeling, Interdiscip. Sci. 9 (3) (2017) 445–458.
[104] M.A.V. Hasanloei, et al., A combined Fisher and Laplacian score for feature selection in QSAR based drug design using compounds with known and unknown activities, J. Comput. Aided Mol. Des. 32 (2) (2018) 375–384.
[105] G. Lambrinidis, et al., Challenges with multi-objective QSAR in drug discovery, Expert Opin. Drug Discovery 13 (9) (2018) 851–859.
[106] C. Fang, et al., Receptor-based 3D-QSAR in drug design: methods and applications in kinase studies, Curr. Top. Med. Chem. 16 (13) (2016) 1463–1477.

[107] K. Roy, Advances in QSAR Modeling: Applications in Pharmaceutical, Chemical, Food, Agricultural and Environmental Sciences, Springer, Cham, Switzerland, 2017.
[108] Danishuddin, A.U. Khan, Descriptors and their selection methods in QSAR analysis: paradigm for drug design, Drug Discov. Today 21 (8) (2016) 1291–1302.
[109] F. Ghasemi, et al., Neural network and deep-learning algorithms used in QSAR studies: merits and drawbacks, Drug Discov. Today 23 (10) (2018) 1784–1790.
[110] T. Usha, et al., Recent updates on computer-aided drug discovery: time for a paradigm shift, Curr. Top. Med. Chem. 17 (30) (2017) 3296–3307.
[111] S. Sharma, et al., Recent trends in QSAR in modelling of drug-protein and protein-protein interactions, Comb. Chem. High Throughput Screen. 24 (7) (2021) 1031–1041.
[112] B.J. Neves, et al., QSAR-based virtual screening: advances and applications in drug discovery, Front. Pharmacol. 9 (2018) 1275.
[113] I. Olier, et al., Meta-QSAR: a large-scale application of meta-learning to drug design and discovery, Mach. Learn. 107 (1) (2018) 285–311.
[114] M. Zivkovic, et al., The application of the combination of Monte Carlo optimization method based QSAR modeling and molecular docking in drug design and development, Mini Rev. Med. Chem. 20 (14) (2020) 1389–1402.
[115] A.A. Toropov, et al., QSPR/QSAR: state-of-art, weirdness, the future, Molecules 25 (6) (2020) 1292.
[116] E.N. Muratov, et al., QSAR without borders, Chem. Soc. Rev. 49 (11) (2020) 3525–3564.
[117] K. Nikolic, et al., Drug design for CNS diseases: polypharmacological profiling of compounds using cheminformatic, 3D-QSAR and virtual screening methodologies, Front. Neurosci. 10 (2016) 265.
[118] H. Haghshenas, et al., Developing a variation of 3D-QSAR/MD method in drug design, J. Comput. Chem. 42 (13) (2021) 917–929.
[119] P.P. Kyaw Zin, et al., Benchmarking 2D/3D/MD-QSAR models for imatinib derivatives: how far can we predict? J. Chem. Inf. Model. 60 (7) (2020) 3342–3360.
[120] S. Ahamad, et al., Designing of phenol-based β– carbonic anhydrase1 inhibitors through QSAR, molecular docking, and MD simulation approach, 3 Biotech 8 (5) (2018) 1–18.
[121] H. Tandon, et al., A concise review on the significance of QSAR in drug design, Chem. Biomol. Eng. 4 (4) (2019) 45–51.
[122] Singh, S.P., et al., QSAR-based drug designing studies on HIV-1 integrase inhibitors. Netw. Model. Anal. Health Inform. Bioinform. 5(1): p. 1-11.
[123] S. Keretsu, et al., Molecular modeling studies of pyrrolo [2, 3-d] pyrimidin-4-amine derivatives as JAK1 inhibitors based on 3D-QSAR, molecular docking, molecular dynamics (MD) and MM-PBSA calculations, J. Biomol. Struct. Dyn. 39 (3) (2021) 753–765.
[124] I. Bera, et al., Current therapy and computational drug designing approaches for neurodegenerative diseases-with focus on Alzheimer's and Parkinson's, Curr. Signal Transduction Ther. 14 (2) (2019) 122–128.
[125] M. Najar Adel, et al., Design, synthesis, pharmacological evaluation and DFT investigation of new bioactive unsymmetrical bi-functional ligand, J. Drug Deliv. Ther. 12 (4) (2022) 73–80.
[126] R. Kumar, et al., Computational drug designing and development: an insight, Drug Dev. Life Cycle 3 (05) (2016) 10–14.
[127] J. Chavda, et al., 3D-QSAR (CoMFA, CoMSIA, HQSAR and topomer CoMFA), MD simulations and molecular docking studies on purinylpyridine derivatives as B-Raf inhibitors for the treatment of melanoma cancer, Struct. Chem. 30 (6) (2019) 2093–2107.

[128] A. Mollica, et al., Combinatorial peptide library screening for discovery of diverse α-glucosidase inhibitors using molecular dynamics simulations and binary QSAR models, J. Biomol. Struct. Dyn. 37 (3) (2019) 726–740.
[129] K.C. Sivakumar, et al., Prospects of multitarget drug designing strategies by linking molecular docking and molecular dynamics to explore the protein–Ligand recognition process, Drug Dev. Res. 81 (6) (2020) 685–699.
[130] K.B. Dar, et al., Modern computational strategies for designing drugs to curb human diseases: a prospect, Curr. Top. Med. Chem. 18 (31) (2018) 2702–2719.
[131] H. Safarizadeh, et al., Molecular docking, molecular dynamics simulations and QSAR studies on some of 2-arylethenylquinoline derivatives for inhibition of Alzheimer's amyloid-beta aggregation: Insight into mechanism of interactions and parameters for design of new inhibitors, J. Mol. Graph. Des. 87 (2019) 129–143.
[132] S. Rai, et al., Recent trends in in-silico drug discovery, Int. J. Comput. Biol. 5 (1) (2016) 54–76.
[133] D. Fourches, J. Ash, 4D-quantitative structure–activity relationship modeling: making a comeback, Expert Opin. Drug Discovery 14 (12) (2019) 1227–1235.
[134] D. Kumar, et al., Understanding the binding affinity of noscapines with protease of SARS-CoV-2 for COVID-19 using MD simulations at different temperatures, J. Biomol. Struct. Dyn. 39 (7) (2021) 2659–2672.
[135] F. Ballante, A.J. Kooistra, S. Kampen, et al., Structure-based virtual screening for ligands of G protein–coupled receptors: what can molecular docking do for you? Pharmacol. Rev. 73 (4) (2021) 1698–1736, https://doi.org/10.1124/pharmrev.120.000246.
[136] A. Balupuri, P.K. Balasubramanian, et al., 3D-QSAR, docking, molecular dynamics simulation and free energy calculation studies of some pyrimidine derivatives as novel JAK3 inhibitors, Arab. J. Chem. 13 (1) (2020) 1052–1078.
[137] C. Fenollosa, et al., SEABED: Small molecule activity scanner web service based, Bioinformatics 31 (5) (2015) 773–775.
[138] J. Zhu, et al., Theoretical studies on the selectivity mechanisms of PI3Kδ inhibition with marketed idelalisib and its derivatives by 3D-QSAR, molecular docking, and molecular dynamics simulation, J. Mol. Model. 25 (8) (2019) 1–14.
[139] H. Abbasi, M. Fereidoonnezhad, Z. Mirveis, Vilazodone-Tacrine hybrids as potential anti-Alzheimer agents: QSAR, molecular Docking, and molecular dynamic (MD) simulation studies, Biointerface Res. Appl. Chem. 12 (1) (2022) 588–607.
[140] P.P. Kyaw Zin, et al., Benchmarking 2D/3D/MD-QSAR models for imatinib derivatives: how far can we predict? J. Chem. Inf. Model. 60 (7) (2020) 3342–3360.
[141] S. Mathew, et al., In silico inhibition of GABARAP activity using antiepileptic medicinal derived compounds, Bioinformation 11 (4) (2015) 189.
[142] Z. Cui, et al., Screening ingredients from herbs against pregnane X receptor in the study of inductive herb-drug interactions: combining pharmacophore and docking-based rank aggregation, Biomed. Res. Int. 2015 (2015).
[143] J. Caballero, The latest automated docking technologies for novel drug discovery, Expert Opin. Drug Discovery 16 (6) (2021) 625–645.
[144] S. Sakkiah, et al., Development of a nicotinic acetylcholine receptor nAChR α7 binding activity prediction model, J. Chem. Inf. Model. 60 (4) (2020) 2396–2404.
[145] S. Razak, et al., Molecular docking, pharmacokinetic studies, and in vivo pharmacological study of indole derivative 2-(5-methoxy-2-methyl-1H-indole-3-yl)-N′-[(E)-(3-nitrophenyl) methylidene] acetohydrazide as a promising chemoprotective agent against cisplatin induced organ damage, Sci. Rep. 11 (1) (2021) 1–23.
[146] D.S. Karlov, et al., MM-GBSA and MM-PBSA performance in activity evaluation of AMPA receptor positive allosteric modulators, J. Biomol. Struct. Dyn. 36 (10) (2018) 2508–2516.

[147] M.A. Sahai, et al., Molecular mechanisms of action of stimulant novel psychoactive substances that target the high-affinity transporter for dopamine, Neuronal Signal. 5 (4) (2021) NS20210006.

[148] A. Lemos, et al., Computer-aided drug design approaches to study key therapeutic targets in Alzheimer's disease, in: Computational Modeling of Drugs Against Alzheimer's Disease, Neuromethods, Springer, 2018.

[149] Y. Zhang, et al., Review of the applications of deep learning in bioinformatics, Curr. Bioinf. 15 (8) (2020).

[150] G. Floresta, et al., A pseudouridine isoxazolidinyl nucleoside analogue structural analysis: a morphological approach, Molecules 23 (12) (2018) 3381.

[151] J. Mao, et al., Quinone–thioether metabolites of hydroquinone play a dual role in promoting a vicious cycle of ROS generation: in vitro and in silico insights, Arch. Toxicol. 93 (5) (2019) 1297–1309.

[152] T. Anwar, P. Kumar, A.U. Khan, Modern tools and techniques in computer-aided drug design, in: Molecular Docking for Computer-Aided Drug Design, Elsevier, 2021, pp. 1–30.

[153] S. Muscat, et al., The impact of natural compounds on S-shaped Aβ42 fibril: from molecular docking to biophysical characterization, Int. J. Mol. Sci. 21 (6) (2020) 2017.

[154] P. Wadanambi, U. Mannapperuma, N. Jayathilaka, Molecular docking and ADMET based study to identify potential phytochemical inhibitors for papain-like protease of SARS-CoV-2, Saudi J. Biol. Sci. (2021).

[155] D.A. Borozdenko, et al., A novel phenylpyrrolidine derivative: synthesis and effect on cognitive functions in rats with experimental ishemic stroke, Molecules 26 (20) (2021) 6124.

[156] Y. Yan, et al., Efficient conformational ensemble generation of protein-bound peptides, J. Cheminf. 9 (1) (2017).

[157] M. del Carmen Salazar-López, et al., Voltage-dependent sodium channel blocker anticonvulsants: an approach to the structure-activity relationship, Med. Chem. 17 (9) (2021) 1023–1045.

[158] T. Djikic, et al., Human dopamine transporter: the first implementation of a combined in silico/in vitro approach revealing the substrate and inhibitor specificities, J. Biomol. Struct. Dyn. 37 (2) (2019) 291–306.

[159] Z. Konyariková, et al., Biosynthesis of galactan in Mycobacterium tuberculosis as a viable TB drug target? Antibiotics 9 (1) (2020) 20.

[160] L. Mojica, et al., Evaluation of the hypoglycemic potential of a black bean hydrolyzed protein isolate and its pure peptides using in silico, in vitro and in vivo approaches, J. Funct. Foods 31 (2017) 274–286.

[161] M.C. Yoon, et al., Selective neutral pH inhibitor of cathepsin B designed based on cleavage preferences at cytosolic and lysosomal pH conditions, ACS Chem. Biol. 16 (9) (2021) 1628–1643.

[162] G.W. Caldwell, et al., ADME optimization and toxicity assessment in drug discovery, Curr. Top. Med. Chem. 9 (11) (2009) 965–980.

[163] Y.F. Xu, et al., PTP-MEG2 regulates quantal size and fusion pore opening through two distinct structural bases and substrates, EMBO Rep. 22 (5) (2021), e52141.

[164] M. Ramesh, et al., Computer-aided drug discovery (CADD) approaches for the management of neuropathic pain, Curr. Top. Med. Chem. 21 (32) (2021) 2856–2868.

[165] M.G. Tirumala, et al., Novel methods and approaches for safety evaluation of nanoparticle formulations: a focus towards in vitro models and Adverse outcome pathways (AOP), Front. Pharmacol. (2021) 2157.

[166] Z. Zhuo, et al., A loop-based and AGO-incorporated virtual screening model targeting AGO-mediated miRNA–mRNA interactions for drug discovery to rescue bone phenotype in genetically modified mice, Adv. Sci. 7 (13) (2020), 1903451.

[167] Z. Cang, L. Mu, G.-W. Wei, Representability of algebraic topology for biomolecules in machine learning based scoring and virtual screening, PLoS Comput. Biol. 14 (1) (2018), e1005929.
[168] B. Tang, et al., Recent advances of deep learning in bioinformatics and computational biology, Front. Genet. (2021) 709–732.
[169] D. Lagorce, et al., Computational analysis of calculated physicochemical and ADMET properties of protein-protein interaction inhibitors, Sci. Rep. 7 (1) (2017) 1–15.
[170] H.T. Ghomi et al., Fibpredictor: a computational method for rapid prediction of amyloid fibril structures. J. Mol. Model. 22(9). DOI: https://doi.org/10.1007/s00894-016-3066-1.
[171] T.R. Van Vleet, et al., Screening strategies and methods for better off-target liability prediction and identification of small-molecule pharmaceuticals, SLAS Discov. 24 (1) (2019) 1–24.
[172] A. Clyde, et al., A Systematic Approach to Featurization for Cancer Drug Sensitivity Predictions with Deep Learning, Arxive, 2020.
[173] D.M. Dambach, et al., Safety lead optimization and candidate identification: integrating new technologies into decision-making, Chem. Res. Toxicol. 29 (4) (2016) 452–472.
[174] S.U. Khan, et al., Sequential ligand-and structure-based virtual screening approach for the identification of potential G protein-coupled estrogen receptor-1 (GPER-1) modulators, RSC Adv. 9 (5) (2019) 2525–2538.
[175] M.M. Mysinger, et al., Directory of useful decoys, enhanced (DUD-E): better ligands and decoys for better benchmarking, J. Med. Chem. 55 (14) (2012) 6582–6594.
[176] A. Cereto-Massagué, et al., DecoyFinder: an easy-to-use python GUI application for building target-specific decoy sets, Bioinformatics 28 (12) (2012) 1661–1662.
[177] S. Lätti, S. Niinivehmas, O.T. Pentikäinen, Rocker: open source, easy-to-use tool for AUC and enrichment calculations and ROC visualization, J. Cheminf. 8 (1) (2016) 1–5.
[178] P.C. Hawkins, et al., Comparison of shape-matching and docking as virtual screening tools, J. Med. Chem. 50 (1) (2007) 74–82.
[179] X. Zeng, et al., NPASS: natural product activity and species source database for natural product research, discovery and tool development, Nucleic Acids Res. 46 (D1) (2018) D1217–D1222.
[180] P.C. Hawkins, et al., Ligand-based methods in GPCR computer-aided drug design, in computational methods for GPCR drug discovery, Methods Mol. Biol. (2018) 365–374. Springer.
[181] A.K. Shiau, et al., The structural basis of estrogen receptor/coactivator recognition and the antagonism of this interaction by tamoxifen, Cell 95 (7) (1998) 927–937.
[182] J. Dundas, et al., CASTp: computed atlas of surface topography of proteins with structural and topographical mapping of functionally annotated residues, Nucleic Acids Res. 34 (suppl_2) (2006) W116–W118.
[183] S.U. Khan, et al., Natural bioactive compounds as a new source of promising G protein-coupled estrogen receptor (GPER) modulators: comprehensive in silico approach, J. Biomol. Struct. Dyn. (2020) 1–12.
[184] H.-P. Sun, et al., Identification and optimization of novel Hsp90 inhibitors with tetrahydropyrido [4, 3-d] pyrimidines core through shape-based screening, Eur. J. Med. Chem. 79 (2014) 399–412.
[185] C. Bologa, et al., Virtual and biomolecular screening converge on a selective agonist for GPR30, Nat. Chem. Biol. 2 (2006) 207–212.
[186] J. Xia, et al., The discovery of novel HDAC3 inhibitors via virtual screening and in vitro bioassay, J. Enzyme Inhib. Med. Chem. 33 (1) (2018) 525–535.

Index

Note: Page numbers followed by *f* indicate figures and *t* indicate tables.

C

T

Kolibri 360 GmbH
Ferdinand-Jühlke-Straße 7
99095 Erfurt, Deutschland
produktsicherheit@kolibri360.de